Feel Good Remedies

Feel Good Remedies

PLEASURABLE SOLUTIONS TO MORE THAN
100 EVERYDAY HEALTH PROBLEMS

VALERIE GENNARI COOKSLEY, R.N.

Reader's Digest

PUBLISHED BY THE READER'S DIGEST ASSOCIATION, INC.

Pleasantville, New York / Montreal

Originally published as *Healing Home Spa* by Prentice Hall Press, a member of Penguin Group (USA) Inc.
Feel Good Remedies is published by The Reader's Digest Association, Inc., by permission of Penguin Group (USA) Inc.

Cover illustrations ©2003 Casey Lukatz.

Address any comments about *Feel Good Remedies* to:

The Reader's Digest Association, Inc.
Managing Editor, Home & Health Books
Reader's Digest Road
Pleasantville, NY 10570-7000

To order copies of *Feel Good Remedies*, call 1-800-846-2100
Visit our website at rd.com

Library of Congress Cataloging-in-Publication Data

Cooksley, Valerie Gennari.
  Feel good remedies : pleasurable solutions to more than 100 everyday
health problems / Valerie Gennari Cooksley.
      p. cm.
Includes bibliographical references and index.
  ISBN 0-7621-0518-6 (hbk.)
  1. Self-care, Health--Handbooks, manuals, etc. 2. Medicine,
Popular--Handbooks, manuals, etc. 3. Herbs--Therapeutic use--Handbooks,
manuals, etc. 4. Traditional medicine--Handbooks, manuals, etc. 5.
Alternative medicine--Popular works. I. Title.
  RA776.95.C665 2003
  613--dc22
                        2003016646

Printed in the United States of America
1 3 5 7 9 10 8 6 4 2

US4559/G

To all caregivers who do so much for others . . . while sometimes disregarding their own individual needs. May you be compelled to nurture your body and soul with sanctity and admiration, putting in service the natural provisions created by God. Be well, be blessed, and teach your children the way.

The way to health is to have an aromatic bath and scented massage every day . . . healing is a matter of time, but is sometimes also a matter of opportunity.

HIPPOCRATES, FATHER OF WESTERN MEDICINE (460–377 B.C.E.)

Acknowledgments

I thank the following inspirational people I have had the joy and honor of learning from. I, too, believe that healing and teaching others to heal themselves is the highest calling. Dr. Joseph Puleo, Dr. Bruce Berkowsky, Dr. Daniel Penoel, Dr. Bruce Lipton, Dr. Kurt Schnaubelt, Dr. Philippe Goeb, Dr. Andreas Marx, Laraine Kyle, Master Chuang Sun, Jan Kusmerik, John Steele, Sylla Sheppard-Hanger, and Peggy Parker.

To all my cherished students: Your inquisitive interest and strong desire to heal yourself and others continue to inspire, affirm, and reward my efforts. You have taught me as well.

I sincerely thank my editor, Debora Yost, who creatively envisioned this book and who was so easy and positive to work with on this project. I am grateful to Kristen Jennings at Avery and Kathleen Stahl for her careful eye while copyediting.

I am indebted to my spiritual friends who offered their emotional support, a listening ear, and, more important, their prayers; my sister Christine and dear friend Bonnie Wood; Avis Allison, Betty Rotta, Pat Neufeld, Lorraine Brown, Nicole Gentry, Herb Young, Sue Keister, Elaine Smitha, Karen Erickson, Ed Thompson, Lora Jansson, Kathleen Hults, and Corinne Commagére.

Lastly, with deep gratitude and blessing, I recognize and thank the Divine Author and Infinite Spirit; and my precious family, for the love and support they bring to my life.

Contents

Introduction

Feel Good Remedies

The Perfect Cure-all

Welcome to *Feel Good Remedies,* the ultimate selection of healing pleasures you can perform safely in your home.

Feel Good Remedies takes you to a new level of wellness, one where you create your own sacred and harmonious healing sanctuary; where you perfect your personal environment and purify your body; where you experience harmony of mind, body, and soul; and, above all, where you learn to respect self-healing and honor self-love.

My hope is that you will find the principles of *Feel Good Remedies* so practical and easy to use that they will become the basis of your personal wellness belief system. I envision hints of them in your kitchen, bathroom, and bedroom—the smell of aromatic candles, the sound of healing music, the softness of massage pillows, the purity of essential oils, the enjoyment of stained and tattered recipes.

Feel Good Remedies is for anyone interested in using natural alternatives to complement conventional medicine: the young mother who desires natural care for her family, the mature woman who recognizes the importance of rejuvenation and renewal, the avid athlete who needs proper refueling and relief from aching muscles, the environmentally conscious person who wants to avoid harmful chemicals, or the stressed-out executive who needs to unwind.

Feel Good Remedies follows the principles of naturopathic medicine: First and foremost do no harm; utilize the healing power of nature; identify and address the cause of the imbalance; care for the "whole" person (bio-psycho-social-emotional-spiritual); and practice prevention through lifestyle, diet, and awareness of thoughts. *Feel Good Remedies* is actually healing harmony in practice.

HEALING HARMONY

Feel Good Remedies is designed to assist the body in balancing itself in order for healing to take place and to maintain a state of wellness. An increasing number of people are now actively participating in their own health care, no longer surrendering their health to others. Nearly half of the acute conditions in the United States are now being treated without direct physician intervention. As a matter of fact, recent trends show that as many as 59 percent of Americans say they are now more likely to treat their own health condition than they were a year ago. And an overwhelming majority—96 percent—say they are confident about the health decisions they make for themselves.

That's where *Feel Good Remedies* comes in. I am a registered nurse who has been teaching and practicing aromatherapy, the art of using essential oils to heal, for more than twenty years. I have witnessed firsthand thousands of "healing miracles" using oils and other pleasure therapies. The therapies I selected for *Feel Good Remedies* are based on personal and client-based case histories and observations, traditional usage, and modern scientific evidence that they work. They all bring pleasure in some way—a massage, bath, or long, slow stretch, for example—are easy to use, and, most important, are safe. They are:

- Aromatherapy
- Breath Work
- Diet
- Herbs
- Hydrotherapy
- Inhalation
- Lifestyle
- Massage
- Salves
- Sound and Music Therapy

- Teas and Tonics
- Yoga and Movement

These therapies have all survived the ages, and many are only now experiencing a reawakening. What better way to experience health and healing than through sensual, natural pleasures.

Now don't misunderstand me. While the twelve tools of *Feel Good Remedies* can be used as a primary treatment of healing, they are not intended to be used as a replacement for your current treatment or in lieu of seeking qualified professional help when it is needed. Rather, it should be considered a fusion of therapies designed to assist your body during the healing process. Success in healing everyday common ailments is found in prevention and early treatment.

The key to using the tools of *Feel Good Remedies* is in their synergy, the way they work together. For example, while aromatherapy oils and herbs are effective working alone, in many instances combining specific oils and herbs in a special blend works even better. Yoga and Breath Work work in perfect harmony, as do Salves and Herbs, and Aromatherapy and Hydrotherapy. I have created hundreds of healing recipes that you will enjoy both making and using.

I urge you to read Part One before you start using the advice and healing recipes in this book. Understanding each of the twelve therapies—how they work and why they work— is important to enjoying the spa experience.

Remember, sound health occurs when the mind, body, and spirit are in perfect harmony and balance.

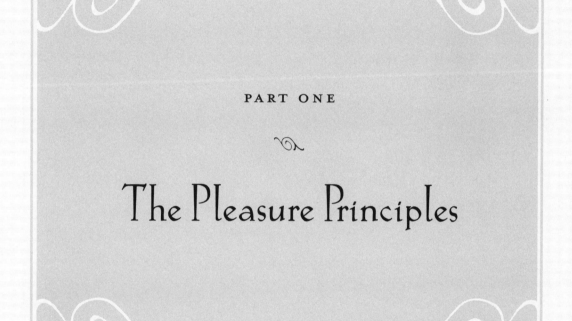

PART ONE

The Pleasure Principles

Aromatherapy

✧

The Essence of Health and Healing

If good things come in small packages, then aromatherapy is Mother Nature's greatest gift to your health.

Aromatherapy is the ancient healing art of using essential oils—highly concentrated aromatic extracts from flowers and plants—to promote physical, emotional, and spiritual well-being. These oils all contain unique healing properties that can both prevent and cure an array of health problems. Some relax, sedate, balance, rejuvenate, invigorate, and even enhance memory. Some possess properties that fight inflammation and infection, ease pain, and battle bacteria and fungus.

Essential oils are so powerful, it often only requires a drop or two of the oil to perform its healing action. To give you an idea of how potent these oils are, consider this: One drop of essential oil equals about thirty cups of herbal tea in terms of concentration.

By definition, *aromatherapy* simply means the "study of scent." If you have never experienced aromatherapy, a whole new world of pleasure awaits you, one that blends ancient knowledge with modern scientific proof of its power to heal the body and nourish the mind. Aromatherapy is considered among the most therapeutic and rejuvenating alternative therapies practiced today.

What Are Essential Oils?

When you brush against a rosemary bush in the garden or sniff a rose growing in the hedgerow you experience essential oils being released into the air. They are the very essence of that particular plant. Essential oils are tiny droplets contained in glands, glandular hairs, sacs, or veins of different plant parts: leaves, stems, bark, flowers, roots, and fruits. They are responsible for giving the botanical its unique scent and energetic imprint.

Essential oils are volatile, which means they readily turn from liquid to gas at room temperature or higher. It also means they are very potent. They aren't actually oily at all, but rather are more of a waterlike fluid. Rupture an essential oil gland or expose it to heat and you will help release these natural, memory-evoking, volatile scents. This is one of the reasons why we experience more fragrances in the summer than in the winter. When the weather is cold and the air dense, molecules move at a slower rate, meaning essential oils are less likely to evaporate.

Not only do individual plants hold unique healing powers, but different parts of the same plants have the ability to heal in different ways. That's because the oils change composition depending on their location in the plant. Take the orange tree, for example. Neroli oil is obtained from the blossoms, orange oil from the citrus fruit itself, and petitgrain essential oil from the leaves of the tree. Each of these oils has different characteristics, scents, properties, and applications.

Essential oils are extracted by several different methods, but the most common process is steam distillation. Steam is forced into a vat of plant material, where it breaks open and ruptures these glands, releasing the precious oil. Following a cold-water bath (cooling phase), the volatile oils are collected and bottled. It can take hundreds and even thousands of pounds of plant material to distill a single pound of the essential oil. That's why these oils are so precious and why they vary greatly in their cost.

Home Experiment

After eating your next piece of citrus fruit, save the rind from the grapefruit, orange, or lemon and perform this simple experiment: Squeeze a piece of the citrus rind by twisting it over a candle flame. You will see tiny fireworks. It's proof that the oils are not only present but that they are also volatile and flammable.

How Oils Enter the Body

Essential oils penetrate the body in four major ways: through the nose (olfactory and respiratory systems) and the skin (integumentary system), as well as internally via the mouth and rectal/vaginal orifices. In this book, I primarily utilize the nose and skin pathways.

The olfactory system—the nose-brain association—is the most direct connection we have with the environment. Think about how sensitive our sense of smell is, approximately ten thousand times more sensitive than any other sensory organ we possess. The fact that our sense of smell is linked directly to the limbic brain where emotions, memory, and certain regulatory functions are seated makes you realize how this important route of absorption is neglected in everyday life. I think in the near future you will begin to see medicine given more and more via this route.

The second way essential oils penetrate the body is through the skin, the body's largest organ. Your skin, which is called the integumentary system, is constantly shedding and renewing itself. It helps regulate the body's temperature by sweating to cool it and shivering to warm it.

Caution: Pregnancy Care

If you are pregnant or think you may be pregnant, be cautious using any essential oils for self-treatment. Essential oils should be used sparingly during the first trimester of pregnancy and should only be used in consultation with your doctor or midwife.

This book contains recipes using essential oils for some side effects of pregnancy, such as swelling and morning sickness. There are also recommendations for use of oils during childbirth. While these are safe formulas I've used successfully for years, you should still have the consent of your doctor or midwife before using them.

Because essential oils are organic in nature and have an inherently low molecular weight, they are easily absorbed through the skin. Unlike synthetic chemicals or drugs, essential oils do not accumulate in the body. When essential oils are applied to the skin via water (bath, compress, facial mist), lotion, or oil, they penetrate through the skin's pores and hair follicles, where they are absorbed by tiny capillaries. Once in the bloodstream, they can affect adjacent organs and structures and circulate throughout the entire body, until they are excreted.

It takes anywhere from fifteen minutes to twelve hours for these essences to be fully absorbed. It takes about three to six hours to expel or metabolize them in a normal, healthy body. One factor that will make this time interval variable is the condition of the skin. Poor circulation, thick toughened skin, or excessive cellulite or fat may slow down the rate of absorption, whereas heat, water, aerobic exercise, and broken or damaged skin will cause

The Skin Patch Test

If you have an allergy to a plant or fruit, most likely you will be allergic to its essential oil because of its high concentration.

Let's say that you are sensitive to the mint family. You pick up a bottle of body oil labeled Herbal Garden Delight. It boasts a combination of twelve pure essential oils but fails to list every essence it contains. This poses a risk to you if it contains peppermint, spearmint, or any menthol-related oils. When you have definite allergies or sensitivities, either make your own blends or get a definitive list of ingredients from any highly complex blends.

To test for an allergic reaction, do a simple skin patch test. Put a drop of oil on a cotton ball or swab and swipe the inside of your arm adjacent to the elbow. Leave it on for fifteen to twenty minutes. If you note any redness or itching within this time frame, wipe it off immediately. This oil is not for you.

increased absorption. Also, the carrier used may affect the absorption rate, since some vegetable oils are heavier than others.

Essential Oil Families

Many essential oils fall into certain classifications according to their healing properties. Here are some basic guidelines to keep in mind when you are first embarking on aromatherapy.

Citrus are mood elevators and stress relievers and include the fruits of bergamot, bitter orange, blood orange, grapefruit (pink and white), lemon, lime, mandarin, and sweet orange.

Florals are mood elevators and relaxants and include flowers such as geranium, helichrysm, jasmine, lavender, neroli, rose, and ylang-ylang.

Grasses are relaxants and skin toners and include lemongrass and vetiver.

Herbals are anti-infectious, stimulating, and balancing and include herbs such as bay, marjoram, oregano, rosemary, and thyme.

Mints are mental stimulants, refreshing and cooling and include peppermint and spearmint.

Spices are energizing and warming and include anise, black pepper, cardamom, coriander, cumin, fennel, ginger, and nutmeg.

Trees are air purifiers and respiratory and breathing facilitators and include black spruce,
cedarwood, cypress, eucalyptus, fir, pine, sandalwood, and tea tree.

How to Know the "Real Thing"

There are several variables that can affect the quality and quantity of a particular essential
oil: the plant variety, time of harvest, soil condition, method of cultivation, and the
process of extraction. Another variable has been added due to recent advances in chemistry: synthetics. And it is done mostly in the name of price.

These cheaper synthetic versions adulterate an oil and compromise its healing action.
This is why dealing with reputable producers and distributors is important. You want to
make sure you are purchasing pure, 100 percent natural oils. They can range in price from
$5 to $30 for a ⅓-ounce bottle. If
you see a shelf full of various oils all
similarly priced, you can bet that
they have been "stretched" or adulterated to lessen the cost. Many, if
not all, aroma practitioners believe
that only the whole essential oil
in its natural form should be used
to ensure its greatest therapeutic
value. Adulterated versions increase the risk of toxicity, allergic
reactions, and skin irritations.

Genuine and authentic essential oils are the highest grade and
purest essential oils produced. They
possess a full, sweet, and mild char-
acter, making it possible to use a

The World's Most Expensive Scent

Bulgarian rose takes approximately four thousand
pounds of handpicked flower petals to make one
pound of oil, making it one of the most expensive
oils that can be purchased. It is often used by professional practitioners for treatment of depression, grief, sadness, and low self-esteem. It costs
roughly $50 to $70 for a 3-ml bottle. In compar-
ison, the very popular lavender yields one pound
of essential oil from every one hundred pounds of
plant material. It costs roughly $8 to $11 for a
15-ml bottle.

minute amount to achieve effective results. Astonishingly, pure and complete oils only
constitute 2 percent of the world's use of essential oils. The rest of the oils are used in food
flavoring, cosmetics and fragrances, and pharmaceuticals.

When you become more experienced with the true essences and use them regularly, you will slowly be able to discern what is the real thing and what is probably not. Your nose will know. If you can detect a gaseous, harsh, alcohol-like odor from the bottle, the oil may have been stretched with an alcohol.

In my workshops, I often pass around synthetic versions of lavender or rose and let the class experience firsthand the differences between them and the true, fine French lavender or Bulgarian rose. Occasionally, the genuine scent surprises them, an indication that we are becoming too familiar with today's artificially scented world. Synthetic fragrances are everywhere—from laundry soap, personal care products, and household cleansers to the new sneakers and women's hosiery you purchase.

CONCRETES AND ABSOLUTES

These highly concentrated fragrance materials are not considered true essential oils, as they are produced by solvent extraction rather than steam distillation or expression. In solvent extraction, chemical solvents such as ethanol alcohol, diethyl ether, and volatile hydrocarbons such as hexane and benzene are used to "pull out" the soluble plant molecules; therefore, they are not pure or complete. While these are less expensive means of extracting the oil, some of the chemicals used are potentially dangerous.

Concretes, which contain plant waxes, fats, and fixed oils, as well as the essential oil, are often more viscous than the pure essential oil. Concretes are then often heated with alcohol to separate out as much of the essential oil as possible, producing the absolute. Both the concrete and absolute are primarily used in natural perfumery rather than essential oil therapy or aromatic medicine.

CHOOSING YOUR OWN OILS

Now that you know the basics, the next step is purchasing a few bottles to get you started. First, decide which essential oils you wish to include in your aromatherapy apothecary. It will not be easy to narrow the choices down to a few, but you are best starting with one, two, or three different types and really getting to know them well before moving on to a multitude. Appendix A has a listing of the botanical names and origins of many essential oils, their common measurement equivalents, and resources where you can buy them. Before you purchase essential oils and blending products, familiarize yourself with these lists.

This section will help you focus on what your intentions are in purchasing them. Before choosing your oils, you will need to keep in mind safety concerns, dilution requirements, and your intended use. As you learn about the many uses of aromatherapy oils—from recipes to treating ailments to simply discovering favorite scents—you will also discover which oils are best for specific purposes.

There are several essential oils I suggest you have in your medicine or spa bath cabinet because they are useful around the house, for personal body preparations, and for self-care treatments. You will find these oils to be multibeneficial, safe, and affordable and are considered my basic "must-haves."

Cedarwood

Eucalyptus

Geranium

Lavender

Lemon

Peppermint

Tea tree

Most essential oils come in ⅓-ounce and ½-ounce amber bottles. This is a reasonable amount to start with and will last quite a while, considering you use only a few drops at a time. However, you can order larger sizes directly from most companies if you wish to order in bulk quantities. Your oils should be stored in amber, cobalt blue, or other colored glass to protect them from the light. Keep them out of direct sunlight and away from any heat source, preferably in a cool, dark cabinet. I have an antique china closet in my office where I keep over three hundred essences. I also keep others in the first aid kit, the kitchen, and the bathroom for convenience.

Because of their potency, oils should be kept away from and out of reach of small children. My children are old enough now to respect these precious bottles that hold the scents they have gotten to know so well.

Another idea for keeping your essential oils safe is to label them. There is nothing worse than finding a bottle not labeled and hence not knowing its exact contents. I find using small labels covered with clear tape protects the label from smearing. Do not use rubber stoppers or rubber eyedropper-type lids to store your pure essences long-term. Over time the rubber parts will be softened and destroyed by the essential oils gassing off in the bottle. Always keep the screw tops on tightly, since the oils do evaporate quickly.

For optimum shelf life it is best to re-bottle your oils if they are below half full, since the air inside the vacant space encourages oxidation or, in other words, a shorter shelf life. Citrus oils are very susceptible to oxidizing, so I find if they are kept in half-empty bottles they do not last nearly as long. When these guidelines are kept and storage is ideal, you can expect most of your oils to last two to five years.

When an essential oil is mixed with a carrier such as vegetable oil, the shelf life of that preparation will equal that of the carrier. For example, let's say you make a wonderful body oil that consists of lavender and ylang-ylang essential oils in a carrier base of sweet almond oil. The sweet almond oil will determine the shelf life of this aromatherapy blend, not the essential oils.

You may also want to keep your aromatherapy collection away from homeopathic medicines, since the high potencies can be affected by strong volatile oils such as camphor, eucalyptus, and mints. Also, be cautioned that essential oils can harm some varnished wood surfaces and some plastics, especially Plexiglas. So if you are mixing oils or using them in a diffuser, it would be safest to do so on glass, ceramic, metal, Formica, stone, or natural wood surfaces, just in case of accidental spills.

Safety and Common Sense

Not all essential oils are beneficial to your health. Some are dangerous. Of the hundreds of oils produced and marketed, about one hundred are commonly utilized by trained aroma practitioners on a regular basis. Of this number, about forty or more are safe, affordable, and readily available for you to use in your home spa with confidence.

Throughout this book I refer to the common names given to essential oils (the plant from which it was derived); however, it is crucial that you refer to the individual listings of each essence on pages 495–497 for the specific botanical name (Latin binomial) to ensure the correct essential oil/plant is used.

Guidelines for Diluting Essential Oils

Because essential oils are highly concentrated and some are known skin irritants, they generally must be diluted in another substance, known as a carrier, to keep them safe for usage. Common carriers include vegetable oil, lotion, and bath salts. There are two ex-

Danger: Stay Away from These Oils

Not everything in nature is safe, and essential oils are no exception. The essential oils listed here are not advised for personal use because they can be harmful to your health. These oils are considered toxic; can be harmful to the skin, kidneys or liver; and some are potential carcinogens. Some essential oils listed have simply not been tested and should be avoided for obvious reasons.

Unless you are an aromatherapy professional, I recommend that you limit your use of essential oils to only those found in this book. Do not exceed recommended dosages. Most important, stay away from the following essential oils. Note: Infusion oil of arnica (not the essential oil; clary sage essential oil, and the herb sage) is safe to use and is recommended in recipes throughout the book.

Ajowan	Clove	Santolina
Arnical	Elecampane root	Sassafras
Bitter almond	Horseradish	Savin
Boldo leaf	Jaborandi	Savory
Buchu	Mugwort	Southernwood
Calamus	Mustard	Tansy
Camphor (yellow	Parsley seed	Thuja
or brown)	Pennyroyal	Tonka bean
Caraway	Peru balsam	Wintergreen
Cassia	Rue	Wormseed
Cinnamon	Sage	Wormwood

ceptions to this rule: Lavender and tea tree oil can be used straight or neat; that is, they can be used directly on the skin in their pure form.

In the recipes I use throughout this book, I've done most of the work for you. For this reason, you should not exceed the recommended amounts. The dilutions used, however, are for the typical healthy adult, except in the chapters that cover childhood diseases and pregnancy. In the chart below, you will find general guidelines for making your own dilutions. Appendix B offers a complete list of carrier oils and further blending instructions for many common therapies.

Preserving Your Feel Good Blends

Antioxidant amounts listed in parentheses in the chart below represent the equivalent of 10 percent of the total carrier volume. This is the recommended amount of antioxidant to add to vegetable oils to prevent them from oxidizing. Adding antioxidant agents such as jojoba oil, vitamin E, or carrot seed oil is optional; however, if you want to preserve your blends for long-term usage, it is highly recommended. For example, if you were making a 1-ounce blend, you have the option of adding ½ teaspoon of a natural preservative to the total carrier amount.

CARRIER VOLUME	ESSENTIAL OIL DILUTION		
	1% Special Populations: children, elderly, and pregnant	2% Typical adult whole-body application	4% Concentrated treatment for local use
½ ounce or 1 tablespoon (¼ teaspoon antioxidant)	3 drops	6 drops	12 drops
1 ounce or 2 tablespoons (½ teaspoon antioxidant)	6 drops	12 drops	24 drops
2 ounces or 4 tablespoons (1 teaspoon antioxidant)	12 drops	24 drops	48 drops or ½ teaspoon
4 ounces or ½ cup (2 teaspoons antioxidant)	24 drops	48 drops or ½ teaspoon	96 drops or 1 teaspoon
8 ounces or 1 cup (4 teaspoons antioxidant)	48 drops or ½ teaspoon	96 drops or 1 teaspoon	192 drops or 2 teaspoons
16 ounces or 2 cups (8 teaspoons antioxidant)	96 drops or 1 teaspoon	192 drops or 2 teaspoons	384 drops or 4 teaspoons

Caution: Children's Dosages
When using aromatherapy for small children, always dilute the normal/adult amount by half or more. This book deals with adult preparations unless otherwise noted, as in the special sections relating to children's ailments.

MANY USES, BIG BENEFITS

Throughout this book you will find numerous creative and simple ways to benefit from using essential oils, from the obvious and most natural ways of enjoying aromatherapy (herb and flower gardens, evergreen forests, live aromatic plants, and fresh cut flowers) to the more subtle ways (using candles, aroma lamps, room mists, aromatic salts, and diffusers). Additional healing spa therapies include aromatic body soaks, footbaths, massage, natural body perfume and lotions, as well as steam inhalations, body wraps, and first-aid compress treatments. They all bring basic methods of preventive medicine into your home for restorative enjoyment and self-care. Your reward will be a much happier and healthier body and mind, increased vitality, and a long and healthy life.

Hydrosols and Floral Waters

A hydrosol is the distillate water from a flower or plant that is extracted during the extraction process used to obtain oils. It contains the water soluble parts or constituents of the plants as well as minute amounts of essential oil.

They are very hydrating, providing moisture and a soothing anti-inflammatory effect on the skin. They are perfect as a skin toner, as they are low in pH and do not dry out the skin like alcohol-containing toners. No emulsifiers are needed, and permeability is increased when these are utilized in spa beauty and skin-care treatments.

Do not confuse with hydrolates or commercial preparations, which are made with alcohol, distilled water, and essential oil. These tend to be drying and may contain solvents, which are a source of irritants for sensitive skin.

Breath Work

✏

Nature's Tranquilizer

As early as the sixth century B.C., the art of rhythmic breathing—what the ancients called *prana,* or life force—was used to achieve perfect health, balance, and eternal youth.

Breath is vital to life—you will only survive a short time without it. But the ancients discovered that it is not breathing itself but the quality of the way we breathe that is most important to our vitality and longevity.

Most of us take breathing for granted. In fact, we pay very little attention to it. Yet, in reality, most of us don't know how to breathe—or at least how to breathe properly. Check your breathing right now. You likely can't even feel your chest expand as you take in a breath. Good? Not at all.

This type of breathing —what most of us do—is shallow breathing. You are not taking in all the oxygen you could and *should* be getting. This is especially true if you are feeling anxious or stressed. It's been found that breathing slowly in a deep and steady rhythm promotes relaxation and inner calm. It's why the science of breath work is called "nature's tranquilizer."

Benefits Are Big

The benefits from long, deep breathing are enormous. Proper breathing retunes your brain, fills your lungs, readjusts your bio-electrical field, and increases the flow of spinal fluid to the brain. Proper breathing increases life-force energy (prana), increases oxygen to your brain and cells, decreases toxin buildup, stimulates brain neurohormones, and purifies the blood. In addition, breath work increases alertness and clarity, cleanses your nerve channels, increases energy and endurance, enhances the healing process, helps conquer addictions, decreases fear and insecurity, reduces pain, and eliminates stress.

Deep breathing is needed to regulate your heartbeat. It acts as a powerful stimulator and eliminator of waste products. It oxygenates and recharges your blood (hemoglobin). The slower and deeper you breathe, the longer your life span is apt to be. Deep breathing encourages calmness, even during stressful and anxious times. It also prevents emotions from blocking communication, gives energy to your psyche, and makes it very difficult to be angry or emotionally intense.

Convinced? Good. Here's how to get started.

Awareness Is Fundamental

This is a technique you can take with you anywhere. Although at first a little awkward, it is deceptively simple. The more you practice it, the more aware you'll become of the mind/body connection. Awareness is fundamental to the breathing process, so you'll need to practice without distraction. Find a comfortable place to relax in whatever position is best for you—lying on a bed or floor, sitting in a chair or on the floor. Before you begin, clear your nasal passages. Relax and focus completely on your breathing.

> ## Fat–Burning Breath
>
> This technique, called Breath of Fire, will help burn fat, detoxify the body, and increase energy. Find a comfortable place to sit, either on a chair or the floor. Take a deep breath through your nose, then exhale forcefully and rather quickly through your mouth. Do this for one full minute, then rest for the same amount of time. Repeat for up to five minutes.

1. Open the rib cage and stretch your spine by stretching your arms over your head as high as possible and slowly lowering them to your side. Or clasp your hands behind your back and lift.
2. Inhale through the nose slowly and in a relaxed manner to a count of three. This allows the air to be filtered, moistened, and warmed.
3. On the count of four, completely exhale.
4. Practice breathing exercises in several positions for varied air distribution.

You can practice this technique three different ways. For upper chest breathing, concentrate on filling the upper chest area with your breath. Place your hands on your chest to focus. For abdominal breathing, concentrate on filling the lower lungs with your breath.

Place your hands on your stomach to confirm the rise and fall. Lateral chest breathing calls for expanding your lower ribs with each breath. Place your hands on each side of your lower rib cage to help focus your attention on this area.

The actual process of respiration is an interesting journey from the environmental atmosphere through your nose and lungs to the circulatory system and finally to each and every individual cell of your body. Make breathing a daily habit, and I promise it will become a pleasure you can't do without.

Diet

A Wellness-Centered Philosophy

It's not the food in your life that is most important but the life in your food.

Feel Good Remedies takes a two-pronged view on healthful eating. One is focused on preventing disease and protecting the body from environmental assaults. The other is focused on overcoming a health crisis.

The preventive diet includes nutriment-based whole foods such as grains, vegetables, fats and oils, legumes, nuts and seeds, beans, fruit, sea vegetables, fermented foods, and a small amount of concentrated proteins. During a healing crisis, the preventive diet is adjusted to increase nourishment and enzymes by eating more sea vegetables and fermented foods and less protein. By eating this way, you will naturally eat more fiber and less fat and sugar. And, I can attest, you will feel enormously satisfied and less inclined to overindulgence.

The Importance of Enzymes

This diet is based on the belief that youthfulness, longevity, and vitality come from nature. Raw foods contain life-giving energy and restore harmony. Studies done at the University of Vienna found that raw foods raise the "micro-electric potential" in living cells—your body. You should eat freshly picked, organic (locally grown if possible) raw fruits and vegetables with every meal.

Enzymes, which are present in raw and cultured vegetables, are essential because they contain *prana,* or "life force." They promote healthy pH balance and aid digestion. There are over six hundred different types of enzymes responsible for virtually all vital processes of your body.

Without enzymes your body cannot break down food to fuel the body. Enzymes help protect you against inflammation, promote healing, dissolve clots and tumors, heal scars, counteract drug reaction, coagulate blood, oxygenate blood and tissues, enhance sexual desire, and prevent premature aging. However, to get the most benefit from these enzymes, raw food must not be heated over 122 degrees, as excess temperatures destroy the enzymes.

Focus on Fermented Foods

The word *enzyme* comes from the Greek word *enzymes,* which means "to ferment or leaven." That's why fermented foods are part of the *Feel Good* diet.

Fermented foods neutralize toxins and aid in predigesting cereal grains, beans, and dairy products. Naturally fermented foods include sour pickles, kim chee, sauerkraut, active cultured yogurt and kefir, raw honey, raw fruit, miso, tempeh, raw grains, and sprouted seeds. Other foods rich in enzymes are sourdough bread, brewer's yeast, rose hips, and kelp.

Tropical raw fruits from the Pacific, such as papaya, pineapple, banana, apple, and melon, are a particularly tasteful part of this diet. Their natural acids, enzymes, vitamins, and fiber contain rejuvenating properties.

You can rejuvenate your entire body by eating these healthful *Feel Good* foods. The more you consume, the healthier and more vital you will be.

The Super Green Foods

Sea plants contain nearly twenty times the mineral content of land vegetables. Although they are still not very common in the United States, for thousands of years they have been used for both food and medicine to prevent disease, enhance beauty, and promote long life.

Sea plants are extremely rich in vitamins and minerals, high in fiber, and low in fat and cholesterol. Seaweed is rich in vitamin K and iodine. It is a staple in the Orient, where it is believed to promote youthful figures, vitality, and sexual vigor. Sea vegetables provide bio-available minerals, including calcium. They detoxify, act as a natural diuretic, regulate the bowel, remove radiation from the body, improve water metabolism, clean the lymphatic system, alkalize the blood and tissues, lower cholesterol, and rejuvenate the lungs and digestive system. Because they are a rich source of iodine, they help keep the thyroid, which is dependent on iodine, healthy.

Edible seaweed is brown, red, or green in color. The most common varieties can be found in Asian markets, natural food stores, and through mail-order companies. These include agar, dulse, hijiki (my favorite), kombu (also known as kelp), limu, nori, and

Dining Out Delight

If you live near a large city, chances are you are in proximity to a health spa or vegan restaurant that serves "spa cuisine" or raw foods. It's one of my favorite ways to dine out.

Spa fare is luxuriously presented, fresh, light, and nutritious meals based on raw fruits and vegetables, salads, and sprouts with or without sources of protein. A typical meal usually includes a fresh greens salad, a light vegetable-based soup or consommé (broth), a small-portioned entrée (which could include chicken or fish), and a fruit-based dessert.

The dining experience itself is relaxed and peaceful, with or without calming background music. The soothing atmosphere aids digestion and encourages family conversation and connection. To fully appreciate the experience, I suggest you eat slowly to fully taste the food and enjoy the texture. Going to a spa restaurant when you are really hungry will enhance the experience even more.

wakame. Most sea vegetables need to be soaked for five to ten minutes prior to cooking to soften them (save the water for facial mists and masks, body wraps, and baths). Soaking decreases the natural sodium content and rehydrates them.

Because sea vegetables are so concentrated, you do not need to eat great quantities to enjoy their nutritious and detoxifying benefits. Seaweed can be added to salads and soups and used in powdered form as a condiment.

Pure Water Wanted

Water, water everywhere—but what is fit to drink?

In my mind, the only safe water is purified or pure spring water. It is advisable to drink at least eight to ten glasses of pure water daily, depending on your individual or physiological needs. Check the labels on bottled waters, choosing natural spring or mineral water over artesian well or filtered municipal water. Also look for low sodium content. It is first and foremost in the *Feel Good* diet when it comes to promoting perfect health.

The dangers of tap or municipal water have been widely researched and documented, and, although it is considered safe to drink, you may want to know these often unpublicized facts about your drinking water. Municipal (public) tap water is recycled "toilet" water, containing as many as forty thousand carcinogens. A few of the major chemicals known to be cancer-causing are aluminum, which is added to get feces, leaves, and dirt to fall to the bottom of the reservoir; chlorine, to kill off the harmful bacteria; and fluoride, which is added to counteract the effects of the chlorine. Considering water's critical role in your wellness, it is evidently clear that you must choose the best source of it for drinking, cooking, and bathing. Investing in a good water filter for the shower is a good idea.

Organic: The Only Way to Go

Buying or growing organic foods is a high priority in the *Feel Good* diet. It is tantamount to healthful eating.

By eating organic you avoid toxic pesticides and benefit from a higher nutrient content. It is the only way you will be able to avoid genetically modified organisms (GMOs), especially in light of the fact that there is no legislation to date mandating that GMO-containing foods be labeled.

Also, avoid meats, fruits, and vegetables that have been radiated. It is likely that a lifetime of eating radiated foods is equal to being exposed to one hundred thousand chest X rays! The ill effects of such handling of your food is obvious and should be avoided.

Besides growing your own vegetables, I recommend you look into becoming a member of a local organic farm cooperative. When we moved from our home that had a large vegetable, herb, and flower garden to a home without the space to grow a large amount of our food, I joined an organic coop farm. It was a great experience making the trip to the farm on a weekly basis to pick up our freshly harvested vegetables. I also got to cut my own flowers and herbs each week.

Your local farmer's market is another way to get local, farm-fresh, and safe fruits, vegetables, and plants.

The State of America's Farmland

A staggering amount of synthetic chemicals in the form of additives and pesticides are routinely used on your food.

- Approximately two thousand food additives are approved by the FDA and are permitted in the United States.
- More than four hundred pesticides are licensed for use on foods produced or grown in the United States.
- A staggering 2.5 billion tons of pesticides are used each year, making their way into your food, water supply, and environment.

SPROUTS FOR LIFE

Sprouts are one of the world's most economical and nutritious foods. Biologists confirm that young plants achieve their maximum nutritional content in the first five to ten days. This means sprouts contain the highest amount of enzymes, vitamins, minerals, and protein of all living plants.

It is so easy to grow sprouts that even kids can do it. In fact, it is a biweekly family activity in my house. And it can be done indoors. Some of the ideal seeds to sprout for chlorophyll-rich greens are alfalfa, clover, fenugreek, radish, and sunflower.

Grains and nuts can also be sprouted to increase their digestibility and multiply their nutritional content. They are one of the best quick-energy foods in existence and keep for almost a week refrigerated.

Synthetic Food Additives: Why You Should Avoid Them

Educating yourself is the first step in improving your diet, preserving your health, and creating a *Feel Good* lifestyle. Avoid the following as much as possible as they can create deleterious effects as noted below.

Artificial colorings: Linked to allergies, asthma, and hyperactivity. May cause cancer.

Artificial flavors: Linked to allergies and behavioral problems.

Artificial and hydrogenated fats: Can cause cardiovascular disease, diarrhea and digestive problems, and obesity.

Artificial sweeteners: Linked to allergies and behavioral problems, hyperactivity. May cause cancer.

MSG: Linked to allergies, behavioral changes, chest pains, depression, dizziness, headaches, and mood swings. May be toxic to the nervous system.

Nitrites and nitrates: Possible carcinogens.

Preservatives: Linked to allergies and hyperactivity. Some could be toxic to the central nervous system and could cause liver damage and cancer.

Refined sugar: Linked to anxiety, cardiovascular disease, decreased immunity, depression, digestive problems, hyperactivity, hypoglycemia, mood swings, nutritional deficiency, obesity, premenstrual syndrome, tooth decay, and yeast infection.

Sulfites: Linked to allergies and asthma.

Table salt: Linked to aches, false thirst, high blood pressure, an increase in pain, inflammatory conditions, kidney problems, and tightness in back.

Don't be fooled by the unfamiliarity of sprouting; it can be as easy as soaking your seeds overnight and growing them in a canning jar. There are many books available to get you started.

You should make sprouts a healthy habit by eating them daily, preferably with every meal.

COMPATIBLE EATING

Food combining is based on research that has shown that certain foods, like fruit, pass through the digestive system very quickly, while other types of food, such as protein, commonly take much longer. In order to achieve optimal digestion, you must eat foods that are compatible with one another as they digest. By ensuring that the foods you eat follow your natural digestive cycle, you can expedite digestion and avoid side effects such as putrefaction or fermentation within your body. The three basic rules of food combining are to:

1. Eat fruits alone.
2. Always eat protein with non-starchy, low-carbohydrate vegetables.
3. Eat grains and starchy vegetables with non-starchy vegetables.

Herbs

∂

THE ROOTS OF MODERN MEDICINE

Mother Earth was humankind's first drugstore. Herbs found in the wild have been used as medicine since the beginning of time. They've been known by every ancient culture, and their healing attributes are recorded on tablets, scrolls, and papyrus.

It is believed that the earth produces between 250,000 and 500,000 plants but only a small number—approximately 5,000—have been seriously studied for their medicinal qualities.

The healing potential of herbs is extraordinary, which is why, along with essential oils, they are the foundation of the *Feel Good* philosophy and system. When the two are combined in special formulas (such as those in Part Two), healing potential multiplies.

Herbs work their healing action by encouraging the natural processes of the body to function. They contain properties that fight infection and inflammation, quell pain, cure digestive complaints, protect the heart, strengthen the immune system, soothe emotions, and alleviate allergies. And that's just for starters. Herbs have the potential to remedy a multitude of conditions—in fact, every malady listed in this book can be helped or healed with herbs. For example, you'll find that ginger soothes an upset stomach, shitake mushroom stops cold symptoms, while chamomile and valerian herbs encourage sleep.

As with essential oils, the healing properties are found in various parts of a plant: bark, berries, flowers, fruit, leaves, resin, roots, sap, and seeds. But, unlike essential oils, many herbs work by ingesting them. They can also be used in topical treatments such as salves, poultices, baths, and compresses.

THE ROOT OF ALL HEALERS

Herbal healing, also known as phytotherapy, is the root of modern medicine. In fact, nearly 75 percent of our modern-day drugs have their origins in plants. Aspirin, for example, comes from the herb meadowsweet, codeine comes from poppy, and quinine is derived from the fever tree. Throughout healing history, herbalism was a reputable therapy recommended by alternative and traditional healers. However, during the nineteenth and twentieth centuries, allopathic (conventional) medicine campaigned against herbs and the simplicity of self-healing, and many were convinced to forsake botanical medicine. By 1930, herbalism had nearly disappeared from mainstream America.

Garlic's Heroic History

Garlic has a long history as a healing agent and preserver of human life.

According to herbal lore, French priests, who ate garlic as a staple of their daily diet, were saved from a plague that swept Europe, while English clergy, who shunned garlic, perished.

Throughout early history, garlic was used to treat war wounds, hard swellings, leprosy, whooping cough, asthma, smallpox, tubercular consumption, epilepsy, rheumatism, and to revive the hysterical sufferer.

Today, aged garlic is made into odorless garlic tablets and syrups for medicinal purposes. It continues to be a common dietary staple in many cultures, especially in France and Italy.

But today, I'm glad to say, it is back. And you can even say support for herbal healing is stronger than ever. Numerous scientific studies on hundreds of herbs now verify and authenticate what others believed for centuries. Much of the credit for this is owed to the extensive scientific studies documented and collected over the years by Commission E of the German Federal Health Agency, the world's most advanced system for assessing modern and traditional research of herbal medicines.

Be a Responsible User

Herbs can often work effectively without any side effects when they are used correctly, carefully, and responsibly. Herbs are most effective when combined with other holistic therapies such as aromatherapy and hydrotherapy. Most herbs are utilized in small dosages over an extended period of time.

Here are some basic guidelines for using herbs wisely.

- More is not better. Read labels carefully and do no exceed recommended dosage. Both the common and Latin botanical name should be written on the label, similar to essential oils.
- Dosage recommendations for adults and children are not the same. Follow label directions for children or the guidelines given in this book.
- Check and honor the expiration date and health warnings or cautions.
- When using herbal formulas such as those found in this book, try a small amount or dose first to check for adverse reactions.
- Some herbs are not safe to take during pregnancy. Check with your doctor or midwife before taking anything while pregnant.
- If you are taking prescription drugs, interactions between some drugs and herbs are possible. Check with your clinical herbalist or knowledgeable pharmacist.
- Herbs to be used with caution are chaparral, coltsfoot, comfrey, ephredra (ma huang), goldenseal, and yohimbe, and stimulant laxatives such as cascara sagrada and senna.

Harvest Moon Over the Herb Garden

Herbs are most potent when the plants are fresh and harvested by the full moon. Although this sounds mysterious and perhaps even magical, it is founded in science. The gravitational pull of the moon, which causes tidal changes, also aids in the extraction of the active herbal ingredients.

Many herbalists harvest on the new moon and decant (finish processing) their herbal medicines (such as tinctures) on the full moon. Use wooden utensils (no metal) and glass or ceramic containers when preparing your herbal medicines and home spa treatments.

Ancient Oriental Wisdom for Taking Herbs

According to Oriental medicine, the effectiveness of herbs for certain ailments can be augmented by the time of day they are taken. Here are some guidelines:

- *Acute illness (quick onset):* Take in powdered form—capsule, tablet, pills.
- *Ailments of bones and joints:* Take in the evening after dinner.
- *Arm and leg problems and discomforts:* Take early on an empty stomach.
- *Chest ailments (above chest):* Take after meals.
- *Chronic illness (long-term):* Take in liquid form—syrups, tincture, teas.
- *Digestive complaints (below chest):* Take early on an empty stomach.

Hydrotherapy

⟋⟋

THE HEALING WATERS

Hydrotherapy is another ancient healer that can be traced through the centuries. In the region between the Caucasus Mountain range and the Black Sea, the ancestral line of cave dwellers known as Abkhazians carried their sick to ancient bathing places such as natural hot springs. The Mexican Indians also used hot springs and mineral water for healing their sick.

Man has instinctively been drawn to healing waters to restore and rejuvenate; rivers, lakes, springs, and oceans were common attractions. The ocean, especially, is known for its healing powers. It is rich with minerals (especially iodine), and its perfect balance of briny nutrients made it an ideal Oriental folk remedy and secret method of rejuvenation.

For centuries, seaweed and sea salt baths were used to restore inner harmony and promote self-renewal. The Egyptians, Greeks, and Romans all used the bath as a healing treatment. In some places, such as Sparta, hydrotherapy was made into law, requiring the townspeople to take cold baths frequently. Public baths were a popular form of medicine in Rome for more than five hundred years.

MYSTICS OF THE MISTY WATERS

Today, people are no longer required by law to take public baths, but hydrotherapy has remained intact as a powerful healer. Literally translated, *hydrotherapy* means "water healing." In the home, this form of therapy involves the extended use of baths or showers using hot or cold temperatures or sometimes a combination of both. *Hydrotherapy* can also be defined as the use of water, in any of its forms—solid, liquid, steam, and sauna—in the treatment of disease or trauma, both internally and externally. Hydrotherapy is extremely pleasurable and effective in relieving muscle soreness, inducing relaxation, increasing oxygen uptake, and improving lymphatic flow to promote health and healing in all the body's tissues. In general, it strengthens and cleans out the body.

By manipulating temperatures and using various techniques, hydrotherapy can stimulate every organ in the body. It can help equalize blood circulation, increase muscle tone

Water Cautions

Accurate water temperature is essential to effective healing action. Water that is too hot or too cold can have adverse reactions. I recommend you confirm water temperature with a thermometer (candy or other cooking thermometers work well).

Also, never allow yourself to get to the point of fatigue or chills. In general, it is not advised to use water therapy within one hour of eating. There are a few instances when hydrotherapy should be discontinued: discomfort, extreme skin sensitivity, faintness, headache, nausea, shivering, or palpitations.

and nerve strength, improve digestion, alleviate congestion, stimulate the perspiration glands, and aid in the elimination of toxins and waste via the skin.

Hydrotherapy is easy to use and is pure pleasure. In part 2 you'll find various uses of this healing art: whole body baths, hand and footbaths, sitz baths, compresses, ice application, nasal irrigation, sponging, rubs, friction, steam sauna, and shower.

MANIPULATING TEMPERATURES

Various temperatures have shown specific healing effects on the body. For instance, 97 degrees—nearly the same as the normal body temperature of 98.6 degrees—has a sedative effect because the neutral temperature has virtually no stimulating effect on the skin. Extreme temperatures, either hot or cold, are most often used for a specific reactive effect and are only needed for short durations. Moderate (warm or cool) temperatures are primarily used for a less pronounced, temporary effect and can therefore be prolonged. The warm bath is the most commonly used.

Since hydrotherapy can raise body temperature effectively, be aware that it can cause an artificial fever. An increase in body temperature will achieve the following: sweating, deep breathing, relaxation of muscle tension, elimination of shivering, increase in blood circulation to the skin, increase in white blood cell count, and removal of wastes from the skin. Here are temperature guidelines for safe and effective use:

TEMPERATURE	DURATION	HEALING ACTIONS	CONDITIONS	CAUTION
HOT 100 to 104°F	2 to 20 minutes	Increased body temperature, metabolism, white blood cells; induces sweating; cleanses and detoxifies	Arthritis, muscle spasms	Use only under professional supervision. Not recommended for those with abnormal blood pressure, heart problems, or who are elderly or obese.
WARM 92 to 100°F	20 to 60 minutes	Sedative, relaxing	Insomnia, circulation problems, pain, toxic buildup, hyperactivity, stress	Heart rate can increase by as much as four times the normal rate the first 5 minutes and then will normalize. Follow with cool water.
NEUTRAL 94 to 98°F	15 to 20 minutes	Sedative, relaxing	Hyperactivity, stress, burnout, high blood pressure, irritability	None known
TEPID 80 to 92°F	20 to 60 minutes	Rejuvenating, cooling, anti-inflammatory	Inflammatory conditions such as hives, itching, sunburn, swellings, and rashes	None known
COOL 70 to 80°F	Several minutes or less	Gently stimulating, reviving, invigorating	Debilitation, sluggishness, fatigue, fever	Use for short duration only. Do not allow yourself to become chilled or uncomfortable.
COLD 55 to 70°F	Several seconds or less	Strongly invigorating, stimulating, restorative, tonifying, constricts blood vessels	Acute joint pain, bursitis, sprains, and other first-aid treatment	Use only under professional supervision. Not recommended for those with abnormal blood pressure, heart problems, or who are elderly or obese.

Bath Enhancers

Hang a pleasing aroma around your faucet by making a Victorian-style bath sachet wrapped in muslin. A wide variety of herbs, flower petals, and grains such as oatmeal can be mixed together according to your personal preference.

Select four to six tablespoons of a combination of herbs, flowers, oatmeal, and/or milk powder and add it to a muslin or organza bath bag. If you like, add six to ten drops of essential oil to the herb and grain mixture.

Seaweed, sea salt, and Epsom salt can also be added to these sachets. These have drawing-out properties and are deep cleansers. Other fine ingredients for the spa bath are baking soda, cornstarch, and powdered ginger.

Hang the sachet from the faucet spout while the bath is filling. Use hot water to steep the herbs and then allow to cool to desired temperature before immersing yourself. The sachet can be dried and reused.

Another way to include aroma to a bath is to add fresh or dried herbs and flowers such as chamomile, lavender, lemon balm, lemon verbena, and rose petals. Not only do they smell wonderful but are also soothing to the skin. Additionally, citrus peels from grapefruit, lemons, mandarins, and oranges possess uplifting and refreshing aromas and are also welcomed in the spa bath.

Inhalation

RESPIRATION, PURIFICATION, INSPIRATION

The health of the respiratory system is crucial to your quality of life. You want to keep it clear, pure, and free of irritants so you can enjoy all the benefits of deep breathing. While inhaling and exhaling are the two basic rhythms of this system, a whole host of other chemical exchanges takes place with each and every breath you take. Since the respiratory system (including the olfactory, or nasal, system) is in direct contact with the external environment, the quality of the air you breathe is extremely important.

The respiratory system includes the nose and sinuses (upper respiratory) in addition to the bronchial tubes and lungs (lower respiratory). As air is inhaled with each and every breath, it becomes moistened in the nasal cavity and large airways. This moist air then comes into contact with the alveoli, which is where the oxygen and carbon dioxide exchange takes place in the lungs. As we exhale, we expel this gas waste from the body.

The airway passage below the larynx (the voice box) is relatively sterile, which is why there is a major difference between the upper and lower sections of this tract. The secretions present in this lower tract contain natural antimicrobial substances that the body produces under healthy conditions. These substances kill invading micro-organisms, neutralize harmful bacteria and toxins, and activate the immune system. There is a plentiful blood supply that is in close contact with the lining of the lungs. An increase in blood supply in this area means that the immune defense system—white blood cells, macrophages, and lymph—is readily available when needed.

When your health becomes compromised through stress, poor nutrition, and other negative lifestyle habits, your immune defenses go down and open you up to a whole host of respiratory problems and infections.

Synergy in Motion

Inhalation is a perfect example of the synergistic effect of the *Feel Good* system. Since inhalation usually involves steam or vapors, it is a form of hydrotherapy. This inhalation method is used because it has the ability to get deep within the respiratory system, where it can carry the essences of aromatherapy and herbs to aid in healing. So, it's possible to experience four of the major *Feel Good* techniques in combination: inhalation, hydrotherapy, aromatherapy, and herbal healing.

In this book you'll find many examples of how inhalation can work. And it works not only to fight disease but also to promote wellness. It's one method that can affect multitudes of people at once, a technique called indirect inhalation.

For example, one popular method you'll get familiar with in *Feel Good Remedies* is misting—disbursement of healing oils or herbs in a water mist. Indirect inhalation devices include diffusers, humidifiers, aroma lamps, misters, aromatherapy candles, light bulb rings, clay aromatic pots, scented plants, incense, potpourri, pomander, sachets, and herbal pillows. Depending on the health or healing goal, some of these aromatic applicators are more effective than others.

Direct—one to one—methods of inhalation include facial steams, personal inhalers, aromatic smelling salts, aromatic jewelry, and infused tissues, handkerchiefs, blotting paper, cotton balls, and scent strips. This book is filled with practical and economical ways to use inhalations. Use them freely.

Lifestyle

❧

The Basis of Mind/Body Balance

A lifestyle that promotes wellness and prevents mind/body imbalances is core to the *Feel Good* philosophy. I believe our state of health must be addressed holistically to be truly wellness centered, as opposed to the classic Western way of thinking that prefers to attack the symptom and ignore the cause.

A very basic interpretation of the holistic approach to wellness is to imagine spokes of a wheel. Each spoke plays an important role in the strength and working condition of the wheel. If one or more spokes weakens, the wheel becomes unbalanced and, with time, will no longer work properly. Preserving health entails balance in all "spokes" of your life: diet, breathing, water intake, physical activity, relaxation, sunshine, sleep, sexual activity, emotional well-being, positive outlook, and personal environment, among others. If one or more of these factors is stressed or compromised, it will affect the whole you!

The *Feel Good* lifestyle is an integrative and holistic approach that includes personal empowerment for making positive life choices, sensory balance, a natural and harmonious living environment, preventative and nurturing self-care, effective stress relief practices, meditation, connection to a higher power, a raw foods–based diet, and a strong connection to family and community.

HEALING SOLITUDE

Scientific studies have found that the ability to sustain a meditative state has numerous health benefits. Among them, it helps lower blood pressure; reduce blood cholesterol; relieve anxiety, depression, and stress; improve memory; relieve chronic pain; enhance immunity; and prolong life.

Meditation is anything you want it to be as long as it is something that offers you quiet and solitude. There is a part of you that desires this every day. You need time to be alone and think, explore your inner self, and pursue personal passions.

There are several ways to meditate. It can be as simple as lighting a candle, focusing your attention on your thoughts, then gradually creating a space between your thoughts and the outside world. It is in this dynamic plane that creativity, insight, and intuition are nurtured.

Walking can be another form of meditation, especially if you tend toward more active forms of contemplation. Labyrinths are particularly good for this, as well as quiet walks in nature, following narrow paths through the woods or park. The fresh air and beauty of nature are nourishing to your soul. Art can be another effective way to reflect, as well as listening to the subtle sounds of nature (or nature recordings) or your favorite music. Dancing is one of my favorite ways to ruminate and is an active form of movement that can be quite profound.

Many believe, and anecdotal evidence confirms, that prayer has the power to heal. Current research is confirming that people who have faith or a strong belief recover faster from illness and have lower rates of depression compared to those who do not pray. Intercession—praying for others—is also a spiritual intervention that seems to have merit in its connection with family and community. Prayer is also helpful because it encourages stillness, peace, and quiet (which counteracts stress) by dramatically inhibiting the release of specific brain stress hormones (cortisol, epinephrine, and norepinephrine). Prayer has shown positive benefits in illness prevention and coping with severe and chronic illness and stress as well as fostering a rapid recovery from illness or surgery.

GENERAL HEALTH RECOMMENDATIONS

Feel Good Remedies favors a lifestyle that is based on actively doing what you can to support and nurture your body, mind, and spirit, thereby creating a foundation for well-being. Ponder this: When you really love (cherish and delight in) yourself, you will make the time to do nurturing things that demonstrate that you value and respect all that you are—body and soul. Health is your birthright.

The *Feel Good* lifestyle is aimed at a harmonious balance between mind, body, and spirit. Its main practices include:

Environment: Peaceful and harmonious surroundings; pleasing scents; nature sounds; music; color and sensory stimulation; art, personal and meaningful objects; health promoting, sacred spaces; cleanliness and order; use of natural products that do not harm the environment

Hygiene: Clean body through bathing, skin brushing, and use of natural products

Mind/body balance: Positive, loving thoughts; intimacy and sexual health; self-discipline and control; awareness and harmony with self, others, God, and nature; spiritual balance; supportive relationships; community involvement; and sensory balance

Movement: Daily exercise or physical work; walks in the fresh air; breathing exercises; dance, yoga, gardening, all forms of exercise, outdoors as much as possible

Nourishment: Natural, organic, health-giving foods; drinking pure water; breathing fresh air day and night; and getting adequate sun exposure

Proper elimination: Raw vegetables and grains; adequate hydration; and prevention of body toxification

Rest and relaxation: Adequate rest; sound sleep; stress management; quiet and alone time; aromatic baths; appreciation of nature; yoga, massage, meditation and prayer; self-reflection; pleasant music; and sound therapy

Healing with Touch

When it comes to attaining superior health, touch is as important as diet and exercise. It is so important to life that it is the first sense to grow in the womb and one of the last senses to diminish in old age.

Neurologically, we are wired for touch and thrive best when we receive sufficient doses of loving and playful stimulation. Although instinctively we know this to be true, research confirms that we need touch on a daily basis to maintain good health.

THE BENEFITS OF TOUCH

The skin is the largest organ of the body, taking up approximately twenty square feet, or one-quarter of our weight. Within the skin are specific channels or ducts, known as meridians, that extend internally to every organ in the body. Gentle pressure on these meridians is the basis for the soothing modality called massage therapy.

Scientific studies overwhelmingly confirm the numerous benefits of massage therapy. It is best known for its ability to ease pain and melt stress. It has been successfully used in controlling cardiovascular and neurological ailments and correcting gynecological imbalances. Massage is capable of relieving headaches, jaw problems, muscle spasms, and swelling from fractures and injuries, as well as promoting recovery from illness and surgery.

In general, massage increases lymphatic and blood circulation, stimulates the production of natural pain-relieving hormones called endorphins, and helps correct posture. Some of the long-term benefits of touch include reduced stress, increased circulation and organ function, improved muscular and skeletal endurance, improved skin texture and immune response, and elimination of toxins. Massage nourishes the skin by increasing the flow of life-giving oxygen to the tissues.

Routine massage treatments promote body awareness, boost self-confidence, improve concentration, and encourage the positive flow of bio-electric energy throughout the body. Hospital studies show that massage also greatly benefits infants and children as well as the elderly.

THE KNEAD TO KNOW: MASSAGE STROKES

There are several types of therapeutic massage commonly practiced in the United States, many of which require a skilled and licensed massage therapist. I've limited the techniques used in this book to those you can learn and use on your own or with a partner. Done properly, they will elicit a healing response. However, I encourage you to experience a professional massage. Getting a massage on a regular basis is better yet. It is the ultimate in pleasure and relaxation.

When using massage at home, the most important thing to be aware of is the direction of the stroke. Different strokes and directions promote different healing responses. There are numerous good books and videos with easy-to-follow directions for massage. Here are the basic strokes:

- *Clockwise motion:* Releases tension, calms the body, and decreases physiological activity.
- *Counterclockwise motion:* Activates energy and stimulates physiological response. Follow with clockwise motion.
- *Effleurage:* Gliding movements with palms and thumbs. Used for relaxation.
- *Friction:* Small circular movements made with heel of hand, fingertips, or thumb. Breaks up and releases fibrous areas, adhesions, and connective tissue.
- *Petrissage:* Kneading and squeezing strokes with hands and fingers using rhythmic, gentle pressure. Relaxes major muscles and improves circulation.
- *Tapotement:* Percussionlike movement using tapping, clapping, cupping, and light slapping. Stimulates deep muscles, nerves, and tendons; aids circulation and metabolism. Can be relaxing or stimulating, depending on tempo used.
- *Vibration:* Swinglike movement that shakes or vibrates the body. Used to stimulate or relax.

FULL-BODY TREATMENT

For a first-time massage, I recommend you get a full-body aromatherapy massage. It usually comes in either a sixty- or ninety-minute session. Its main effect is to be relaxing and nurturing. It's a wonderful experience.

Massage therapists use special tables in their practice, but a futon or padded floor area will work at home. A bed isn't firm enough and makes it awkward for the masseuse. A large bath or beach towel covered with a cotton bedsheet works well for either the floor or futon method.

You will be asked to remove your clothes and slide under a warm towel or blanket, either facedown or faceup. Professional massage tables have an opening in which to place your face. The masseuse may place a hot-water bottle under your feet. The room will be sufficiently heated, the lights dim, and the surrounding environment quiet. Soft background music or nature sounds will be heard in the background. An aromatherapy candle may be lit.

Dry Skin Brushing: An Oriental Secret for Youthful Skin

Dry skin brushing is an ancient healing art that removes dead layers of the "scarf skin," or surface skin, to revitalize nerve endings and bring about a youthful appearance.

Your skin contains a vast network of blood vessels, lymphatic vessels, nerve tissue, and intercellular fluid. Skin also supports small channels called meridians that supply the body with bio-energy. This invisible energy flowing beneath the skin's surface is an important immunity and energetic "force" field that acts as a barrier to harmful bacteria, environmental pollutants, and adverse climatic conditions.

Body brushing increases venous blood and lymphatic circulation, enhances vital force energy, supports skin health and beauty, and promotes the renewal of new skin cells. Skin brushing also strengthens collagen and elastin fibers to aid in scar healing and removes uric acid crystals and mucous residues. One of the most dramatic results of regular dry skin brushing is toning and tightening of the skin, thus helping to prevent cellulite. Skin brushing benefits aging skin by improving circulation, increasing moisture, and strengthening skin pores and sweat and oil glands.

Skin brushing should be performed daily as part of a detoxification program or once or twice per week as a routine health maintenance program. I recommend doing it in the morning so you can feel its invigorating effects all day.

- Use only a natural vegetable bristle brush. Be aware there are look-a-likes on the market made of synthetic nylon of the same color. These irritate and scratch the skin, causing harmful rather than healing effects.
- Use gentle pressure and increase as tolerated.
- Brush toward the heart to encourage blood and lymphatic flow.
- Pay special attention to the soles of your feet, often neglected nerve endings (meridians) corresponding to other parts of the body.
- Brush the whole body (except the face, genitals, nipples, and open/irritated areas).
- Follow with a bath or shower.
- Follow your bath or shower with an aromatherapy lotion or oil for the best skin rejuvenating and moisturizing full-body treatment.
- Wash your brush every few weeks by rinsing in warm water with a few drops of grapefruit seed extract or five drops of lavender or tea tree essential oil. Dry before reusing.

The masseuse will begin working on your body starting with the hands or feet and work from the extremities toward the heart or body center. This encourages blood flow back to the heart. Each area of the body will be swathed with a warm oil before kneading begins. You should remain quiet and relaxed, with eyes closed, and clear your mind of all thoughts. Concentrate instead on what is happening to your body. Strokes will be slow and gentle, light and sensitive, each movement blending into the next.

Do not drink any stimulants for several hours prior to the massage and empty your bladder before the massage begins. Eat lightly before the massage and drink plenty of water afterward. A full-body massage should be avoided if you have the flu or a fever.

On Your Own

If you or your partner find a full-body massage too much to handle at first, you may want to practice back massages. They are much easier to do and don't take as long. Give special attention to the lower back and neck area where you tend to store tension and stress. The skin on your back is evenly distributed and thick, making it a perfect area for application of essential oils and herbal infusions and vegetable oils. This part of your body is often neglected because it is so difficult to reach yourself. Regular massage and nurturing (non-sexual) touch are pleasurable, valuable, and influential in maintaining beautiful skin, emotional balance, and vital health.

Salves

Direct Healing Action

Salves are herbs that you wear instead of ingest. In fact, they work best when dressed in full ensemble: oils, herbs, water, and soft, clean, white cotton.

Salves, also known as ointments and unguents, are semisolid preparations that are applied directly to the skin. Beeswax is added to the preparation to provide firmness to the salve and to enhance the absorption of the healing substances. When applied to warm skin, the salve softens and melts.

Salves are typically protective, emollient, healing, nourishing, and nonirritating. They are made with various oils or fats and beeswax to form a coating over weakened or soft areas of skin that need extra protection to heal. They are a perfect first-aid treatment for bites, stings, and wounds.

Age-Old Solution

In ancient times, herbs were heated in animal fat to make primitive ointments and salves for a wide variety of skin irritations and wounds. Common ingredients in modern salves are aloe vera, beeswax, calendula, chamomile, comfrey, olive oil, St. John's wort, and vitamins. Raw honey, which possesses healing qualities, is also used to bind a salve.

Salves can be made on your own (my preference) or purchased as ready-to-use, semisolid creams. They can be found in natural-health stores, pharmacies, and beauty supply stores.

Sound and Music Therapy

Healing in Harmony

No doubt you can attest firsthand to the ability of music to lift your mood and guide your emotions. What you may not have experienced is the ability of sound and music to help cure your physical ills.

People have been using sound and other forms of music for thousands of years to heal the body, promote fertility, aid birthing, and expand awareness. It is very possible that dance and song preceded spoken language, making these the original forms of communication.

Today, the practice of sound and music therapy is gaining in popularity as a serious alternative healing art form. Used as an adjunct to other natural healing practices, it has been found to help reduce pain and speed healing. Music has been proven to reduce stress and improve productivity and communication in the workplace as well as effectively balance and harmonize the most stressed persons in schools, hospitals, and nursing homes.

The Sounds of Healing Music

Among the many and varied forms of music and sound therapy are chanting (Sufi, Mongolian, and Gregorian), toning, mantras, Tibetan singing bowls and bells, and Chinese gongs. However, musical sounds made by the human voice, such as chanting, have the most power to heal. When you combine the human voice (frequency) with focused intention, you will actualize a degree of healing.

Music is considered a universal communication tool. Tones and chants are said to synchronize your brainwaves, thereby affecting your state of consciousness. Primitive tribes used resonant sounds in their mantras. Music can be used either to insulate and deny feelings or to reveal and release them.

Research studies have explored the body/mind effects of meditation and deep relaxation states during healing. Music is a supreme relaxant and can serve as a type of meditation. Music has the ability to harmonize, balance, and heal through its vibratory sounds and rhythms.

Music reduces stress by producing natural painkiller and feel-good hormones called endorphins and peptides. Music can also increase energy and enhance creativity. Just by actively listening to music that is high in harmonics, you can stimulate the cortex of your brain, decrease your heart and respiration rates, and slow down brainwave activity. This is identified as the relaxation response, which is greatly beneficial to health.

Sound healing as part of an integrated approach to wellness can be effective in treating digestive and intestinal disorders, emotional and psychological imbalances, gynecological ills, respiratory problems, bone and joint disorders, neurological problems, and other more specific ailments such as fatigue, headaches, high blood pressure, chemical addictions, insomnia, stress, anxiety, asthma, circulation problems, depression, hyperactivity, and mental exhaustion.

Good Vibrations

Sound is basically changes in air pressure as it moves through the atmosphere. Your ears pick up this information, and your brain processes it into harmonic/sound information. You also receive vibratory information through your skin as it is picked up in nerve endings. In fact, every cell in your body can be considered a vibratory or sound resonator. Because your body has a high content of water, it is able to conduct sound very easily. It is likened to a deep massage on a molecular level.

Vibratory sound has an effect on cells, tissues, and organs. You absorb these energies as they subtly alter your breathing, pulse rate, blood pressure, skin temperature, and muscle tension. Music is a combination of these sounds into a lyrical blend of pitch, melody, rhythms, relationships, proportions, and harmonies. It is a profound and essential part of *Feel Good Remedies*.

Beethoven's Babies Bill

To encourage early childhood brain development, a bill was passed in Florida requiring state-funded child-care centers to expose children to classical music during the day. The intention of the bill is to ensure that children are offered an environment that will enhance language and music.

HOME SPA LISTENING GUIDE

Lie on a flat surface, preferably somewhere comfortable like a bed, or sit in a comfortable position with legs and arms uncrossed. The room should be warm and the window opened or cracked for fresh air. Remove jewelry and tight-fitting clothing. Close your eyes and become aware of your surroundings and breath.

Concentrate on enjoying the sound therapy and exploring its healing power. Listen not only with your ears but also with your heart and your whole body.

A listening session should be at least fifteen minutes daily and not directly after eating (digestion uses up as much as 80 percent of your bio-energy). Many different kinds of music can be therapeutic. Mozart's music in particular has been called a prescription for health, since its effects on humans have been well studied.

MUSIC OF LIFE

Generally speaking, deep sounds have a calming and grounding effect and will relax and heal, enveloping you like a warm, safe blanket. High sounds and fast frequencies aid in clearing, revitalizing, and refreshing you and recharging your brain. Different musical instruments are known to affect particular aspects of your mind and body. For example, brass, percussion, bass notes, and most electronic music affect the physical body. Wood-winds and strings can cause changes in your emotional state, while strings can also affect your mind. Throughout history, the soul and spirit have been reached by harp and organ music as well as wind chimes and high strings. Tuning forks are used in sound therapy, as well as Tibetan bowls, bells, chimes, and gongs.

Different composers and musicians have been known to create certain kinds of music that affect most individuals in a specific way. Mozart's music, for example, is complex and is considered therapeutic for the higher brain center's activities. In contrast, repetitive, more primitive sounds will have the opposite effect. Gregorian chant is considered excellent to study and meditate by and may help reduce stress. Broadly applied, religious and sacred music can ground and center you, promoting a feeling of deep peace and calmness. Sacred music may also aid in releasing emotional pain.

Music by Mendelssohn tends to calm tense and agitated persons and brings in healing energy. Most of Mendelssohn's compositions revive lethargic, sick, and lonely individuals with its soothing and serene sounds.

Romantic music, on the other end of the musical spectrum, most often highlights feelings and emotional expression. It typically enhances feelings of sympathy, compassion, and love. Jazz, blues, soul, and reggae have an uplifting and inspiring quality that often aids in releasing joy or sadness. Where does rock music fit in? Rock and roll is known to prompt physical activity and release emotional, mental, and physical tension. However, rock music may also have the ability to create tension, stress, or pain if you are not in the mood to be energetically stimulated.

During meal times, concertos for flute can aid digestion. Sounds and melodies of nature as well as new age music are generally relaxing and soothing and can also be played throughout the day to create a sacred environment and harmonious home spa.

And let's not forget the joyful sounds of children, nature sounds (birds, waterfalls, rain, animals), laughter, and, of course, the profoundly healing power of silence. Silence can be a comforting and therapeutic healing balm for the body, mind, and spirit.

Teas and Tonics

✍

INNER CLEANSING

More and more people are getting behind the new popularity of tea drinking as the health benefits of herbal teas, infusions, and tisanes over coffee are becoming more publicized. I'm pleased to say I'm one of them.

Not that there is anything about tea that wasn't known centuries ago. The emperor Shen Nung of China discovered the actual tea plant known as Oolong tea, also called black or green tea, in 2700 B.C. For thousands of years since, the healing plant has been gathered and brewed into medicines to soothe discomforts and heal disease.

Tea has now reached a new popularity, thanks to the renewed interest and acceptance of alternative cures, and the market is now brimming with herbal and fruit blends that range from simple organic options to exotic varieties.

Concocting herbal teas and tonics in your kitchen is easier than you think and is actually quite pleasurable and relaxing in and of itself. You will need to choose the highest quality ingredients you can find, preferably organic or wild crafted, to customize your own home spa remedies. You can purchase tea from your local natural-food store, wild craft your own from clean fields, buy them from reputable mail order companies, or opt to grow your own.

THE ART OF BREWING

The varieties of herbal teas you can prepare and enjoy in your home spa are endless—from warming teas sweetened with aromatic honey for long, cold wintry days to cool summer citrus infusions made with edible flowered ice cubes. In the simplest form, herbal teas are called infusions. These can be either hot- or cold-water macerations (immersions) of fresh or dried plant parts. Pure water is used to extract the herbal properties.

Infusions are most appropriate for delicate and aromatic plant parts such as flowers, leaves, and fragrant fruits. Weak and much diluted herbal infusions are called tisanes. You should use two to three teaspoons of dried, or one to two tablespoons of fresh, chopped plant material per cup of water. Bring the water to a near boil first and then add the plants and immediately remove from the heat. Always cover them and steep for three to five minutes for tisane and ten to twenty minutes for infusion. Strain the tea mixture and enjoy the aroma, color, and taste.

A cold infusion is made by adding the herbs to cold water and allowing them to stand for several hours. Decoctions are made from hard plant material such as woody herbs, seeds, nonaromatic roots, and barks. Considerable heat is necessary to extract the flavor, aroma, and healing properties of these solid botanical parts. The herbs must be simmered in water over low heat for ten to twenty minutes. Use the same ratio of herbs to water as infusions (two to three teaspoons dried to one to two tablespoons fresh). The difference is in the simmering.

Tonics are frequently used in Chinese and Ayurvedic medicine. Tonics are made with tonic herbs to build energy or bitter herbs to prevent disease. Tonics may also contain other ingredients such as aloe vera, lemon juice, and vinegar for medicinal purposes.

In general, when preparing teas and tonics, roots are boiled gently, while leaves and flowers are infused. Always use pure water—spring water is ideal—and glass, enamel, or stainless steel pots. Never use aluminum, Teflon, or chemically treated pots.

The Caffeine Comparison

Approximate amount of caffeine per cup of tea and coffee.

Herbal infusions	0
Decaf coffee	2–6 mg
Green tea	35–75 mg
Black tea	60–90 mg
Coffee	150–200 mg

PROTECTIVE POWERS OF GREEN TEA

Green tea has preventive powers due to its flavonoid and phytochemical compounds. Scientific studies have found that it can help prevent stroke, heart disease, obesity, cancer, and dental problems.

The difference between green and black tea is the way the leaves are processed after harvesting. When the leaves are quickly steamed and packaged, it is called green tea. It contains very little caffeine. Black tea is exposed to air before packaging, which accounts for its darker color and high caffeine content. Both forms possess significant levels of antioxidants.

SWEET SUBSTITUTES

Stevia is a natural herbal sweetener and is the perfect option to white sugar and artificial chemicals. I recommend it throughout *Feel Good Remedies* as a sweetener for my recipes. It has no calories, is sweeter than sugar, and is safe for those with diabetes. I also recommend raw honey and Vanilla Honey (see recipe on page 221).

Other natural sweeteners include amasake, barley malt, brown rice syrup, date sugar, fruit juice, fruit juice concentrate, maple sugar and syrup, and molasses.

Ginger Honey

Ginger honey is the most frequently used aromatic in our home. It has powerful
healing benefits, especially for digestive and respiratory ailments. It can
be put in warm milk, herbal tea, hot apple cider, or rice pudding.
It's made by heating whole ginger in raw honey. The heating process extracts
the ginger oil and combines it with the honey. It has a delightful taste.
If you own a dehydrator, save the ginger slices, sprinkle with sugar,
and dry to make ginger candy. Although hotter than the store-bought
variety, it is very appealing during a cold! Store in a clean glass jar and label.

1½ cups raw honey
2-inch piece fresh ginger root, thinly sliced

Heat the honey over a low setting. Add the sliced ginger and heat gently, taking care not to boil. Excessive heat damages the beneficial qualities of the honey; that is the reason for buying raw and not pasteurized honey. In about 20 to 30 minutes, taste the honey. It should be very flavorful and the ginger slices almost dry. Strain with a slotted spoon.

Herbal Tea for Children

In preparing herbal infusions for children, use the following guidelines for safe and effective treatment:

Children less than 1 year	use 1 part tea to 4 parts water
1 to 3 years	use 2 parts tea to 3 parts water
3 to 5 years	use 3 parts tea to 2 parts water
5 to 10 years	use 4 parts tea to 1 part water

Yoga and Movement

MOVING IN A HEALTHY DIRECTION

To most people, the term *yoga* conjures up visions of white-bearded gurus sitting in pretzel-like poses, chanting weird sounds. But behind the stereotypes, you will find an ancient spiritual practice utilizing time-honored devotionals, meditations, and knowledge based on selfless service, physical health, psychoemotional well-being, and spiritual awareness.

The term *yoga* actually means "union" and is a popular mind/body integration and harmonization. This rich practice and lifestyle originated in India about 3000 B.C. The basic premise to yogic practice is to unite body and mind through relaxation, proper exercise, rhythmic breathing, a well-balanced and nourishing diet, and positive thinking and meditation. Yogic philosophy is based on the belief that, when the mind is stressed, the body will be compromised as well. It is based on preventive as well as curative medicine. The practice of yoga energizes your physical body while calming your mind. A few of the primary aims of traditional yoga are to produce tranquillity, poise, and serenity.

What Hatha Does

Hatha yoga is comprised of asanas, a variety of postures and physical exercises that creates changes in the body. Originally, asanas, which means "ease" in Sanskrit, were designed to support an easy transition for the body in preparation for meditation practice. Over the centuries, however, yoga has become highly refined, and during the past seventy-five years these postures have become recognized as therapeutic.

Different styles of yoga can range from brief and relaxing regimes to more demanding practices meant to strengthen and invigorate the body. Yoga enhances the health and well-being of the nervous and endocrine systems by toning and stimulating internal organs and nerve plexuses. Circulation is increased to these areas in addition to the beneficial effect of breathing on the nervous system. Hatha yoga requires very little movement; however the mind and breathing are involved in every asana to enhance discipline, relaxation, and awareness. Yoga can draw you from a hectic, stressed-induced life into a quiet, peaceful interlude.

The connection between the breath and the mind is of utmost importance in the practice of yoga. The goal is to calm and focus the mind and actualize a steady and rhythmic breathing pattern. Studies done in Great Britain found that regulating breathing, called *pranayama,* can help digestion, improve heart conditions, and reduce asthma attacks. It's also been found to reduce stress, alleviate anxiety, regulate blood pressure and heart rate, and improve respiration. Daily practice helps to improve memory and intelligence, assist in pain relief, improve motor skills, and heighten visual and auditory perceptions.

Other health conditions benefited by yoga include alcohol and tobacco addictions; arteriosclerosis; arthritis; back pain; cancer; chronic fatigue; diabetes; hemorrhoids; insomnia; menstrual, PMS and menopausal symptoms; migraine; obesity; and ulcers. When yoga is practiced regularly for six months or more, it can increase lung capacity, reduce body weight, and increase resistance to stress.

Go for Motion

Movement is essential in creating a vital body and vigorous health and is why it is part of the *Feel Good* system. While yoga is the ultimate healing exercise, I feel all types of movement are important, such as dance, walking, and stretching. Simple exercises to counteract stress, such as shoulder shrugs, palming, taking frequent breaks at work, gardening, hobbies, and play, are motions discussed and highly recommended. In addition to these forms of exercises and movements are simple and easy to perform yoga postures.

Hatha yoga is suitable for beginners and is limited only by your commitment to practice. In general, yoga consists of five basic poses, with many variations. Standing poses are to enhance flexibility, strength, and stamina, while the seated poses encourage a healthy back and spine, poise, and inner reflection. Forward bends help to calm and nurture, gently massaging the internal organs. Inverted (backward) poses support good circulation and reduce stress. When you perform the exercise along with regulated (conscious) breathing, you begin to foster a deep sense of awareness, relaxation, and energy renewal.

Yoga in Your Home

To experience the wide range of healthful body and mind benefits of yoga, you need a quiet, warm place in your home to practice. A yoga mat or folded blanket is helpful. Yoga should be practiced at least three hours following a meal; therefore, mornings and evenings are ideal. Wear loose clothing and remove your jewelry and glasses. A cushion or pillow, as well as being near a bare wall, will also prove useful for some of the poses.

Healing with Pleasure: An A–to–Z Guide

Acne

ᴖ

We all experience a skin breakout now and then, but when does a simple pimple turn into full-fledged acne?

Acne is caused by the accumulation of too much oil (sebum) or dead dry skin that blocks a pore and becomes infected, resulting in sore and sometimes unsightly red spots. It's a condition that should not be ignored. If not treated properly, it can lead to scarring.

While poor hygiene is often the chief suspect, other external factors can contribute to the problem. Fluctuations in hormones, such as those that occur during puberty, can cause an excess accumulation of skin oils. Hormonal changes are the reason why women who are premenstrual or who take oral contraceptives may experience bad skin outbreaks. Stress and taking certain medications have also been linked to the problem.

Tip: Don't Overdo It

When it comes to skin care, even the best intentions can create unwanted results. Overwashing, harsh scrubbing, and overdrying skin can irritate and complicate the healing process as well as cause scarring. Proceed with care. In the case of acne, what's worth doing is not worth overdoing.

AROMATHERAPY

Aromatherapy has alot to offer acne treatment because essential oils are very potent agents against bacteria and inflammation; in fact, they are unsurpassed by modern medical treatments. Used correctly, therapeutic essential oils are highly antiseptic and gentle to the skin.

Try these oils. Essential oils known to positively affect acne conditions are numerous. My top choices include bergamot, cedarwood, chamomile, clary sage, eucalyptus, geranium, grapefruit, juniper, lavender, lemon, lemongrass, lime, mandarin, neroli, patchouli, peppermint (in low dilutions), petitgrain, rosemary, sandalwood, tea tree, and ylang-ylang.

Carrier oils useful in acne conditions should be light, easily absorbed, anti-inflammatory, and healing. Calendula infusion oil, carrot seed (10 percent dilution or less), hazelnut, jojoba, kikui nut, vitamin E, and wheat germ, and are some useful oils that fit the bill. Avoid mineral oil, petroleum by-products, and lanolin, as these have been shown to block pores and inhibit skin respiration.

Pamper with the perfect toner. This is a powerful yet gentle home-prepared antibacterial, anti-inflammatory astringent toner that can be applied easily by facial mist or with cotton pads. It closes the pores, balances the skin's pH, and acts as an all-in-one toner. You will find it refreshing after a long day.

✍ Nighttime Toner ✍

In the summer keep a bottle of this in the refrigerator for a cool treatment.

4 ounces distilled water
1 tablespoon apple cider vinegar
1 tablespoon witch hazel lotion
1 teaspoon honey
2 drops tea tree essential oil
2 drops bergamot essential oil
2 drops juniper essential oil

Pour the water into a small spray bottle or glass bottle with a tight-fitting lid. Add the vinegar and witch hazel. In a small bowl, add the honey and essential oils and mix well. Add the honey mixture to the water mixture. Cap securely and shake until thoroughly mixed. Label.

Mist over the face after cleansing (keeping eyes closed, of course) or moisten a cotton pad and smooth over the face to remove oils as needed.

❧ Oil-Away Blend ❧

Here's a great acne facial nourishing blend specifically made for naturally oily skin conditions. The vitamin E and wheat germ help prevent scarring.

2 teaspoons hazelnut oil

1 teaspoon jojoba oil

¼ teaspoon wheat germ oil

6 drops rosemary essential oil

2 drops bergamot essential oil

2 drops cedarwood essential oil

2 drops tea tree essential oil

400-international unit capsule vitamin E

In a 1-ounce amber glass bottle with a tight-fitting lid add the hazelnut, jojoba, and wheat germ oils. Add the essential oils. Break or cut open the vitamin E gel capsule and squeeze the contents into the bottle. Cap securely and shake until thoroughly mixed. Label.

Moisten your face. Put a few drops on clean fingertips and spread over your face using upward and circular motions, avoiding the eye area. Apply to the neck, back, or shoulders if needed. Use twice daily, following cleansing or facial steaming.

Cleanse with clay. Another way to rid excessively oily, acned skin of dirt and other impurities is with a clay facial mask. Clay masks are only recommended for oily skin types or for occasional use for combination skin. Since clay absorbs many times its weight in moisture, it can be too drying for flaky and dry skin. For more information on masks and mask treatment, see pages 237 and 379.

Rub and scrub. A finely ground facial scrub can be used to exfoliate dead skin cells and deeply clean pores. Take care not to overly scrub, or it will irritate the skin. A facial scrub is most beneficial for acne that includes flaky dry skin, blackheads, and whiteheads.

⁄σ Farm‑Fresh Facial Scrub ᴏ⟍

The following recipe for an exfoliating scrub will leave your face feeling softer than you can imagine. It is easy to prepare, inexpensive, and yet as effective as any preparation you can buy. Besides petal‑soft skin, you will have a natural rosy glow. I call it Farm Fresh because of all the ingredients used and because it reminds me of the clean, young‑looking skin of a country girl. This scrub is gentle because the exfoliants are oatmeal and cornmeal, which are abrasive yet effective. I recommend below that you use lavender oil, but you may substitute with other mild oils such as bergamot, chamomile, or sandalwood.

1 teaspoon finely ground oatmeal

1 teaspoon finely ground cornmeal

1 teaspoon raw unprocessed honey

1 teaspoon natural active‑cultured plain yogurt

½ teaspoon brewer's yeast (optional)

Mineral or floral water or herbal tea (enough to make a paste)

3 drops lavender essential oil

Combine oatmeal, cornmeal, honey, yogurt, and brewer's yeast (if desired). Add just enough water to make a paste‑like consistency. Add lavender essential oil and mix well. Apply to face with fingertips, massaging very gently in upward and circular movements. Do not rub hard or get the scrub too close to the eyes. Rinse well with warm water.

Tip: Banish Blemish Overnight

Here's a quick and effective treatment for individual blemishes:

Saturate a cotton swab with witch hazel or cider vinegar and then apply a drop or two of cedarwood, lemon essential, or tea tree oil. Be sure to just dab the oils onto the infected area only. Used before bedtime, you can often dry up a pimple and bring redness and swelling down overnight.

HERBS

Know what's helpful. Fresh or dried herbs such as calendula, echinacea, goldenseal, lemon balm, myrrh, peppermint, sage, and yarrow can be used in the form of herbal infusions and mixed with clay masks, scrubs, and toners for their natural antiseptic, healing, and astringent benefits. Facial steams with any of these herbs and flowers can be very useful as well.

HYDROTHERAPY

Take the steamy defense. A facial steam is an excellent treatment for acne because it opens and clears pores and increases circulation by bringing infection to a head.

⟋ Acne Facial Steam ⟍

Feel free to substitute any of the essential oils and herbs mentioned above.
Always begin your facial steam with cleansed skin.

4 to 6 cups simmering water (not boiling)*
1 drop bergamot essential oil
2 drops lemon essential oil

Pour the water into a ceramic bowl large enough to hold the water without spilling while handling. Add the essential oils. Close your eyes and bend over the bowl no closer than 8 inches from water level and place a towel over your head to form a tent. Steam for 15 or 20 minutes or until the water has cooled.

Gently pat your face dry with a clean towel. Follow with a toner or facial spray (floral mists are good) to close the pores and balance the skin's pH.

Caution: To avoid burning the skin, never use boiling water. Water is ready after it comes to a simmer. Also, keep your head at least 8 inches from the water level.

Real-Life Cure

TREY TOOK AN ABOUT-FACE

Trey was fourteen years old when he came to me, stressed and embarrassed, with a nasty case of acne fueled by changing hormones and a bad diet. Nothing seemed to help, he told me, and the medicated soap he was using was only making his problem worse. He wanted to try aromatherapy.

Because his skin was visibly flaky and very dry around the forehead and nose, I recommended a formula including carrot seed, frankincense, myrrh, and sandalwood and taught him how to properly cleanse and treat his skin.

I also had him make changes to his diet. He began by decreasing refined sugars and saturated fats—candy, pastries, chips, and soda. He also became more aware of how much he handled his face, which only worsened his acne and spread infection. To stress the point, I showed him several pictures in one of my professional skin-care books that illustrated the scarring that can result from mistreated acne. That alone was enough to keep his hands away from his face.

With just a few changes to his lifestyle, diet, and skin-care regime, his acne problem started to disappear. Trey continued through puberty experiencing only an occasional minor blemish.

Aging Skin
ᴐ

SMOOTH OUT THE WRINKLES

We are all aging—but then that's the goal, isn't it? The problem is none of us wants to look (or feel) our age.

Aging skin, of course, is a natural occurrence. Premature aging isn't. Our bodies are bombarded daily by natural and man-made elements, a process known as oxidation. Aging and disease proliferate when cells do not receive adequate amounts of oxygen. There are numerous reasons why oxygen deficiency is so prevalent today. Topping the list are sun, alcohol, smoking, and lack of exercise. All of these rob the skin (and body) of oxygen.

Nicotine causes constriction of the blood vessels, which restricts nutrients and oxygen available to the skin. Heavy smokers may be four times as likely to wrinkle as their friends who do not. Sun exposure is the greatest danger to skin changes, including skin cancer. Although you do not observe changes immediately, over time these factors will take their toll. Fluctuations in weight, a nutrient-deficient diet, and various environmental insults also play a part in creating wrinkles or dry skin.

The good news is that there are plenty of pleasurable things you

Toxins That Do the Body No Good

More than fifty different toxic chemicals have been identified as poisonous pollutants that can seep into the body. Samples taken from human fat cells (adipose tissue) confirm traces of anywhere from fifty to one hundred harmful toxins. The long list includes chlorine, bromine, gasoline, additives, pesticides, herbicides, wood preservatives, heavy metals (lead, cadmium, etc.), household chemicals, residues of prescription drugs, and mercury (from amalgam fillings).

Thank Your Lucky Genes

Who is most likely to defy aging skin? People with oily skin, dark complexions, and dark hair will generally retain a more youthful appearance than those with fair skin, freckles, and light-colored hair.

Why is this? Typically, people with darker skin and hair experience oily skin conditions. More oil (sebum) means fewer wrinkles. Wrinkles are basically the skin folding in on itself. The skin's collagen becomes hard and crisscrossed, greatly diminishing its ability to hold moisture.

The areas of the body prone to the signs of aging are those parts exposed to the weather, such as the face, neck, and hands. So protect these as much as you can.

can do to rejuvenate your skin and keep you looking younger than your biological years. Herbs, flowers, vegetable oils, and essential oils are the perfect softening agents for mature and wrinkled skin. They soften, nourish, moisturize, tone, firm, and protect the skin. Even if you already are seeing signs of aging, it's not too late to start.

AROMATHERAPY

Essential oils are marvelous anti-aging agents because they work at the deepest level by reaching the tiny blood vessels of the skin and feeding new emerging cells. To counteract wrinkles and dry, mature skin, essential oils are combined with vitamin-rich plant oils to soften and nourish the skin. Nutrient-packed nut and seed oils are carriers for the essential oils to aid in moisturizing and protecting delicate tissue.

Remember your carrots . . . Essential oils that are the best for mature, aging, and dry skin conditions are the highly nutritive oils such as carrot seed, clary sage, fennel, frankincense, geranium, jasmine, lavender, mandarin, myrrh, neroli, patchouli, rose, sandalwood, and ylang-ylang.

. . . and your plants. Botanically rich oils such as plant, nut, and seed oils are great anti-agers. Topping the list are black currant, borage, evening primrose, hazelnut, kikui nut, macadamia nut, rose hip seed, St. John's wort, vitamin E, and wheat germ.

It Doesn't Happen Overnight

It takes time to develop wrinkles, so you shouldn't expect to get rid of them overnight. Since skin cells replenish every twenty-eight days or so, I suggest you use the remedies suggested here for at least a month or longer in order to see improvement. Your skin will begin to appear smoother, firmer, and moister. If you perform regular facial massage, you will multiply the effects. Be careful not to overuse essential oils or overwork the skin, and follow the recipes and frequency in accordance with your skin's particular needs.

Moisture is a must. Floral waters and facial mists, professionally known as hydrosols, are ideal for aging skin and preventing signs of aging because they add moisture to the skin. The best time to use them is during the day.

They should also be part of your regular skin-care regime. Misting adds a layer of moisture to the skin's surface and gently tones the skin. Use them prior to applying moisturizers and facial oils because they provide glide and make application easier. This is crucial, especially in aging skin conditions, since we do not want to pull, rub, or overmanipulate delicate face tissue.

Rejuvenating hydrosols for aging skin include carrot, chamomile, lavender, rosemary, sage, sandalwood, and thyme. Avoid using alcohol-containing toners, which are too harsh.

Get your royal dew. After using this recipe for a few months, you may want to start calling it your fountain (or bottle) of youth! Of all the recipes given in this book, this particular blend may be the most costly to make, but it's worth it; it contains some of the finest ingredients known to help with aging skin. I consider it the "royal" treatment because it contains both rose (the queen of flowers) and jasmine (the king of flowers) essential oils, renowned since ancient times for possessing anti-aging properties. It just may be the best that aromatherapy has to offer for youthful beauty.

∽ Royal Oil ∽

2 teaspoons hazelnut oil

1 teaspoon avocado oil

10 drops carrot seed essential oil

10 drops rose hip seed oil

5 drops evening primrose oil

3 drops rose essential oil (Bulgarian preferred)

3 drops clary sage essential oil

2 drops jasmine essential oil

2 drops frankincense essential oil

In a 1-ounce amber glass bottle combine the hazelnut, avocado, carrot seed, rose hip, and evening primrose oils. Cap securely and shake well. Add the rose, clary sage, jasmine, and frankincense essential oils. Cap and shake gently to mix well. Label.

To apply, moisten your face and neck with floral water and place 2 to 4 drops of this blend onto your fingertips. Work the blend upward, avoiding the eye area. Apply twice daily.

Renew mature skin. For aging and wrinkled skin that is dry and undernourished, replenishing masks that offer moisture and nutrients are a must. This moisturizing and soothing facial mask is perfect for mature skin. Be sure to use plain, natural yogurt with live cultures in order for this mask to be most beneficial. The geranium essential oil helps to balance and rejuvenate dry and mature skin. Frankincense and myrrh oils are both gentle and effective in replenishing moisture.

⁄𝒪 More-Than-Skin-Deep Treat ⟁

A real softening treat for skin that has seen the test of time.

1 teaspoon natural yogurt with live cultures
2 teaspoons honey (raw or unpasturized honey preferred)
1 vitamin E capsule
2 drops geranium essential oil
2 drops frankincense essential oil
1 drop myrrh essential oil
1 teaspoon oat flour (or finely ground oatmeal)

In a shallow bowl, combine the yogurt and honey. Cut open the vitamin E capsule and add the contents to the mixture. Add the essential oils and mix completely. Add the oat flour and mix to make a smooth paste. Adjust the flour as necessary.

Apply the mask to the entire face and neck area with circular strokes, avoiding the eyes. Lie down and relax while the mask is on for at least 20 minutes. Rinse with warm water to remove. Follow with a floral water or facial mist.

The Real Wrinkle Cure

Here's an instance where egg on your face is what you want!

This firming mask literally masks the signs of aging—perfect for those special occasions, such as a high school or college reunions, when you want your skin to look its youthful best. It works by temporarily tightening pores and firming facial tissue.

Wrinkles seem to disappear. The egg whites are the protein that accounts for this "magic."

∞ Cinderella's Secret Mask ∞

Remember, this is good for only an evening.

2 fresh large egg whites, well beaten
Pinch or two of powdered clay (purchase at natural-health store)
½ to 1 teaspoon oat flour (enough to form a paste)
3 to 5 drops petitgrain essential oil (total)

Make sure the egg whites are fresh. Beat the egg whites in a shallow bowl. Add the clay and stir. Gradually add the oat flour a pinch at a time until you form a smooth paste. Because the egg size is so variable, it is hard to judge how much oat flour it will take to make a paste. Adjust accordingly. Add petitgrain essential oil and mix well. Apply with small spatula or fingers. Keep on for 15 minutes. Remove with a cold, wet cloth, being careful not to scrub.

BREATH WORK

Take a deep breath. Oxygen is good for the body and helps improve circulation. It is especially helpful as an anti-aging tool because it is a great stress reducer, oxygenates cells, increases circulation, and gives your skin a healthy glow. So take several deep breaths several times a day.

Diet

Feed your face with water. Since dry skin is a major cause of shriveled skin it only makes sense that you want to keep it well hydrated. Drinking plenty of pure water—at least eight 8-ounce glasses a day—is one of the best things you can do. I carry a bottle of mineral water wherever I go to make sure I get enough fluid throughout the day. And I mean water. Soft drinks containing caffeine and salt are dehydrating.

Get your vitamins and minerals. The antioxidant vitamins A and E, as well as beta-carotene and the mineral selenium, have been proven to be true age defiers. Make sure to get plenty in your diet.

Vitamin A is best known for feeding collagen, which is responsible for giving the skin its elasticity. It's abundant in the orange-colored fruits and vegetables: butternut squash, cantaloupe, carrots, mangos, pumpkin, and sweet potatoes. Selenium, an important mineral for silky smooth skin, is found in brazil nuts, clams, cooked oysters, crab, lobster, and whole grains.

Detox your body. Two little-known yet powerhouse youth enhancers are the underwater sea plants kelp and algae. Both are heavy-duty detoxifiers; they "sponge up" and carry heavy metals out of the body. You can find them in capsule form in natural-food stores.

Seaweed is used abundantly in skin-care products because of its many youth-enhancing benefits. But it is also good for you to eat. Buy it at natural or Asian markets in the form of dulce flakes, hijiki, toasted nori, and wakame. You can learn to cook with it, or eat it in snack form. See my recipe for Wholesome Sea Green Soup on page 389.

Learn to love cilantro. Another great detoxifier is the herb cilantro. It has been found to help escort mercury out of the body. A pungent herb, it is not to everyone's liking, but it does come in capsule form.

Eat lemon to aid your skin. Vitamin C, plentiful in lemons and limes, aids in the manufacture of collagen, which helps maintain the elasticity of the skin.

Eat fiber foods. Avoid constipation by eating plenty of fresh fruits and vegetables and fiber-rich grains. Constipation accelerates aging because toxins and waste products are not excreted in a timely manner and are reabsorbed by the body.

HERBS

Start a youth garden. Some herbs known for their rejuvenating benefits are calendula, comfrey, elderflower, German chamomile, ginkgo biloba, horsetail, lavender, licorice, oats, parsley, rosemary, and rose petals. They can be used in herbal teas or added to floral waters and facial steams as plant infusions.

HYDROTHERAPY

Give your face an herbal bath. An herbal facial steam, using nature's best anti-aging herbs and flowers (listed above) is a gentle, healing, and rejuvenating treatment. Choose 2 to 4 tablespoons of any single herb or combination, or simply add 1 to 2 drops of the essential oils known to prevent aging skin. Adding hydrogen peroxide (3 percent solution) is optional but highly recommended to boost the oxygen content of this treatment.

∿ Herbal Steam ∿

Vital defense for aging skin.

2 to 3 cups hot water (not boiling)
2 to 4 tablespoons fresh or dried herbs
(from the Youth Garden list above)
¼ cup hydrogen peroxide, 3 percent
solution (optional)

Bring the water to a near boil in a pot large enough that the water won't spill while handling. Add the herbs. If desired, add the hydrogen peroxide. Remove the pot to a place where you can comfortably sit over it. Hold your face 8 inches from the pot and place a towel over your head to create a tent. Steam for 10 to 15 minutes. When you're finished, splash your face with cold water followed by a floral mist or gentle toner. Follow with a facial nourishment oil or cream.

Turn the faucet to cold. End your shower with a cold water spray. Use the coldest setting you can tolerate and turn your face upward so the water runs over your face, neck, and shoulders. The cold will help tighten and tone your skin. This is one of the best beauty treatments known. Not only does it promote a healthy and radiant complexion, it helps avoid wrinkles.

LIFESTYLE

Live life to a healthy hilt. You've heard it before but it's well worth repeating.

- Stay out of the sun, especially at the beach, when the sun is hottest: between 12:00 P.M. and 3:00 P.M.
- Get plenty of sweat-producing exercise at least three times a week. The moisture is great for your skin, but you must make sure to replenish the water lost.
- Eliminate stress. There are plenty of ideas starting on page 457.
- Don't smoke or drink.
- Eat healthy foods.
- Maintain a healthy weight.
- Get a good night's sleep.

Tip: How to Get Your Beauty Sleep

If you wake up in the morning with sleep lines on your face, you could be asking for wrinkles before their time. Sleeping on your side, or worse, your face, creates creases in your skin from long hours of hugging your pillow. Over time it gets harder and harder for these lines to "spring back" after a few minutes of wakefulness. Try sleeping on your back or without a pillow. Satin pillows are best.

Allergies

THE ESSENCE OF RELIEF

An allergic reaction is Mother Nature's way of telling you that something "out there" doesn't agree with you. It can be something in the environment like pollen, something in your home like dust, your neighbor's cat, or something you ate.

When you get in the path of one of these enemies, your body's immune system comes to the defense by acting in an exaggerated or abnormal way. While this may be good for keeping you out of harm's way, many scientists believe that people with allergies are more susceptible to common viral and respiratory infections as a result of this defect in the immune system.

When a body gets in contact with an enemy allergen, it reacts by producing extra histamine, a chemical compound housed in the immune system. Over time, repeated exposures and allergic responses can cause tissue damage to the lymph, nervous, and digestive systems.

Many symptoms and conditions are considered to be allergy related. These include asthma, runny nose, hay fever, cough, tonsillitis, sore throat, sneezing, catarrh, sinusitis, fatigue, hyperactivity, learning disabilities, ear infections, and headaches. Many skin conditions such as eczema, itching, redness, and hives are allergy related.

Common environmental allergens include paint, solvents, glue, adhesives, heavy metals, smoke, chemical gases, pollen, perfume, dust, and animal dander. Food allergens vary greatly from person to person;

> ### Tip: Is It an Allergy?
>
> How do you know if that runny nose is an allergy or the sign of a cold or sinus problem? When your nose is draining a clear liquid and you don't have a fever or other signs of infection, it's likely that something in the air is causing the problem. This is especially true if this happens during a seasonal change.

however, some common ones are wheat, milk, chocolate, citrus, eggs, fish, shellfish, nuts or peanuts, and chemical food additives (dyes, preservatives).

AROMATHERAPY

Choose an oil to match your symptom. Bergamot and lavender are the essential oils of choice when it comes to allergies. These oils, among others listed below, are recommended for their general tonifying properties. Since most allergies involve an inflammatory response, anti-inflammatory essential oils such as cypress, German chamomile, lavender, and peppermint are helpful. Lemon is one essential oil I often include with allergy remedies because it is purifying, antitoxic, and antibacterial.

To relieve itching, which is a common symptom in many allergies, use essential oils of chamomile, lemon, and peppermint. Rose has been used traditionally for many types of allergies, while hyssop is specific to the respiratory tract.

When used correctly and in moderation, essential oils can strengthen your respiratory, immune, and nervous systems.

Safety First—Do a Patch Test

If you are prone to allergies, it's possible that you could get a reaction to essential oils. To find out, perform this simple patch test before trying any new essential oil:

Apply 1 to 2 drops of a single essential oil to the inside of your forearm. Observe the area for the next several hours to see if there is any adverse reaction. For more scientific testing, especially for those testing for sensitization, apply 2 drops of the oil to a Band-aid (without antiseptic) and place on the inner forearm area. Check it in 24 to 48 hours.

Irritation—that is redness, itching, or swelling—means the test is positive and you should avoid the essential oil.

Scents for stress. Almost always, stress plays a major role in aggravating allergies. Aromatherapy is extremely effective for preventing and relieving stress. Essential oils that promote relaxation are typically included in allergy-related treatment programs. For the most effective remedies, see Stress on page 457. I also recommend the Thymus Thump on page 180 to strengthen your immune system.

Diet

There are no known foods that you can eat that will eliminate allergies. But there are a few dietary habits that can help strengthen your immune system.

Squeeze some lemons. Drink fresh lemon juice daily in warm water to purify and detoxify the body. Be sure to drink plenty of pure water, too! Antioxidants with high levels of vitamin C like lemons may also help in prevention, and, of course, stay away from the foods that cause problems for you.

Slurp some soup. The Old-Fashioned Garlic and Onion Soup I recommend for bronchitis on page 137 and the Wholesome Sea Green Soup on page 389 are excellent choices to include in your diet. They are both immune strengthening and fortifying recipes.

Inhalation

Clean the air. For general use for people with allergies, I recommend this aromatic blend, which can be diffused in the air several times per day. The healing benefits of the oils will help control airborne allergens and germs and help purify the air. The scent is also wonderfully rejuvenating.

✒ Aromatic Air Spray ✒

This recipe calls for a large amount so it can be stored and used in a diffuser.
Alternatively, you can place several drops in an aroma lamp, potpourri
burner, or pan of hot water on the stove, wood stove, or radiator.

5 parts lavender essential oil

2 parts bergamot essential oil

1 part lemon essential oil

1 part juniper essential oil

1 part peppermint essential oil

Using an eyedropper or teaspoon, measure out each oil and add one at a time to an amber glass bottle. Cap securely and shake gently. Fill the diffuser according to the appliance instructions. Diffuse this essential oil blend three to four times daily for 10 to 15 minutes duration each time.

LIFESTYLE

Get proactive. If you have airborne allergies, there is plenty you can do to relieve your symptoms in your own environment. In the great outdoors, you can get active in any local or regional environmental groups. Starting at home, here's what you can do:

- Use a HEPA air filter for your vacuum cleaner.
- Fill your house with clean air plants such as dracaena, peace lily, and spider.
- Keep pets out of your bedroom.
- Close windows during peak pollen times.
- Clean filters on air-conditioning units regularly. Sprinkle with eucalyptus essential oil for a refreshing and purifying aroma.
- Use natural cleaners such as vinegar and baking soda. Commercial cleaners commonly contain chemical allergens.
- Stay indoors during extremely high pollen times.

- Avoid cigarette smoke and other respiratory irritants.
- Dust often with a damp cloth (use vinegar mixed with water as a natural antiseptic).
- Vacuum floors; don't sweep or mop (mopping can cause mildew, and sweeping encourages more dust).
- Keep grass, weeds, and hanging plants away from windows and doors so pollen won't get into the house.

MASSAGE

Clear your head. To ease most head-related allergic symptoms, including headache, congestion, and fatigue, the following essential oil blend can be used with positive results. Use it whenever you feel symptoms coming on.

Clear-Head Blend

For maximum benefit, make sure to do the final step.

1 drop Bulgarian rose essential oil
1 drop peppermint essential oil
3 drops lavender essential oil
1 tablespoon olive oil or arnica infusion oil

In a small amber bottle, combine the three essential oils. Add the olive oil. Cap securely and shake gently. Label.

To use, simply apply a few drops of the blend to your fingertips and massage into the scalp, temples, and cervical neck area using small, circular motions. Inhale essences from your hands, take a few deep breaths, close your eyes, and relax.

Side Effects from Common Allergy Drugs

People often complain that the side effects of allergy drugs, both over-the-counter and prescription, are worse than the symptoms. No wonder so many people opt for the misery! Here's what these drugs have in store for some people:

- *Antihistamines:* drowsiness, loss of alertness, poor coordination, heart risk
- *Cromolyn sodium:* headache, sneezing, nosebleeds, stinging nasal passages
- *Decongestants:* drowsiness, eye irritation, dry mucous membranes, swelling of nasal passages
- *Steroid nasal sprays:* high blood pressure, nose dryness, nosebleeds, increased chance of yeast infection

The best alternative to misery? Natural remedies.

Anosmia

✍

PIQUE YOUR SENSE OF SMELL

What in the world is anosmia? Unless you have this condition, you've probably never even heard of it.

Anosmia is the inability to smell. Approximately 1.5 percent of the American population—more than 2 million people—experience this unpleasant condition. The numbers are even greater if you include those who have a reduced ability to smell (hyposmia) or a distorted sense of smell (parosmia).

Smell is a chemical phenomenon. Aromatic molecules attach themselves to the olfactory hairs in the nose and are transmitted directly into the brain. The ability to smell varies from person to person. Our age, genes, state of health, lifestyle habits, environment, and medications we take are among the many factors that affect how well we can smell—all of which is why smell is so difficult to study. Until recently, in fact, the sense of smell has been underrated and practically ignored by mainstream scientific and health researchers. Amazing when you consider that as much as 90 percent of what we taste is actually smell-related.

We depend on our sense of smell to fully enjoy life's pleasures—food, flowers, and the ocean, for example—and to protect us from danger—like rancid food, fire, and gas. It's a wonder that it has taken so long to recognize its importance!

Many people who have lost their sense of smell also suffer from depression, a decreased interest in sex, weight gain, and a greater risk for accidents. It's hard to realize how important our sense of smell really is because it's impossible to imagine life without it.

There are many medical conditions that can affect the sense of smell such as colds, allergies, flu, sinus infections, nasal polyps, overgrowth of adenoids, deviated nasal septum, and deficiencies in vitamin A or B_{12} or zinc. Fortunately, in most of these cases, the problem is only temporary. Other, more serious conditions can alter the sense of smell more permanently such as head injury and other neurological problems, endocrine disorders, liver disease, kidney disease, stroke, and Parkinson's and Alzheimer's diseases.

In some cases, we create the problem on our own. Smoking (including breathing secondhand smoke) and recreational drug use (most notably cocaine) have been linked to temporary or permanent damage to the olfactory system. Medications such as nose drops, antibiotics, blood pressure medications, anticoagulants, antihistamines, and cancer chemotherapy have all been linked to a decrease in the ability to smell as have some dietary supplements.

Environmental factors include exposure to toxic agents such as silicon, aluminum, arsenic, cadmium, hydrogen sulfide, formaldehyde, lead, mercury, and trichloroethylene. These chemicals cause inflammation of the nasal lining and destroy nerve tissues, which prevent the smell message from getting to the brain.

AROMATHERAPY

Make scents with frankincense. It may sound a bit odd to recommend aromatics to someone with a reduced sense of smell, but certain aromatherapy oils can help nourish the delicate nasal mucous membrane lining and protect nerve endings in this area.

Frankincense is the essential oil of choice because it has a low evaporation rate, is antiseptic, and is a gentle expectorant. It is most useful in chronic, slow-to-change conditions. Frankincense is also a mood elevator and therefore helpful to those who feel stressed or depressed as a result of suffering from anosmia.

Become a "sens-abled" sniffer. The following formula is gentle in nature, and, with long-term use, you should notice a positive effect. These oils all contain vitamins and protective antioxidants. Sesame oil was chosen for its calming and balancing effects. Wheat germ oil is richest in antioxidant vitamins. St. John's wort has anti-inflammatory qualities and is of benefit to nerve endings. Mullein also has anti-inflammatory properties and is helpful in nerve-related conditions.

Sense-able Nasal Oil

5 teaspoons natural sesame oil (natural, not toasted)

1 teaspoon wheat germ oil

¼ teaspoon St. John's wort infusion oil

¼ teaspoon mullein infusion oil

1 drop frankincense essential oil

Combine all the ingredients in an amber glass bottle. Cap securely, shake well, and label. To use, dip your little finger in the oil and insert it into one nostril. Hold the other nostril closed with your index finger and sniff or inhale. Switch nostrils and repeat. Use once or twice daily.

HERBS

Go for the green and mineral-packed. There are a multitude of mineral-rich herbs that aid and restore the sense of smell. Among the most noted in this category are the "green" herbs such as alfalfa, chlorella, dulse, kelp, spirulina, and other sea vegetables. Other important herbs are bilberry, dandelion root, echinacea, ginkgo biloba, horseradish, mullein, nettles, plantain, pumpkin seed, and yellow dock root. These herbs can be easily made into a tea or taken in capsule or tincture form.

Unplug Your Sense of Smell

If you experience a residual loss of smell immediately following a cold or flu, try supplementing your daily diet with lecithin or fish oil. You can add 1 to 2 tablespoons of lecithin grains to your yogurt, cereal, or health drink. Omega-3 oils found in fish such as salmon, swordfish, and mackerel can be added to your diet several times a week or taken in supplement form. Both have been found to help improve nerve cell transmission in the olfactory system. Be forewarned: Fish oil has a very pungent odor.

The sea vegetables, such as dulse, kelp, nori, and wakame, can be purchased in most Asian and whole-food markets. They are a bit unusual to the beginner; however, they make excellent additions to salads and soups and can be used as condiments.

Take delicious advantage of these foods as often as possible. Try the Wholesome Sea Green Soup recipe on page 389.

Tip: For Smokers Only

Here's just one more of the many reasons to stop smoking. Many people who successfully quit smoking report that one of the biggest benefits is that food never tasted so good.

Tip: This Mint's Not Meant for You

Avoid the use of large amounts of peppermint essential oil because it contains high amounts of menthol and menthone and can alter the sense of smell or be too harsh for the delicate nasal mucosa.

When to Call the Doctor

Detecting a decrease in the sense of smell is not that easy to do unless, of course, it happens suddenly. Most of the time it doesn't. Some people also experience the inability to detect only certain odors—like gas, for example.

True anosmia can't be treated naturally on your own. You need to see a doctor. If you notice your sense of smelling is fading, discuss it with your doctor. Check your medications for any side effects. If you have sinus problems or excessive snoring, see an ear, nose, and throat specialist to rule out a nasal deformity such as polyps or a deviated septum.

Anxiety

🖎

CAREFREE ANTIDOTES

Anxiety is a general feeling of apprehension, panic, or downright fear. It can cause your breath to tighten, your heart to race, and force you to break out in a sweat even on a cold day. It can interfere with rational thinking, make you nervous and irritable, and generally make your life (and the lives of others) miserable.

Doctors have an easy solution for anxiety: drugs. Antianxiety drugs such as Valium and Xanax are among the most commonly prescribed drugs in America. These drugs are all listed as controlled substances. In addition to coming with a long list of side effects, they are also habit forming.

But there is a much easier way to control the harrowing symptoms of anxiety. Follow my suggestions and it will be a pleasure trip the whole way.

AROMATHERAPY

Rely on these oils. Essential oils useful in relieving anxiety and panic states predominantly come from the flowers and wood/bark of a plant. The flowers aid in balancing the mental state by uplifting and providing nurturance, while the heavier scents from tree bark assist in grounding us and finding our center point. These include basil, bergamot, cedarwood, chamomile, clary sage, cypress, frankincense, geranium, hyssop, jasmine, juniper, lavender, lemon, marjoram, melissa, neroli, orange, petitgrain, rose, sandalwood, and ylang-ylang. They all have the potential to alleviate anxiety if used properly.

Are You an Adrenalizer?

Do you tend to forget priorities and operate with a scattered and racing mind? Then you are "adrenalizing"—that is, creating pressure, suspense, and chaos by overscheduling and underpreparing yourself. Practice the ideas suggested here and make it go away.

The most effective ways to use aromatherapy for anxiety are through inhalations, aromatic baths, and massage.

BREATH WORK

Inhale nature's tranquilizer. Breathing is one of nature's simplest and most profound tranquilizers. Long, deep breathing stimulates the brain's production of endorphins, well-documented feel-good chemicals. Breathing therapy also helps cleanse the blood and increase alertness and clarity.

When used correctly, deep breathing can help dissolve anxiety by relieving stress. During tense or anxious moments, pause and become aware of your breath. Consciously breathe more deeply and in a relaxed manner, counting to ten if that helps you focus. Breathe slowly and deeply for several minutes to help create calm and oxygenate your entire body.

Diet

Kick the caffeine habit. Avoid stimulants such as caffeine, alcohol, and cola drinks, which have the ability to keep people on edge even when they are not anxious. It will go far to conserving energy and preventing the burden that these substances have on your body and emotions.

Get your Bs. Supplement your diet with vitamin- and mineral-rich foods, especially the antistress B vitamins, vitamin C, and the antioxidants. These will nourish your nervous system and keep your body in balance.

Bach Delivers Emotional Release

Bach Flower therapy is a fairly recent (early 1930s) alternative healing method designed for emotional healing. Like aromatherapy, the remedies are derived from flower and plant extracts. They can be purchased in liquid solutions and used daily according to package directions. Anxiety-related problems and their Bach Flower remedies include:

Anxiety: agrimony, aspen, cerato, cherry plum, chicory, crab apple, elm, heather, larch, mimulus, red chestnut, rescue remedy, rock water, white chestnut

Fear: aspen, cherry plum, mimulus, red chestnut, rescue remedy, rock rose

Insecurity: aspen, larch, mimulus, wild oat

Worry: agrimony, aspen, crab apple, elm, gentian, mimulus, mustard, oak, red chestnut, rescue remedy, white chestnut

---

Herbs

Herbs are serious stress soothers. Some of the most effective herbs and botanicals that aid in overcoming severe states of stress are bee pollen and royal jelly, black cohosh, chamomile, ginkgo biloba, kava kava, kelp (sea vegetables), lady slipper root, oatstraw, and valerian root. Other herbs that calm the nervous system are cowslip, dill, hops, lemon balm, and vervain. These helpful herbs can be taken in capsule, tea, or tincture form according to the product labeling and instructions.

HYDROTHERAPY

Sink into a warm, safe place. Separate your mind and body from life's daily insults with this comforting bath. Take your time and allow the deeply soothing essences to permeate your being.

❦ Antianxiety Aromatic Bath ❦

A carefree, cocooning experience.

5 drops lavender essential oil
3 drops ylang-ylang essential oil
2 drops bergamot essential oil
½ cup sea salt or Epsom salt

Add the essential oils to the salt and mix. After drawing the bathwater, add the bath salts to the full warm bath. Imbue yourself for as long as you wish.

INHALATION

Sniff some peacefulness. This recipe was specifically designed for anxiety, and I love it! Put the blend of oils in a diffuser and spray it around your home or office three times a day. Or put it in an aroma lamp.

To get maximum effectiveness, take a few minutes each hour to stop and breathe slowly as suggested above. This recipe specifies the ingredients in parts so that large amounts can be made for diffuser use.

✺ Worry-Free Oil ✺

6 parts lavender essential oil

5 parts ylang-ylang essential oil

3 parts sandalwood essential oil

3 parts marjoram essential oil

In an amber glass bottle, count out each oil using an eyedropper or teaspoon, depending on the total amount you wish to prepare. Cap securely and shake well to mix. Label. Fill the diffuser with the desired amount, according to the appliance instructions. Alternatively, you can place several drops in an aroma lamp, potpourri burner, or pan of hot water on the stove or radiator.

Hurried Habits of the Anxious Person

Do any of these behaviors describe you?

Black-and-white thinking

Jumping to conclusions

Keeping secrets

Perfectionistic expectations

Suppressing your feelings

Taking things personally

Winging it (avoidance and lack of preparation)

If you answered yes to any of the descriptions above, you may have an anxiety-prone personality.

MASSAGE

Feel human contact. Human contact and nurturing touch send signals of assurance to someone feeling anxious. A simple back massage or gentle hand and forearm massage can do wonders for calming someone down.

To make a good thing feel even better, use this massage oil. It is concentrated and not designed for whole-body massage. I think it's best for foot or hand massages.

Caress–Away–Anxiety Oil

2 tablespoons sesame oil or vegetable oil
12 drops lavender essential oil
6 drops ylang-ylang essential oil
4 drops frankincense essential oil
3 drops clary sage essential oil

In an amber glass bottle, add the sesame and essential oils. Shake gently to mix well. Label. To use, warm the oil by placing the bottle in a hot water bath or by rubbing a few drops between your hands. Apply in light, gentle strokes.

SOUND AND MUSIC THERAPY

Lie down and listen. Music soothes—if it's the right kind of music. While musical taste is very individual, studies show that specific harmonics can restore calm, promote relaxation, and deliver you to a more balanced state. Performing slow, deep breathing while you listen to the music will compound the centering effects. A few of my favorites are:

Halpern-Kelly—*Ancient Echoes*
Stivell—*Renaissance of the Celtic Harp*
Lee—*Celestial Spaces for Koto*
Copland—*Quiet City; Appalachian Spring*
Vivaldi—*Oboe Concertos*
Bach—*Brandenburg Concertos*

Handel—*Water Music*
Mozart—*Vesperae Solemnes de Confessore;
Ave Verum Corpus*
Environments—*Psychologically
Ultimate Seashore; Optimum Aviary*

Five Ways to Be Free of Worry

Matthew 6:25 teaches us about worry. Here is a simplified teaching from my pastor, Wendell Smith.

1. Celebrate life.
2. Feed the birds.
3. Plant some flowers.
4. Pray.
5. Let tomorrow worry for you.

YOGA AND MOVEMENT

Make like a corpse. The classic yoga pose to create relaxation is the corpse pose. It appears deceptively simple; however, it is one of the most difficult postures to master and takes practice to develop. But it's worth it. Among its numerous benefits: It reduces energy loss, alleviates stress, lowers respiration and pulse rates, and basically provides rest for the entire system.

To perform the corpse pose, lie on your back, feet spread apart (approximately 18 inches) and your hands about 6 inches from your sides with the palms facing up. Make sure your body is in alignment and symmetrical. Allow your thighs, knees, and feet to turn outward in a relaxed manner. Close your eyes and breathe deeply, fully expanding your lungs by raising your abdomen. Count to five and release slowly. This is called abdominal breathing. You should notice your abdomen rise and fall with each breath when done correctly. Stay in this pose for at least 5 minutes, and longer as you become practiced (15 to 20 minutes is a good goal).

See also Depression *and* Stress.

Arthritis

A Joint Resolution

Here are the painful facts: There are more than one hundred joint disorders, including many forms of arthritis. The most common kinds are osteoarthritis, rheumatoid arthritis, and gout.

These share common characteristics such as pain, swelling, redness, and stiffness of the joints. Arthritis can involve just one joint—as in gout, where the big toe is affected—or several.

Osteoarthritis is the most common form of arthritis and is caused by prolonged wear and tear on the joints. Which is also why, if we live long enough, we'll eventually come down with some arthritic annoyance somewhere in our bodies. Eighty percent of people over fifty years of age suffer from some form of arthritis.

Osteoarthritis is also the easiest to treat and responds well to self-help remedies, which is why I am addressing this form exclusively.

Aromatherapy

The essences of pain. The essential oils that respond well to osteoarthritis are those that are primarily detoxifying, anti-inflammatory, and analgesic in nature. They include cedarwood, chamomile, clary sage, cypress, eucalyptus, ginger, juniper, lavender, lemon, marjoram, myrrh, peppermint, petitgrain, pine, rosemary, sandalwood, and spruce. These essential oils are often used in massage oils, compresses, baths, and hand soaks.

Chronic pain-causing provisions. The following foods and additives have been connected to an increase in some types of pain, including osteoarthritis: alcohol, caffeine (coffee, soft drinks, black tea, chocolate), dairy products, drugs (many over-the-counter), meat, nightshade vegetables, sugar, aspartame, wheat (especially white flour), nuts, citrus fruits, margarine and other hydrogenated fats, MSG, poultry, and eggs.

Edibles that ease pain. Plenty of fish, alkaline grains (amaranth, millet, quinoa, buckwheat), dark leafy greens, fruits (except citrus), most land vegetables, sea vegetables, seeds (flaxseed, sesame, pumpkin, etc.), organic soy products, green tea, herbal teas, fresh vegetable juices, vegetable oils such as flaxseed, olive, and walnut.

Herbs

Follow ancient history. Traditional herbs that have known healing effects on arthritis include alfalfa, aloe vera, barley grass, black cohosh, burdock root, calendula, cayenne pepper, celery seed, chaparral, chlorophyll, comfrey, devil's claw, feverfew, kava kava, kelp, licorice root, meadowsweet, prickly ash, thyme, white willow, yarrow, and yucca.

Meet the allium brothers. The allium family members garlic and onion have been found to be helpful arthritis fighters because of their ability to promote circulation. Use them freely in cooking. Additionally, you will want to make the soup recipe on page 137 called Old-Fashioned Garlic and Onion Soup. Not only is it good for what ails you, it tastes yummy!

Make an herbal master plaster. A poultice or plaster using fresh or dried ground herbs is a simple and very effective way to soothe red, swollen, and painful joints. Calendula, comfrey, yarrow, or any of the herbs listed above can be used singly or in combination to provide relief for this ailment. You may want to add 2 to 4 drops (total) of the essential oils helpful with osteoarthritis together with the ground herb in this treatment.

🕉 Herbal Plaster 🕉

4 tablespoons dried or fresh herbs (enough to cover affected area)
3 tablespoons aloe vera gel or witch hazel lotion
1 tablespoon vegetable oil

Combine all ingredients in a blender. Process until smooth. Add additional aloe vera or witch hazel lotion if needed to form a thick paste. Apply a thick coating (approximately ¼ inch) of this herbal mixture to the arthritic joint. Cover with plastic wrap. Optional: Place ice pack or hot water bottle over the herbal plaster for extra pain-relieving benefit.

HYDROTHERAPY

A cold compress is ideal. The cool temperature of the compress helps decrease inflammation and acts as a temporary analgesic, delivering the therapeutic essential oils into the local tissues via absorption through the skin. By elevating the affected joint (above heart level), circulatory drainage will be encouraged—for example, for a compress treatment to the knee, elevate the knee on pillows while lying down. Hands and feet can also be elevated.

Compress for Creaky Joints

1 cup cold water
3 drops chamomile essential oil
3 drops hyssop essential oil
2 drops cypress essential oil

Pour the cold water into a large bowl or clean basin. Add the essential oils and stir well to disperse. Soak a piece of flannel or a washcloth in the aromatic water. Wring out the cloth until it is very moist but not dripping wet. Apply to the affected joint. Lay a sheet of plastic wrap over the moist compress and then cover with a towel. Alternatively, put an ice pack over the plastic wrap to keep it cool longer.

Once the compress becomes dry or warm, replace it with a fresh one. Leave the compress on for 15 to 20 minutes. This may be repeated two to three times per day for severe pain and swelling.

Soak those limbs. Hand baths and footbaths offer very soothing pain relief to arthritic conditions of the finger joints or ankles. For general aches and pains, use warm (92 to 100 degrees) to tepid (80 to 92 degrees) water. If redness or severe swelling is present, use cold (55 to 70 degrees) water.

✥ Limber–Limb Bath ✥

*For a total soothing experience, follow your bath with
an application of the Arthritis Rub on page 89.*

2 drops juniper essential oil
1 drop lavender essential oil
1 drop cypress essential oil
1 drop rosemary essential oil
2 tablespoons Epsom salt

Fill the tub with warm water. Add the drops of essential oils to the Epsom salt and mix. Add the aromatic salt to the water and stir with your hand. Soak the affected limb for 15 to 20 minutes.

Submerge completely. When you ache all over, a full aromatic warm bath is the best choice for you. This bath recipe has been used with favorable results by persons suffering from fibromyalgia, an arthritis-related condition that affects the entire body.

A warm bath temperature encourages relaxation of the muscles and helps increase circulation and absorption of the essential oils. There are several good bath carrier choices that you can use for this recipe, such as sea salt, Epsom salt, and baking soda. However, the Oxygen Spa Soak is highly recommended (see page 95). Epsom salt, which is magnesium sulfate, aids the body in detoxification and relieves muscular tension.

✥ Easy–on–Arthritis Bath ✥

For all-over aches and pain caused by arthritis.

4 drops juniper essential oil
2 drops lavender essential oil
2 drops cypress essential oil
2 drops rosemary essential oil
½ cup carrier of choice
    (Epsom salt, Celtic Sea salt, or baking soda)

Blend the essential oils together with the salt or baking soda. After the bath has been filled, add the mixture and stir into the bathwater. Soak for 20 to 30 minutes. Pat dry and apply the Arthritis Rub to any local areas that need special attention. This bath salt can be used daily or as needed.

MASSAGE

Rub the ache away. Many people who have used this balm proclaim its soothing, pain-relieving, and cooling benefits. An avid golfer once told me she would not think of playing a game without it!

The oils in this blend work synergistically to provide safe and effective pain relief. Most have dual benefits as anti-inflammatory and analgesic agents. The juniper and carrot seed aid in eliminating fluid and toxin accumulation in the joint and surrounding tissue.

The carrot seed oil is an essential oil; however, it is used in 10 percent dilutions in a vegetable oil base. It is very helpful in healing damaged tissue caused by trauma and surgical procedures. You can make a much simpler version by using two or three different essential oils and omitting the carrot and St. John's wort oils.

⟋ Arthritis Rub ⟋

This is a concentrated oil blend and is designed for local application only.

14 drops lavender essential oil
10 drops rosemary essential oil
8 drops peppermint essential oil
6 drops juniper essential oil
1 teaspoon carrot seed oil
2 tablespoons St. John's wort oil
2 tablespoons vegetable oil

In a 2 ounce amber bottle, add the essential oils and mix. Add the carrot seed, St. John's wort, and vegetable oils. Cap securely and shake gently to mix well. Label.

To use, put a few drops in your hands and gently rub into painful or swollen joints. Apply two to three times per day.

TEAS AND TONICS

Drink tea with C. Drinking a citrus-laced herbal tea daily will be helpful in alleviating pain. This recipe uses raw apple cider vinegar and fresh lemon juice as the primary cleansing, pH-balancing, and anti-inflammatory agents.

Arthritis is known as an acidic condition, so it is imperative to balance the blood and body chemistry (pH) when you can can.

✍ Herbal Citrus Tonic ✑

1 teaspoon chamomile flowers
1 teaspoon meadowsweet herb*
1 cup hot water
1 teaspoon fresh lemon juice
1 teaspoon apple cider vinegar
1 teaspoon honey or Ginger Honey (page 48)

Put the chamomile flowers and meadowsweet in a cup or small teapot and pour the hot water over them. Steep for 5 minutes. Strain into a cup and add the lemon juice and vinegar and stir. Add the honey to taste. Drink warm or allow to cool.

Note: If you are allergic to salicylates, omit the meadowsweet. It contains naturally occurring salicylate, which some people are allergic to.

YOGA AND MOVEMENT

Keep moving on. Gentle, nonweight-bearing exercise, such as swimming or yoga, is ideal to keep joints flexible. A minitrampoline is a gentle way to exercise without causing weight-bearing damage to compromised joints. Easy stretching exercises and flowing, classical dance movements are also great choices. Hand and foot rotation exercises are beneficial as well.

Real-Life Cure

PAINFREE AND ACTIVE

Ted, a seventy-year-young man with a history of osteoarthritis, had already undergone a total right knee replacement and did not want to take pain medication. He was very active for his age and, though bothered by his arthritis, continued to work in his garden growing flowers, herbs, and vegetables to sell to restaurants. He depended on his ability to work the land and needed the function of both legs to get his daily chores completed.

When his left knee started to act up, Ted came to me for some advice. His knee was especially stiff in the early morning and grew increasingly swollen and sore by day's end. He didn't want to go through another surgery or take expensive medicine. I told him to apply the Arthritis Rub to his knee daily, first thing in the morning.

Instead of his pain and stiffness getting worse as the day went on, Ted actually felt it ease. He particularly enjoys his evening Arthritis Bath. He says, "I'm taking my oils and getting clean at the same time!"

Asthma

BREATHE DEEPLY AGAIN

People with asthma do not take air for granted. That's because, at any given moment, something could suddenly get in the way of the air and their ability to breathe it in.

Asthma is an allergic disorder characterized by spasms of the bronchial tubes—the airway passages—of the lungs. The result is wheezing, coughing, tightness in the chest, and a very scary sensation that the next breath will be hard to find.

Many things can cause an allergy attack: Springtime tree pollens, summer grasses and weed pollens, animal dander, dust, molds, and fungus are among the most common. Sudden exposure to certain chemicals, smoke, and cold air can also induce an attack. In some people, physical exertion can bring on an attack, a condition called exercise-induced asthma.

There is now some evidence linking this condition to emotions and how we deal with them. I, for one, believe there is a connection, and it is based on my many years of watching aromatherapy work. As you read on, you'll understand how.

AROMATHERAPY

Take an integrative approach. Aromatherapy is not a substitute for asthma medication, but many people who have asthma and have made lifestyle changes incorporating aromatherapy are able to decrease their medications and improve their overall health.

Essential oils are a therapeutic support for asthma because they induce relaxation, purify the air, and generally support the respiratory system. The essential oils that are effective against asthma are basil, cedarwood, chamomile, cypress, eucalyptus (especially *E. radiata* and *E. smithii*), geranium, hyssop, lavender, lemon, mandarin, marjoram, melissa, neroli, patchouli, peppermint, pine, and rosemary.

Be carefree but careful. You can safely and easily use the recipes suggested later in this section along with your present health regime to ease symptoms. However, any essential oil has the potential of triggering an attack. So exercise caution and moderation. People with asthma, as with any allergy, are more prone to sensitivities and allergies and should consult with a doctor before using aromatherapy.

BREATH WORK

Get into the rhythm. Rhythmic diaphragmatic breathing is perhaps one of the most important aspects of breathing there is for someone with asthma. The average person uses the chest muscles rather than the diaphragm to breathe. Such breathing is typically shallow, rapid, and irregular. Diaphragmatic breathing, however, brings more air and oxygen to the air sacs in the lungs and into the bloodstream.

You can practice this simple, highly beneficial breathing exercise lying down on a mat, sitting, or standing, whichever is most comfortable. Place one palm at the center of your chest and the other at the lower edge of your rib cage where the abdomen begins. As you

---

Zap an Attack

I have observed people with asthma having more frequent attacks in public where they have less control over their environment. And, rather than pull out an inhaler, some people take out a vial of aromatic liquid and inhale it.

I recommend a combination of lavender and neroli essential oils because of their relaxing effect. You can also try chamomile, geranium, marjoram, patchouli, and sandalwood essential oils.

If you have asthma, find your favorite and carry an emergency vial with you.

---

inhale, the lower edge of the rib cage should expand and your abdomen rise. As you exhale, the opposite will happen. Your chest should have relatively little movement.

When you become proficient at this part of the exercise, practice cultivating a harmonious rhythmic breathing. With practice, this type of breathing can become habitual and automatic, and you will reap its many benefits.

DIET

Fill a shaker with oregano. This staple of Italian cooking has been useful as a homeopathic medicine for asthma-related and other respiratory conditions.

Pay attention to dietary triggers. Investigate your diet for any foods that could trigger an attack. Keep a food diary, if necessary, to zero in on a culprit. Common food triggers are dairy, food preservatives, nuts, shellfish, soy, and wheat.

Avoid dairy products. Dairy products are known to increase mucus production and therefore are best avoided.

Get your vitamins and minerals. Eat more foods rich in vitamins B_6, C, and E, or supplement your diet with them as they have been shown to reduce the occurrence of bronchitis and respiratory problems. Vitamin C is also a natural antihistamine and protects the lungs. Due to their anti-inflammatory effects, essential fatty acids also may be helpful supplements.

Herbs

Pick from this field of choices. Herbs that are known to promote healthy respiration are elecampane root, ginseng, grindelia, licorice, lobelia, marshmallow root, mullein, pleurisy root, and yerba santa leaf.

Specific herbs are known to aid and support mucous cleansing and include chlorella, elecampane, fenugreek seed, marshmallow, and mullein. Botanical sources that may help your body neutralize pollutants are alfalfa, aloe vera, bee pollen/royal jelly, chlorophyll, fenugreek seed, goldenseal root, kelp/sea vegetables, lobelia, and Siberian ginseng.

Hydrotherapy

Splash your face with this special formula. This very refreshing and cooling remedy is one of my favorite recommendations. It is extremely simple yet very effective for mild to moderate asthma conditions, as these essences possess antihistamine-like properties. Hydrogen peroxide (3 percent solution) is an optional ingredient. It is highly beneficial for asthma conditions as it safely and effectively raises the oxygen content of the water.

Remember to keep your eyes closed during the facial splash, as all essential oils are volatile and can irritate the eyes. This recipe can also be made into a facial mist and kept in the refrigerator. See the General Treatment Blending Chart on page 501 for facial mist proportions.

✍ Aromatic Face Splash ✍

> Cold water
> 1 drop chamomile essential oil
> 1 drop lavender essential oil
> ¼ cup hydrogen peroxide, 3 percent solution (optional)

Clean your bathroom sink thoroughly and fill it with cold water. Add the essential oils and, if desired, the hydrogen peroxide, and swish the water to disperse. With eyes closed at all times, splash your face with the aromatic water several times. Pat face dry with a towel.

Wait a minute or two, and then repeat the same process again. This can be done several times during the day.

Note: This is not recommended for small children.

Take a full body plunge. Asthma is one ailment that traditionally has been treated naturopathically with peroxide baths and oxygen spa soaks. During times of detoxification and rehabilitation, and as a regular part of your spa regime, oxygenating baths have much to offer in therapeutic benefits. Also known as peroxide bath, this spa treatment aids in the removal of toxins from the body and promote balance. Oxygen soaks have been used to treat skin problems, lung afflictions, as well as arthritic conditions. The typical pharmaceutical grade hydrogen peroxide you purchase at the drugstore, which contains 3 percent active H_2O_2, is fine for external use, such as in the spa bath. When added to water in a bath, the hydrogen peroxide reacts by creating a high concentration of oxygen, thereby producing a highly effective oxygen bath treatment that is both invigorating and relaxing. One pint of 3% hydrogen peroxide is equivalent to ten pints of oxygen! Oxygen spa soaks stimulate the mind and relieve stiffness and soreness of muscles. Most people experience a significant increase in their energy a few days following this spa treatment.

❧ Oxygen Spa Soak ❧

Warm water
1 to 2 cups hydrogen peroxide, 3 percent solution

Fill your bathtub with warm water—ideally, 98 to 100 degrees. Add 1 to 2 cups of hydrogen peroxide. Cases of arthritis, lethargy, poor circulation, muscle soreness, stress, and fungal infection benefit best from use of the higher amount. Soak in the bath for 20 to 30 minutes.

INHALATION

Feel the forest from home. I do not advise the use of steam inhalation for patients with asthma because it can trigger symptoms. Instead, I recommend inhalation with an aroma lamp or a diffuser. An electric diffuser is best; there is no heat involved in the process, which can be undesirable in asthma treatments.

This inhalation blend is intended for mild forms of asthma. If you have the time, do your breathing exercises while the diffuser is on. This will help remind you to do them, and you will benefit from the deep inhalation of the essential oils.

This blend has a very pleasant scent reminiscent of a clean, primeval forest rather than the typical medicinal odor you might expect of a respiratory blend. Notice all three oils in this recipe are derived from tree sources. Put a few drops of this blend on a tissue or a few cotton balls and keep in a plastic bag to carry with you for inhaling.

✆ Scent-of-the-Forest Spray ✆

1 part pine essential oil
1 part cedarwood essential oil
1 part sandalwood essential oil

In a 1-ounce amber glass bottle, add the oils one at a time, using an eyedropper if you are using small amounts. If possible, get ⅓-ounce bottles of the oils. Cap and shake to blend the oils. Label. Hook the bottle to your diffuser. Diffuse for 10 to 15 minutes, three to four times daily.

Oxygenate and hydrate the air. A cool mist humidifier can be very helpful for those with asthma. To increase the oxygen as well as hydrate the dry indoor air in your home, pour ½ to 1 cup of hydrogen peroxide (3 percent solution) into 1 gallon of water in your humidifier. It's estimated that 1 pint of hydrogen peroxide (3 percent solution) contains approximately 10 pints of oxygen!

You can also place 10 to 20 drops of the respiratory-enhancing essential oils into the machine as well, according to the manufacturer's directions. Typically there is a reservoir to hold the oils, or place them directly in the water.

LIFESTYLE

Steer clear of problems. Lifestyle changes are crucial to the success of any asthma prevention and wellness program. Avoiding the known irritants is an obvious change that must be considered. Here are some of the common irritant and allergen inhalants that should be avoided when possible:

- Pollens (weeds, grasses, some trees)
- House dust, molds, and fungal spores (including athlete's foot fungus)
- Feathers and animal hair
- Paint, gasoline, and industrial chemicals
- Tobacco smoke, cold air, and air pollutants

Spring clean year round. If you have asthma, the traditional spring-cleaning routine is not enough. Keep your home as clean as possible at all times. Use only natural cleaning products, since many of the chemicals added to commercial-brand cleaners are synthetic in origin and are irritating to many people in general, but especially to those with a sensitive respiratory tract.

Use a vacuum that does not recirculate dust and molds. Remember to ventilate your home regularly, even in the winter months. Additionally, clean air plants can be used for their air-filtering capability. For a list of these plants, see page 72.

Look for emotional roots. Not all people with asthma have an emotional component to their illness; however, it deserves exploration since there is a correlation between the two. I recommend that you read the "Mind over Matter" box on the next page, which highlights common emotions and psychological states and the relating essential oils to balance them. Decreasing levels of stress are beneficial to everyone and particularly to those with health challenges.

MASSAGE

Back to basics. This blend should be applied to the entire back area from the base of the spine up to the base of the neck. Also apply these oils to the feet and ankles. The feet are effective areas for aromatic massage, especially for respiratory ailments such as asthma.

The lavender and peppermint essential oils were chosen for this recipe for their general tonic effect on the entire body. Eucalyptus is included for its well-known respiratory benefits. I include ylang-ylang essential oil for its effect on the emotions, specifically anger, fear, and anxiety, with which asthma has a strong correlation. Together these essential oils create a synergistic blend that has been very effective for many people with asthma.

Mind Over Matter: Aromatherapy for Your Emotions

Use the following list as a guide to personalizing your sacred space and enhancing your mood. You will find throughout Part Two of this book that essential oils are recommended for stress, depression, hyperactivity, lethargy, insomnia, mental and nervous exhaustion, SAD, and pollution, as well as for lifestyle and other integrative approaches to balance and wellness.

Alertness: basil, eucalyptus, peppermint, rosemary, and spruce

Aphrodisia: ambrette seed, black pepper, jasmine, rose, and ylang-ylang

Anger: chamomile, melissa, rose, and ylang-ylang

Boredom: lemon and lemongrass

Confusion: basil, grapefruit, juniper, and rosemary

Depression: bergamot, clary sage, jasmine, lavender, lemon, neroli, and rose

Euphoria: clary sage, marjoram, and ylang-ylang

Hyperactivity: chamomile, clary sage, lavender, marjoram, sandalwood, vetiver, and ylang-ylang

Meditation and prayer: cedarwood, frankincense, myrrh, and sandalwood

Positive energy: bergamot, lavender, neroli, orange, petitgrain, rose, rosewood, and vetiver

Promotion of security: fennel, frankincense, hyssop, juniper, lavender, lemon, sandalwood, and vetiver

Purification: cedarwood, eucalyptus, juniper, lavender, lemon, pine, and rosemary

Sedation: chamomile, clary sage, lavender, marjoram, neroli, sandalwood, and ylang-ylang

Stimulation: basil, cypress, ginger, juniper, lemon, peppermint, pine, rosemary, and thyme

ᴏ Asthma Oil Blend ᴏ

16 drops lavender essential oil
3 drops peppermint essential oil
3 drops eucalyptus essential oil
3 drops ylang-ylang essential oil
2 tablespoons vegetable oil

In a clean amber glass bottle, add the essential oils. Cap securely and shake to mix. Add the vegetable oil and shake gently to mix thoroughly. Label.

To use, pour several drops of the oil on your hands and rub your hands together gently to warm the oils. Apply to the upper back area and the front of the upper chest. Inhale from your hands with several deep and relaxed breaths. Apply three times per day. This practice sends healing vibrations to the lung areas.

SOUND AND MUSIC THERAPY

Hum. To balance and clear the lungs, healing sounds called toning can be made by taking a deep breath of air and making the sound "hum" while exhaling. Repeat this three times daily.

TEAS AND TONICS

Brew a cup. This herbal tea will help strengthen and support the respiratory and immune systems.

ᴏ Your-Lungs-Will-Love-It Herbal Tea ᴏ

3 parts peppermint herb
2 parts anise seed, ground
1 part thyme herb
1 part sage herb

Mix the herbs together. Store in a clean glass jar and label with instructions for use. Use 1 teaspoon per cup or about ¼ cup per quart of water and simmer for 3 to 5 minutes. Remove from the heat and let steep, covered, for 10 minutes longer. Strain. Drink warm or at room temperature, up to three cups daily. Keep stored in the refrigerator for later use. Flavor with honey, lemon, or stevia herb if desired.

Real-Life Cure

SHE OUTSMARTED HER ASTHMA

When Angela, a beautiful, active young woman, developed asthma, she worried it would ruin her active lifestyle. Although her symptoms were occasional and mild, she feared they would eventually get worse.

This needn't happen, I told her, if she kept the symptoms at bay. I shared with her information on air purification and aromatherapy treatments that could help prevent and alleviate her symptoms. Her aromatherapy regimen included diffusing essential oils during the day at regular intervals. She substituted most of her cleaning products with nonchemical options.

Angela loved the aromatic baths I told her to take, which made her feel more relaxed. She performed breathing exercises daily, as well as cut out dairy products in her diet. She used my Aromatic Face Splash recipe (see page 94) as soon as she felt her chest tightening and her breathing becoming slightly labored. She religiously used the Asthma Oil Blend (see page 99) on her back and feet and found it very helpful.

Today, Angela feels as happy, healthy, and active as ever, and her asthma is totally under control. Attacks are mild and few and far between. Best of all, she is confident that her condition will not get worse as long as she continues to pamper herself and prevent the condition.

Athlete's Foot

Step in the Right Direction

There is fungus among us—everywhere. But is there fungus afoot near you?

If you've ever had athlete's foot, you know that it can be the itch from hell. Toe and nail fungus can also be unsightly and sometimes painful.

The term *athlete's foot* is actually a misnomer. Anyone can get it. You can pick up this minute parasitic infection by walking barefoot on contaminated moldy, spore-laden floors in swimming areas, gyms, public restrooms and shower areas, hot tubs, steam rooms, and even your own shower stall.

In severe cases of athlete's foot, the infection can lead to open sores or blisters. Unfortunately, once a person contracts nail fungus (onychomycosis), it is difficult to eradicate. Oral medications are often required. But don't let it get that far. Try these sweet treats for your feet.

Aromatherapy

Aromatic options. There are many natural botanical essences that are known to have antifungal properties. Some essential oils have shown to be very effective for *Tinea pedis* (the typical foot fungus), as well as having general antifungal properties. They are angelica, basil, bergamot, black spruce, cedarwood, citronella, clary sage, coriander, cypress, eucalyptus, fennel, geranium, German and Roman chamomile, helichrysm, lavender, lemon, lemongrass, marjoram, myrrh, neroli, palmarosa, patchouli, pine, rosemary, sandalwood, spikenard, tea tree, and thyme (wild, geraniol, and thymol types).

> ## Tip: Forget the Cornstarch
>
> Cornstarch is a common home remedy for athlete's foot, but I strongly advise against it. Not only does it cake easily but it's rich in nutrients that feed fungal spores. It could make the problem worse.

Say the secret word: clay. A foot powder, rather than an oil or lotion, is most effective for athlete's foot because it promotes dry skin and absorbs moisture. Powdered clay (not cornstarch!) is the basis for this foot powder recipe. Many different powdered types of clay are available, and any of them will work for this recipe. Clay is best because it absorbs more than two hundred times its weight in moisture!

The antifungal essential oils are simply added to this moisture-absorbing powder to increase its effectiveness.

⟨⟩ Sweet–Feet Foot Powder ⟨⟩

This is so sweet-smelling and effective it can double as a foot deodorant.

3 ounces powdered clay

1 ounce arrowroot powder

1 ounce powdered goldenseal herb

1 ounce rubbed sage leaves, finely ground

1 ounce baking soda

25 drops lavender essential oil

10 drops tea tree essential oil

10 drops geranium essential oil

10 drops cypress essential oil

5 drops eucalyptus essential oil

In a blender, add the powdered clay, arrowroot, goldenseal, sage, and baking soda. Blend on pulse until well combined. Add the essential oils and pulse again.

Store in a container with a lid that allows the contents to be shaken out. For example, a recycled spice jar works nicely, especially the type that has holes in the inner lid that allows for sprinkling. Label and keep in a dry, cool place.

Sprinkle onto feet and in between toes daily. You can also shake some into your socks and shoes.

HERBS

Grow your own. Herbs known to be helpful against foot fungus are aloe vera, basil, black walnut, calendula, fennel, garlic, rosemary, savory, and thyme. Use them liberally in your recipes and in your herbal teas. Other traditional but non-palatable herbs useful for fungal problems are horsetail, myrrh, olive leaf, Oregon grape, and pau de arco. These are often taken in capsule or tincture form. See product labeling for directions for use.

HYDROTHERAPY

Soak fungus away. To relieve itching and discourage fungal infection, a footbath is an effective treatment. The recipe below is made with antifungal and healing oils that discourage fungus growth. This particular recipe contains baking soda and Epsom salt as the carriers. Alternatively, you may add ¼ to ½ cup hydrogen peroxide (3 percent solution) to the foot soak, as it oxygenates the water. Oxygen discourages the growth of yeast and fungus. Dry your feet or use a hairdryer after treatment to fully inhibit moisture.

Try the Tip–Top Toe Treatment

Place several drops of geranium or tea tree essential oil onto cotton balls and tuck them between your toes. Or drop the oil onto small pieces of pure cotton or 100 percent wool yarn and wind it loosely between your toes.

Cotton and wool are naturally absorbent and will wick the moisture out of the area. Without moisture the fungus cannot survive.

❧ Athlete's Foot Bath ❧

2 drops tea tree essential oil
2 drops geranium essential oil
2 drops cypress essential oil
2 tablespoons baking soda
2 tablespoons Epsom or sea salt

In a small bowl, add the essential oils, baking soda, and salt and mix. Fill a foot basin or tub with warm (92 to 100 degrees) to tepid (80 to 92 degrees) water. Add the ingredients and swirl around to mix. Soak your feet for 15 minutes. Dry your feet thoroughly.

SALVES

Salve solves serious problem. For stubborn and serious cases of foot and nail problems, try this potent concentration of essential oils mixed in a calendula-infused oil base. You can purchase calendula ointment at your local health-food store.

∽ Fungus-Fighting Salve ∽

½ ounce calendula ointment
2 drops cypress essential oil
4 drops lavender essential oil
6 drops tea tree essential oil

Real-Life Cure

HE GOT TO THE BOTTOM OF HIS PROBLEM

Athlete's foot seemed to follow Keith, a thirty-three-year-old avid runner, wherever he went. His toes were constantly cracked and sore, and the itching drove him to distraction—and to me for help.

Since he was not one to be bothered with "fancy cures," I told him to try an antifungal soap made with essential oils. Since he was either in sneakers or enclosed shoes most of the day, I advised him to switch shoes frequently to give the moisture in the shoes time to dry. I also mixed up a batch of Sweet-Feet Foot Powder and asked him to give it a try. He even agreed to take footbaths.

After years of complaining about athlete's foot, his condition cleared up in just two weeks. Now, he says, no cure is too fancy for his feet!

If you are purchasing store-bought salve, use the same container (make certain it is at least ½ ounce in size to add the amounts of essential oils above). You can make larger amounts if you wish—just be sure to keep the same ratio of oils to ounces of ointment. Label. Apply with a cotton swab to clean, dry areas that are affected.

Teas and Tonics

A mild diuretic and antifungal herbal tea can be easily made from horsetail herb (*Equisetum arvenses*). It is useful for all fungal conditions, including athlete's foot, Candida albicans, ringworm, and thrush. Horsetail tea can also benefit the kidneys by restoring their function. The herb is an excellent source of calcium and other minerals such as potassium, iron, and magnesium.

Horsetail Tea

2 tablespoons horsetail herb
1 quart pure water

Simmer the herb and water for 10 minutes in a ceramic, glass, or enamel pot. Strain and drink during the day. You may flavor the tea with honey or stevia if you wish.

Backache

HEALING WITH PLEASURE

It's workplace nuisance number one.

Back pain, more specifically lower back pain, is the most commonly reported medical complaint when it comes to calling in sick or requesting sick leave. Lower back pain is a common problem in jobs that require heavy lifting or prolonged standing. In fact, eight out of ten people will experience lower back pain at some point in their lives.

But you just can't blame your job for causing your pain. Poor posture, weak muscles due to lack of exercise, and being overweight are major causes of back pain. Medical conditions such as arthritis and degenerative disc disease can create pain that feels never ending. But it's tension, whether created on or off the job, that causes most of us to wince in pain. When we're feeling stressed, tension builds in the neck and/or back muscles. As tension builds, the muscles tighten, creating spasms. Constant contraction inflames the muscles, setting you up for misery that's hard to ignore. Luckily, this is the kind of pain that is a pleasure to cure.

AROMATHERAPY

Spasm no more. The goals of aromatherapy treatment are to relieve muscle spasm and the resulting inflammation. When the muscles relax and adequate circulation can resume, the inflammation will subside. Therapeutic essential oils with anti-inflammatory, antispasmodic, and analgesic properties are the perfect means to a pain-free ending. Chief among them are bergamot, black pepper, chamomile, clary sage, cypress, eucalyptus, fennel, hyssop, juniper, lavender, marjoram, neroli, peppermint, rosemary, and sandalwood.

Use them in compresses, baths, and massage oils.

Tip: The Temperature Gauge

Think cold for sudden muscle spasms and pain that comes on suddenly, what's known as acute pain. Think heat for chronic backache. Sometimes, such as in pain caused by a fall, you want to use both. The rule of thumb is to always start with cold, followed by heat on the second day. If in doubt, check with your doctor.

HERBS

Herbal menders. There are numerous herbs available for a variety of muscular problems. For lower back pain I recommend the following because of their unique antispasmodic and muscle relaxing properties: cramp bark, hops, kava kava, passionflower, valerian root, wild lettuce, and wood betony. These botanicals can be prepared as herbal infusions or taken as herbal extracts or in capsule form.

HYDROTHERAPY

First sign of pain, think cold. For acute (sudden) back pain and spasm, reach for an ice pack or cold compress. Cold helps reduce swelling, which often is all you need to get relief. Put crushed ice in a plastic pack and wrap it in a towel (you don't want to apply it directly to the skin) and rest it against the site of the pain for 15 to 30 minutes. Repeat every hour, or until the pain disappears.

When to seek heat. For those long-lasting aches and pains due to chronic ailments caused by poor posture, being overweight, or stress-induced tension, moist heat may provide greater relief. Apply a hot-water heating pad covered with a towel directly on the irritated or painful muscle. Leave the hot pack on for 15 to 30 minutes at a time.

Soothe the pain away. Treat yourself right, and treat your back with this hydrotherapy treatment combined with essential oils.

❧ Aromatic Backache Blend ❧

For this you'll need a bowl, plastic wrap, and two towels large enough to cover the pained muscle and the immediate area surrounding it.

> 2 to 4 cups warm water (or more, as needed)
> 3 drops chamomile essential oil
> 2 drops rosemary or black pepper essential oil
> 2 drops clary sage essential oil
> 1 drop peppermint essential oil

Pour the water in a bowl large enough to soak the towel. Add the essential oils and stir well to disperse. Soak a towel, then wring until just moist. Apply directly to the painful area and the immediate surrounding area. Cover with plastic wrap (to help keep the towel warm and moist) and a second, dry towel. Optional: Place a cold ice pack or hot water bottle over this if it's available. The cold pack will aid in the alleviation of any swelling. Lie with your knees and hips flexed to take pressure off the lower back. Leave on for a total of 20 to 30 minutes. Moisten the compress as needed.

For a thoroughly enjoyable experience, do the breathing exercise on page 19.

LIFESTYLE

Watch how you move. The way you handle your everyday movements is a huge factor in controlling and preventing back pain. Simple changes in your daily habits can erase pain almost entirely. Take these actions immediately:

- Avoid prolonged sitting, standing, or walking. This includes sitting while driving long hours. Stop and take frequent breaks to walk and stretch.
- Learn to stand straight (most people don't). Practice in front of the mirror. In profile your shoulders should be straight back, your abdomen tucked in, and your knees unlocked.
- If you stand for long hours, especially on cement floors, appropriate shoes with additional cushion and support can be very helpful. Rest at regular intervals and take frequent breaks when possible. You should also consider orthotic foot supports.
- Lift correctly by bending down, not over! This assures your legs, not your back, do the work.

Sleep on it. Sleeping on a firm mattress or futon can help. My father used to sleep on a piece of plywood under the mattress for additional mattress support. If excess weight is a contributing factor, then losing weight will help.

Stress factor. As mentioned earlier, stress plays a major role in some forms of backache, and a good stress-relief program is needed. Refer to "Stress: The Big Chill-Out" (page 457) for effective aromatherapy and other integrative approaches. It would be a good idea to place a diffuser in your work area or inhale relaxing essential oils from a tissue throughout the day for stress prevention.

MASSAGE

Soothe away tension. Massage oil can be applied on a periodic basis to ease back pain and can be used regularly for chronic backache. You can do this treatment on your own, but you will increase the pleasure quotient if another person applies it for you.

Backache Massage Oil

This useful blend of oils, designed for simple lower backaches,
may be applied prior to strenuous activity that could
exacerbate backache, or afterward if pain is detected.

10 drops lavender essential oil
6 drops rosemary essential oil
6 drops sandalwood essential oil
3 drops geranium essential oil
2 tablespoons vegetable oil
(or a half and half combination
of arnica and vegetable oils)

In an amber glass bottle with a tight-fitting cap, add the essential oils and mix well. Add the vegetable oil, cap the bottle, and shake gently. Make sure all the ingredients are thoroughly mixed. Label.

To apply, warm a small amount in your palms by rubbing your palms together for a few seconds and gently massage it into the painful areas using small, circular motions. Or you can add 1 tablespoon of this blend to a warm bath to help soak away the pain. The oil blend tends to float on the surface of the bathwater but will envelope your body as you step into the bath.

Caution: When giving a massage, do not apply pressure directly on the spine.

YOGA AND MOVEMENT

Roll it out. To keep your back muscles stretched and exercise your abdominal muscles, perform this fun and easy maneuver, called the Roll Back exercise. Another benefit of this routine is that it relaxes and calms your mind. The rocking movement should be steady and rhythmic in order to alleviate any stiffness in the spine and gently massage the spinal vertebrae, back muscles, and ligaments. The goal is to roll as smoothly as possible along your spine to gently stretch and elongate the muscles. Do about ten to twelve repetitions, which only takes a few minutes.

Sit on a mat or thick carpet with your knees up and your feet flat on the floor. Imagine your head is being pulled to the top of the ceiling by an imaginary string.

While still in this sitting position, place your arms around your shins and hold in your abdomen.

Hold in That Tummy

Where do your abdominal muscles stand in the support zone?

Strong abs are important because they serve as a muscular corset to support the lower back. This is one of the reasons why poor muscle tone, being over-weight, and bad posture contribute to lower back pain.

Stretch and exercise regularly to keep the abdominal and back muscles toned, fit, and flexible. Try the exercise The Wall Butterfly Pose on page 266 for a great yoga exercise that helps alleviate most back discomfort.

Breathe in slowly as you curl your pelvis and tuck your chin to your chest. Gently roll back on your spine, going as far as you can on your shoulders. To roll back up, breathe out slowly, using your stomach muscles to assist you.

Come back to the sitting position after completing your breath. Again, imagine lengthening your spine to the ceiling while in this sitting position.

When to Call the Doctor

If, as a result of a fall or accident, you experience severe back pain that doesn't improve after one to two days, see your doctor for an evaluation. If you experience difficulty in controlling your bowels or bladder, numbness, or weakness in your pelvis or lower limbs, seek medical attention immediately. This could be a sign of a nerve injury.

Bad Breath

∿

KISS IT GOOD-BYE

Only a good friend will tell you: *You have bad breath!*

Bad breath, or halitosis, can be an embarrassing problem because it has the ability to bother everyone except the offender himself!

Occasional bad breath is common, especially after eating notorious offenders like garlic and onions. But habitual bad breath can be a sign of something awry elsewhere in the body. The chief suspects include poor digestion, food allergy, a highly acidic system, infection, or simply bacterial overgrowth from poor oral hygiene. Certain medications and dietary habits can also cause bad breath.

What Does Your Breath Say?

The Eastern alternative medical systems of oriental medicine and Ayurveda have long used breath odor as a diagnosing tool for determining a patient's state of health. They have long known that conditions like diabetes (sugary, sweet odor), kidney-related problems (uric acid or urine odor) as well as digestive problems can produce a change in breath scent. They consider simply getting close and smelling a patient's breath a legitimate diagnostic tool.

Now alternative health practitioners in the United States as well as researchers in Great Britain are getting in the act, but in a more upscale way. They are employing highly sophisticated computerized equipment that can perform "breath analysis" to diagnose these and other illnesses such as cirrhosis of the liver, stomach ulcers, lung cancers, and other diseases known to produce significant changes in breath odor.

There is no reason, however, that bad breath should be your ban. Even some of the most stubborn cases respond to natural remedies.

AROMATHERAPY

Mint is most essential. An easy and effective mouthwash is all you need for the occasional bad breath or, used daily, for prevention and good oral hygiene. Peppermint essential oil is best known for its beneficial effect on the digestive system and most notably for bad breath. It is no coincidence that many oral-care products, including mouthwashes, breath sprays, toothpaste, and candies, incorporate mint flavorings. My recipe, however, has no preservatives, harsh chemicals, or artificial colors. I've added the lemon juice to help balance pH.

Traditionally, garden sage (*Salvia officinalis*) in tea form was used for a mouthwash, which is why I offer it as an alternative to the distilled water in this recipe. The honey, which has anti-inflammatory and antibacterial properties, acts as the carrier for the essential oils, since they do not dissolve in water. Sage honey gives this recipe even more power, especially if you have a sore throat. To make Sage Honey, turn to page 446.

✍ Kiss–Me Mouthwash ✍

If you find you like this mouthwash as much as my family does, you'll be making it regularly. I recommend mixing up a large amount of the pure essential oils separately in an amber bottle. You can multiply the essential oil drops by 10 or simply measure them out in full droppers, being sure to keep the same ratios (2:2:1). Then, when it's time to make more, just count out 5 or 6 of the premixed drops. For optimum freshness, ymake enough to last no more than a week.

> 1 teaspoon raw honey or Sage Honey
> 2 drops peppermint essential oil
> 2 drops spearmint essential oil
> 1 drop anise seed essential oil
> 1 teaspoon fresh lemon juice (optional)
> 1 cup warmed distilled water or sage herbal tea

In a 2-cup measure, add the honey, the essential oils, and, if desired, the lemon juice. Mix well. Add the warm distilled water or herbal tea to the blend of honey and oils. Stir until completely dissolved. Pour into an amber bottle. Cap and label.

Before each use, shake well. Pour about 2 to 3 tablespoons into a glass and swish it around your mouth for 30 to 60 seconds. Spit out. No need to rinse.

Choose your flavor. In addition to peppermint, other essential oils that aid digestion and erase bad breath are nutmeg, rosemary, and spearmint.

Sweeten your toothbrush. Place 1 drop (no more) of peppermint or anise seed essential oil on your toothbrush along with your tooth-paste before brushing your teeth, for extra kissable breath!

Herbs

Get your share of breath-friendly flavors. Herbs and spices that not only taste good but also make your breath smell good include anise, basil, cardamom, cinnamon, clove, coriander, dill, eucalyptus, fennel, ginger, parsley, peppermint, rosemary, sage, spearmint, and turmeric. All of these can be made into an herbal infusion and used as a mouthwash base. Use them liberally in cooking.

Be sure to buy organic when possible—at least make sure they are chemical free—and grow your own when spring season comes.

Chew on this. In many Eastern and European countries, seeds of specific plants are chewed following a meal to aid in digestion and prevent bad breath. It is the essential oils inherent in the seeds that make them effective. So the next time you go out to your favorite Italian restaurant for a spicy, garlic-laden meal, reach for the Sweet-Breath Seed Mix instead of the candy. Your friends and coworkers will appreciate it.

Mints Too Many to Count

In nature, there are around three hundred species of peppermint, but only two or three are used in commercial industry, with the majority utilized by the dentifrice manufacturers who use peppermint oil to flavor and scent toothpaste, mouthwash, toothpicks, and dental floss.

ᴓ Sweet–Breath Seed Mix *ᴓ*

I keep this mix on the ready in a decorative jar on the kitchen counter.
Keep a supply handy in your purse and office desk drawer.

1 part anise seed
1 part fennel seed
1 part caraway seed

Combine the anise, fennel, and caraway seeds in a bowl. Store openly in a dish or small jar.

Enhance your oral health. Botanicals that are warming, astringent, slightly antibacterial, and healing for connective tissue are the ones to use for maintaining an all-around healthy mouth. These include calendula, chlorophyll, cinchona bark, echinacea, goldenseal, prickly ash bark, and turmeric. You can find some of these herbs in natural, holistic mouthwashes and teeth-cleaning products. Other natural food ingredients for oral health are aloe vera, bee propolis, sesame oil, and wheat germ oil.

Stay lemon fresh. If you smoke, drink alcohol, or have several cups of coffee per day, keep plenty of fresh lemons on hand. Fresh lemon juice helps neutralize acids and is a powerful antibacterial agent.

Lifestyle

If you can't brush . . . Swish your mouth with water. Rinsing after meals with water is the next best thing for good oral hygiene when it is inconvenient to brush. Water acts as a natural mouthwash. This is a good practice to teach your children: Brush morning and night and rinse after every meal.

Brush your tongue. In Ayurvedic medicine, part of good oral hygiene includes tongue-scraping with the use of a flat, wire instrument. It is believed that the tongue collects a coating of toxins and metabolic waste, especially after a night's rest when many toxins are eliminated.

Alternatively, you can brush your tongue effectively using an ordinary toothbrush. Gently brush to get rid of any coating present. Be sure to rinse your toothbrush well afterward and allow it to dry. If you are fasting or on a detoxification program, examine your tongue regularly, and if there is very little coating, it is a good sign of health and complete cleansing.

Bites and Stings

ᴏ

No More Tears

Flies, fleas, mosquitoes, bees. They sure do have a nasty way of introducing themselves! I bet there is no one among us who hasn't experienced the stinging bite (and subsequent itching) of an insect or the startling sting (and subsequent swelling) of a bee, yellow jacket, hornet, or wasp.

Insects have an extremely sensitive olfactory system (sense of smell). It is what guides them to specific plants and other insects in what is a complex interrelationship. Certain plants emit aromatic molecules (essential oils) to attract particular insects to aid in self-preservation via pollination, while others can emit specific aromatic molecules to ward off or deter specific insects for self-protection.

Often, as they go about their business, you get in the way. It could be the perfume or colors you're wearing. Or an arm or foot gets in the wrong place at the wrong time. As a result, commercial bug repellents are big-time business. Many of these products contain irritating chemicals that are potentially harmful and should not come into contact with the skin, eyes, or mucous membranes—or be inhaled, for that matter. This is why I recommend that you go the natural course. Everything I recommend here is safe, and it works.

> ### Tip: Stinger Free in Seconds
>
> The best way to get rid of a stinger is to scrape it out. Using your fingernail or the edge of a credit card, gently scrape under the stinger and flip it out.

Except for removing the stinger, if left behind, the treatment for insect bites and bee stings is relatively the same. Here's how to get the ouch out—naturally.

AROMATHERAPY

Nature's first-aid oils. Essential oils that help relieve the pain, itch, and swelling of bites and stings are basil, bergamot, chamomile, eucalyptus, lavender, lemon, lemongrass, melissa, niaouli, patchouli, pine, and tea tree.

Take it straight. Lavender and tea tree essential oils can be applied directly to the bite or sting by applying 1 drop neat, which means undiluted. These are a few oils that can safely be used this way. All the others mentioned above must be diluted.

Or use a little mixer. Moisten a cotton swab with fresh lemon juice, apple cider vinegar, or witch hazel, then add 1 or 2 drops of essential oil. Dab it onto the skin. It will give you a cool, soothing tingle. Apply as often as necessary.

Bug Off! A Natural Repellent

Citronella is a well-known active ingredient in bug repellents and is frequently found in outdoor candles. It is the scent familiar in many products, including Ivory soap and Avon's Skin-So-Soft lotion, the latter well known for deterring bugs. Citronella, however, has a very strong odor and can be quite overpowering if used in too high a dilution.

I like this blend because the other oils mask the strong odor of citronella but the bugs are none the wiser!

❧ Bug-and Bee-Free Lotion ❧

My kids won't go camping without this. Use a plastic bottle, which is convenient to carry.

> 5 drops cedarwood essential oil
> 4 drops lemon essential oil*
> 2 drops geranium essential oil
> 1 drop citronella essential oil
> 2 tablespoons vegetable oil

In a plastic squeeze bottle, add the essential oils. Cap and gently shake. Add the vegetable oil and cap again. Shake vigorously before using. Apply a few drops onto exposed skin. A little goes a long way to keep bugs away!

Caution: Omit the lemon essential oil if you plan on being in the direct sunlight, as lemon oil is phototoxic and can cause a sunburn if put on immediately prior to sun exposure. Instead substitute lemongrass, rosemary, or eucalyptus for the lemon oil.

Age-Old Enemies That Work

Mother Nature gave certain plants specific aromatic oils to help attract insects for pollination and to repel other insects that could do them harm. The following essential oils are tried and true aromas that provide effective defense in keeping those offensive insects away from you:

Ants: Peppermint
Fleas: Cajeput, lemon, and pine
Houseflies: Citronella, geranium, and juniper
Mosquitoes: Basil, cedarwood, citronella, geranium, juniper, and rosemary

Spice up your sleeping bag. Put a few drops of essential oil on your clothes, sleeping bag, hat, and tent. It doesn't have to be on your skin to keep the bugs away!

HERBS

Feast on garlic. Most insects hate garlic! Eat plenty of it and it's likely they'll fly right by you and settle on someone else for lunch.

Keep Out!

Certain herbs and essential oils are very useful in repelling insects and are relatively safe and natural alternatives—but only if used properly. Pennyroyal herb has been used for centuries in this way, and the essential oil made from that plant is used extensively in many commercial preparations. However, this oil can be dangerous, especially for pregnant women, if used improperly, and is not recommended for personal use. In addition to pennyroyal, stay away from southernwood, tansy, and wormwood. A complete list of hazardous essential oils can be found on page 15.

Spread mint around. Another kind of herb distasteful to insects is mint—any kind of mint. Perhaps that's why mint juleps used to be the classic outdoor party drink.

Other herbs that are picnic perfect are useful as insect repellents are garlic, lavender, lemon balm, all types of mint, pennyroyal, southernwood, tansy, and wormwood. (Be sure the later list is in the form of the herb and not the essential oil.)

Spray them away. Here's an insect repellent spray that you can use on your skin or as a room spray. You'll like the smell, but bugs are guaranteed to hate it! An herbal tea spray can be made from various herbs (dried or fresh, but not the essential oil) to be used as a room mist or to apply on clothing and the skin.

∽ Torment–Them Tea Spray ∽

Note: This is made into a tea spray from the fresh or dried herbs, not the essential oil!

> 2 tablespoons lavender flowers
> 2 tablespoons pennyroyal herb
> 2 tablespoons southernwood herb
> 2 tablespoons tansy herb
> 2 tablespoons wormwood herb
> 1 cup boiling water

Combine the flowers and herbs in a large pot and pour the boiling water over them. Allow them to steep for 15 minutes or longer. Cool, strain through a fine sieve, and pour into a small spray bottle. Label contents with directions for use. Spray into the air or onto exposed skin, avoiding the eyes and mouth.

Powerful pastes. A paste made from baking soda, meat tenderizer, or clay powder can be used to relieve the discomfort of a bite or sting. To make a paste, add 1 to 2 drops of the listed essential oils (basil, chamomile, lavender, and tea tree are my favorite choices) to the above ingredients (singly or in combination). Apply this aromatic paste to the bug bite or sting as a first-aid treatment.

HYDROTHERAPY

Rub it with ice. This is the first thing you should do when you have a bug bite or sting. Rubbing an ice cube over the area that has been stung is helpful in relieving immediate swelling and pain.

LIFESTYLE

Prevention means being aware. Campsites, hiking trails, picnic rest areas, and even your own backyard are common hangouts for stinging and biting insects. Yellow jackets, for example, nest on the ground and are often stepped upon by unwary persons who may be barefoot. Therefore, you should wear shoes or sandals while at such places. Also be aware that bees are attracted to bright clothing, sweet smells, and perfumes.

A Camp-Out Strategy That Works

My oldest son liked to camp a lot as a teenager and found what worked best by trial and error. To successfully keep away mosquitoes, he soaked strips of cloth with a blend of citronella and geranium essential oils in a vegetable oil base. He tied the cloth strips around trees surrounding his camp. It worked! No mosquitoes.

Alternatively, he would burn dried herbs and certain tree barks in his campfire to keep the bugs away. His favorite scents (growing up in the Pacific Northwest) were cedar branches and bark, juniper, and pine needles and cones.

Get Medical Attention Now!

A bee sting can be a dangerous allergen. It can even be deadly. If you or someone in your presence experiences chest tightness, wheezing, a swollen face or tongue, or any other severe symptom, it could be a sign of an allergy that potentially could lead to fatal anaphylactic shock. People who know they are allergic should carry an insect sting kit. If no kit is available, apply an ice pack and head for the emergency room.

Bleeding Gums

RINSE TO THE RESCUE

Healthy gums do not bleed. So bleeding gums means something is unbalanced somewhere.

When dentists hear the words *bleeding gums,* the first thing that comes to mind is gingivitis, an inflammation that, left untreated, can lead to more serious gum disease. In addition to bleeding, early signs of this include redness, swelling, and a receding gum line.

But before jumping to conclusions, there are less problematic reasons why gums bleed. The word we use for this is *trauma.* Gums are delicate tissues and are easily wounded. Smoking can irritate the gums and cause them to bleed. So can plaque buildup, vigorous brushing, or an overly stiff toothbrush.

And then there are braces. Children (adults, too!) challenged to care for their gums properly due to the steel ware have shown early signs of gingivitis.

Besides direct trauma, bleeding gums may be a symptom of an underlying weakness in the immune system or a nutritional deficiency.

Tip: Aspirin and Gums

Taking aspirin on a long-term or continual basis? If you see red on your toothbrush in the morning, aspirin could be the reason why. Aspirin acts as a blood thinner, making tender gums prone to bleed more freely against vigorous brushing. Check it out with your health-care practitioner just to make sure.

The following remedies are excellent for helping the healing process, but the underlying cause must be addressed for true healing to take place.

AROMATHERAPY

Age-old antidotes. Myrrh resin and sage herb have been used traditionally for all mouth and gum disorders. Both the sage and myrrh are healing and astringent in general and help strengthen the gums. Eucalyptus and lemon essential oils are effective in halting bleeding. Other essential oils that combat gum disease are clary sage, fennel, geranium, juniper, rosemary, and tea tree. Use them in mouthwash preparations or look for natural tooth-pastes that contain them.

Rinse the problem away. The following all-natural mouth rinse is considered one of my best recipes by many. I've been told it is almost miraculous in healing and stopping bleed-ing gums. Cleanse the mouth well by gently brushing with natural toothpaste or my tooth powder recipe, especially following meals, to decrease bacterial growth.

Valerie's Miracle Mouthwash

This is best made fresh daily and used warm but can be made ahead of time and stored in the refrigerator. For optimal freshness, make no more than a week's worth at a time.

1 cup warm sage herbal tea
1 tablespoon distilled witch hazel (optional)
1 teaspoon raw honey
2 to 3 drops tincture of myrrh
1 drop lemon essential oil
1 drop eucalyptus essential oil

Pour the sage herbal tea into a small bowl and, if desired, stir in the witch hazel. In a separate bowl, combine the honey, myrrh, and the lemon and eucalyptus oils. Add the honey mixture to the tea and stir to combine. To use, pour 2 to 3 table-spoons in a glass. Thoroughly swish the mouthwash, holding it in your mouth for as long as you can (preferably 30 to 60 seconds). Rinse your mouth with this oral wash several times per day, particularly following meals and prior to retiring at night.

H-mmm *good.* Place 1 drop of fennel or myrrh essential oil on your soft-bristle tooth-brush for an effective and pleasant-tasting gum treatment while brushing. Each of these oils can be used with a natural toothpaste or by itself.

D<small>IET</small>

Sage is for more than stuffing. Since sage (the herb *salvia oficinalis*) is such a great mouth defender, I suggest incorporating it into your diet as much as possible. Experiment with it in your recipes. Use it in your tea. Get it in some form daily or at least several times a week.

> ### Tip: Be a Green-Tea Fan
>
> Among the many healing discoveries of drinking green tea: Its amazing antioxidant qualities may help prevent cavities.

Start the day with a lemon drink. Lemon is healthy for the gums due to its alkalizing and antibacterial properties. I suggest that you take it daily as fresh juice in hot water every morning before the morning meal. Squeeze the juice of half a lemon into 1 cup of warm water and drink first thing in the morning.

Crave those cranberries. Studies have found that cranberries may help prevent plaque from adhering to the teeth and is presently being studied. So eat them often.

> ### Real-Life Cure
>
> HIS GUMS ARE SORE NO MORE
>
> Kevin, a bright-eyed seven-year-old boy with a history of swollen gums and occasional bleeding, used this recipe with great success. His mother stated that when his gums got red and sore, he refused to brush at all, sometimes for days. The doctors she had taken him to see could not find the cause of the bleeding gums. As soon as he tried Valerie's Miracle Mouthwash he felt considerable relief from the soreness and swelling, and the bleeding decreased. By the second day, he was able to brush his teeth, eat without discomfort, and be examined more completely by his dentist, which was not possible earlier. When he uses this mouth rinse regularly, he has absolutely no complaints and his gums stay strong and healthy!

Body Odor

ℴ

Natural Germ Killers

A Natural Scent

Today our culture seems almost obsessed by a new fear: body odor. At least, that's how it appears to me as witnessed by magazine and television advertising. My, how the pendulum has swung since 1820s England, when soap was considered unhealthy! It's time, I say, to find a healthy medium.

I believe the overuse of skin cleansers is stripping the body's natural protective coating (film of sebum) and washing it right down the drain. This natural moisturizing covering on the skin's surface is crucial to keeping our skin—the largest sensory organ of the body—in good working order.

Between our cultural stigma and our state of health, body odor can have quite a different meaning. A malodorous body smell can be caused by bad hygiene, or it can be a sign that something's not right somewhere in the body. In fact, the military service in Japan used to disqualify men who presented abnormally strong body odor, believing it an outward sign of general ill health.

Body scent has an aura of mystery about it. It plays a role in newborns recognizing their mother. There is evidence that suggests body odor is part of the attraction of one person to another. It's said that Napoleon Bonaparte sent a note requesting that his wife, Josephine, not wash for three days prior to his return from battle because he loved her natural body odor and knew his desire for her was strongest when she did not wash.

Body odor isn't always bad. Perspiration by itself does not cause an odor problem as long as good health is maintained and adequate hygiene is practiced. Body odor only becomes a problem when improper hygiene, ill health, or abnormally high bacterial growth comes into play. Bacteria can multiply on the skin's surface, primarily in moist places like the armpits, groin, under the breasts, and on the feet, and cause body odor. This is the most common cause of body odor and the type I'm addressing here.

But first I want to give you some of my personal thoughts. I think it's good for the skin to sweat and perspire; after all, this is a cleansing effect of the body (lymphatic system) and skin. I don't recommend the use of antiperspirants or commercial deodorants. Most of them contain unhealthy chemicals and metals that have been linked to liver damage and Alzheimer's disease.

AROMATHERAPY

Use the right soap. As I said, it is normal for the body to sweat, and we should not interfere with this elimination process. However, there are a few essential oils known to help with excessive perspiration and sweat that do not halt the natural function of the body but rather aid in regulating overproduction and overstimulation of the sweat glands. They are cypress, lemongrass, petitgrain, and pine. They are astringent and tone the skin's pores.

Wash with a mild olive oil–based soap containing these essential oils. You can find them in natural health stores. You'll also find them in body sprays and splashes, body lotions or oils, and aromatic bath products.

Use only skin-friendly oils. Almost all essential oils have antibacterial benefits; however, there are some essences that are stronger than others. Keep in mind that only skin-friendly essential oils should be used on the skin. These include bergamot, clary sage, cypress, eucalyptus, grapefruit, juniper, lavender, lemon, lemongrass, mandarin, neroli, patchouli, peppermint (in low dilution), petitgrain, pine, rosemary, sandalwood, and tea tree.

Personalize and deodorize. Make your own natural body deodorant spray and customize it with your own combination of essential oils. Don't fret about smelling like vinegar; the vinegar odor fades after a few minutes.

Note: Do not apply essential oils under the arms. The heat and moisture in this area decrease the ability of the oils to evaporate and can cause skin irritation or sensitization. This recipe is a gentle body deodorant spray for general use.

⁓ (Fill in Your Name) Body Scent Spray ⁓

7 ounces floral water, herbal infusion, or mineral water
1 ounce raw apple cider vinegar

2 teaspoons raw honey

60 drops (total) essential oil (from the selection below)

10 drops grapefruit seed extract (optional)

In a fine mist spray bottle, add the water and vinegar. Put the honey in a small bowl and add the essential oils one by one, mixing as you add each. Add the grapefruit seed extract if desired. Add the mixture to the water. Shake well. Label. After showering or bathing, or for use during the day, simply spray over the entire body, avoiding the eyes and under the arms. Shake well before each use.

Clean options. Do you want the feel of being in a garden? Would you prefer the crisp clean scent of citrus? Or do you like the down-home aroma of herbs? Each of the following combinations has a distinctive aroma and will have a characteristic feel on you. Experiment to discover which is uniquely you. Your natural deodorant can be as individualized as you are.

Soft Floral

7 ounces rose floral water

40 drops lavender essential oil

14 drops mandarin essential oil

4 drops clary sage essential oil

2 drops patchouli essential oil

Fresh Citrus

7 ounces orange blossom water

20 drops grapefruit essential oil

20 drops lemongrass essential oil

15 drops bergamot essential oil

5 drops cypress essential oil

Caution: Avoid use in direct sun, as citrus oils can increase your chance of sunburn.

Light Herbal
7 ounces lavender floral water
20 drops rosemary essential oil
20 drops sandalwood essential oil
5 drops eucalyptus essential oil
15 drops juniper essential oil

HERBS

Antiseptic herbs. Any combination of these herbs can be made into an infusion (tea) and used in place of floral water in the body spray recipe given above. You should also use them liberally in your daily diet. They are basil, lavender flowers, lemon balm, marjoram, oregano, peppermint, sage, and sweet thyme.

HYDROTHERAPY

Beat body odor with baths. Full aromatic baths can be taken several times weekly to kill odor-producing bacteria and naturally deodorize the skin. Add a total of 8 to 10 drops of any of the essential oils mentioned above to 2 cups of apple cider vinegar and pour into the bathwater.

The vinegar naturally balances the pH of the water and is slightly acidic to discourage bacterial growth. Rose Petal Perk Me Up on page 216 can also be used in the bath to eliminate body odor.

Sweet-feet solution. If your body odor is coming from your feet, then an aromatic foot-bath is very helpful. Add the following essential oils to the Detoxifying Bath Salts recipe. Mix 4 to 6 drops of cypress essential oil in about 1 to 2 tablespoons of the bath salt and add to the basin. Soak your feet for 15 to 20 minutes. Follow with the Sweet-Feet Foot Powder recipe (on page 102), which aids in keeping the feet dry and odor free. You can substitute any of the essential oils listed in this section in the foot powder recipe so it will be extra deodorizing for this problem. You can also use other essential oils of your choice in this bath salt recipe for other purposes.

∾ Detoxifying Bath Salts ∾

1 teaspoon baking soda
2 teaspoons Epsom salt
3 teaspoons Celtic Sea or Dead Sea salt
1 teaspoon powdered kelp or clay (optional)
6 to 12 drops essential oil of your choice

Mix the dry ingredients together in a small dish. Add the essential oils of your choice and stir well. Add to the bathwater.

LIFESTYLE

Go into body combat. To win the battle against odor-causing bacteria, do the following as part of your daily routine:

- Use only pH-balanced soaps and body shampoos.
- Avoid over-the-counter antiperspirants and chemical deodorants.
- Make your own natural body sprays and splashes.
- Decrease consumption of dairy products and sugar.
- Get plenty of zinc in your diet (good sources are organic eggs, pumpkin seeds).
- Detoxify your body as needed (at least yearly, spring cleaning with tonics).
- Promote friendly flora in your diet (raw cultured vegetables, kefir, probiotics).
- Eat plenty of fiber (fruits, vegetables, whole grains, or supplement).
- Hydrate your body to flush out toxins (8 to 10 glasses of pure water daily).
- Eat natural, health-promoting foods (sea vegetables are highly recommended; avoid chemicals, preservatives).

Boils

❧

AN ANTIBACTERIAL BATH

Blocked and infected pores may be annoying but are still a fairly superficial skin condition. But a boil, quite literally, will get under your skin.

Often painful and unsightly, boils bore deep in the skin and often involve hair follicles and surrounding tissue. Boils are caused by infection, usually bacterial in origin. Symptoms include redness, swelling, heat, blisters, or pus-filled lumps.

Do not attempt to squeeze boils, as this will encourage the bacteria to spread to surrounding areas and will injure the tissue, very possibly causing scarring. Very gentle treatment is necessary, as suggested here.

AROMATHERAPY

Welcome pore help. Essential oils are very effective for healing boils because they are strong antibacterial and anti-inflammatory agents. They are highly concentrated as well as safe and gentle to the skin. Oils of choice are bergamot, carrot seed, chamomile, clary sage, eucalyptus, geranium, lavender, lemon, myrrh, neroli, patchouli, rose, and tea tree.

Dress with care. If a boil opens (hint: it will ooze), a sterile dressing should be applied immediately to prevent spreading the infection. A simple Band-Aid is sufficient. Soothe the sore by putting a few drops of lavender or tea tree essential oil on the dressing before covering the open wound.

Change the bandage three times daily, as drainage will continue. Make sure your hands are clean. A sterile environment is essential.

Once the wound has healed and is completely closed (with no signs of infection), use the Scar-Diminishing Preparation on page 415, especially important if the boil is on your face.

DIET

Watch your A and E. Vitamins A, C, and E and the mineral zinc are helpful to healthy skin. Make sure you are getting plenty in your diet.

HERBS

Fight infection from the inside out . . . Keep your body active against infection with echinacea, garlic, goldenseal, and onion. All can be taken internally.

And the outside in. Herbs that can be used topically (on the skin) are aloe vera, chickweed, comfrey, and parsley.

Old Folk Cure: Onion

I've never tried it, but this old folk cure for boils is well documented. A softly baked onion cut in half and applied to the boil will help draw out and bring the infection to a head.

HYDROTHERAPY

Compress it. Here is a soothing and aromatic compress made with hot sea water, Epsom salt, and essential oils that will encourage the infection to surface and be released from the body.

✍ Hot Compress for Boils *✍*

2 cups hot water*
2 tablespoons sea salt
2 tablespoons Epsom salt
4 drops chamomile or lavender essential oil
2 drops tea tree essential oil
2 drops lemon essential oil

In a bowl or very clean basin, add the hot water. In a small dish, add the sea and Epsom salts. Add the essential oils to the salts and mix well with a spoon. Add the aromatic salts to the hot water and stir. Soak a piece of flannel cloth in the water solution, wringing it out until it is moist.

Put the hot compress over the boil and cover with plastic wrap and a towel. Replace the compress with a fresh, hot one when it has become cool or dry. Leave on for 20 minutes. Repeat three times daily until the infection comes to a head and is released. Optional: Cover the dressing described above with a hot water bottle to prolong heat therapy.

Caution: Water that is 100 to 104 degrees is detoxifying and increases circulation. Measure water temperature carefully with a thermometer to prevent skin burns.

Backside relief. If you have a boil on your backside or other location that makes compress therapy difficult, take a full bath using the Detoxifying Bath Salts recipe on page 128.

Drink, drink, drink. Drink plenty of pure water—8 to 10 glasses a day—and herbal teas to help cleanse the body from the inside.

Drink a lemon aide. Here's another way to wash away infection: Add the juice of half a lemon to 1 cup of warm water. Drink daily, up to three times a day if desired.

Take long hot showers. Avoid taking baths once the boil has opened to prevent the infection spreading to other areas.

When to Call the Doctor

If you find yourself continually developing boils or infected pores, it may be a sign of a weakened immune system, poor diet, inadequate hygiene, or diabetes. Repeated exposure to environmental pollutants may also be the cause. See a health-care professional who is knowledgeable in natural alternative medicine to identify the underlying cause.

Take an ocean swim. According to medical folklore, swimming in salt water helps heal skin infection. It is worth a try and a great excuse for taking a vacation!

Breast–Feeding Problems
✺

BABY THOSE SORE NIPPLES

Painful bliss sounds like an oxymoron—unless you're a new mom with dry or cracked nipples. To make this blissful time of your life less painful, try the following.

AROMATHERAPY

The essence of relief. Essential oils are naturals for cracked and dry nipples because they are natural healers and moisture savers. The most helpful oils are typically from roots and flowers. The best oils are benzoin, frankincense, geranium, German and Roman chamomile, jasmine, lavender, myrrh, neroli, patchouli, rose, sandalwood, and ylang-ylang. Niaouli and tea tree can also be included for their healing and antiseptic benefits, especially if there are deep fissures present.

MASSAGE

Baby your breasts. This aromatic massage oil is extremely effective in soothing sore nipples. Massage the breasts in a circular motion from the center (midline of chest) outward in a counterclockwise direction. This stroke direction encourages lymphatic drainage away from the congested breasts to the lymph nodes under the arms.

✺ Baby-Your-Breast Oil ✺

4 drops orange essential oil
2 drops geranium essential oil
2 tablespoons vegetable oil

In a 1-ounce amber glass bottle, add the essential oils. Add the vegetable oil, cap securely, and shake well. Label. Apply once a day or as needed.

Note: This should not be used immediately prior to breast-feeding. The best time to apply is after nursing.

Call in the breast guard. For nipples that are very sore and cracked, a more potent medicinal may be needed. The healing balm is well worth the time to prepare. You can make your own infusion oil (see recipe on page 206), or, to cut down on preparation time, you can purchase the calendula infusion oil already made.

◎ Mother's Breast Balm ◎

4 (200 IU) vitamin E capsules
4 drops German chamomile essential oil
8 drops tea tree essential oil
20 drops lavender essential oil
10 drops sandalwood essential oil
2 ounces calendula infusion oil

Mix the vitamin E and essential oils into the base oil. Open the vitamin E capsules by cutting the ends and squeezing their content into the base ointment. Blend well and label. Apply a small amount to the affected areas. Wash hands well. Be sure to wipe off the nipples just prior to breast-feeding if the balm has not completely absorbed.

Breast Tenderness

✺

A Soothing Support System

Do your breasts these days feel too heavy to handle?

For most women, "these days" are PMS days when fluctuating hormones race through our bodies, causing a variety of uncomfortable symptoms, the most common being swollen and painful breasts. But it usually takes pregnancy to realize just how uncomfortable this feeling can be. And the agony can last for weeks. Here's how to make the best of it.

Hydrotherapy

Cool, calm, and collected. I have recommended this compress to moms-to-be many times, and it always gets high ratings. The cool temperature of the aromatic water feels especially good on swollen breasts.

✺ Best Breast Compress ✺

For large breasts, tube socks are a good alternative to washcloths.

Cool (70 to 80 degrees) water
2 drops orange essential oil
1 drop geranium or German chamomile essential oil

Fill a bowl or very clean basin with cool water. Add the essential oils and stir with your hand to mix into the water. Soak two washcloths (or two large tube socks) in the aromatic water. Wring the cloth until it is moist but not soaked. Wrap the washcloths or socks around each breast. Drape a towel over the washcloths, lie down, and relax. Leave the compresses on until they become too cool or dry, then replace with fresh ones. Leave on for 15 minutes, one to three times daily.

Take a cold shower. At the end of a shower, turn the spray to cool and let the water run over your breasts. Do this for as long as you are comfortable.

Lifestyle

Get the support you need. The increasing weight and stretching of the breasts during pregnancy can become very uncomfortable. Wearing a good support bra that fits properly is key. This is also especially good advice for large breasted women going through PMS. However, I do not recommend wire bras due to their restriction to the lymphatic system.

Bronchitis

Nature's Clearinghouse

By definition, bronchitis is an inflammation of the bronchi, the large passageways in the lungs that transport air toward the bloodstream to create the life-sustaining process known as breathing.

By experience, bronchitis is a miserable, aching feeling and deep, hacking cough that just won't stop. Phlegm that turns ghoulish shades of gray or green is the big tip-off that your common cold has progressed to bronchitis.

Acute bronchitis can follow a cold, flu, or sinus infection and is most common in the wintertime. Environmental air pollutants, such as inhaling cigarette smoke, noxious gas fumes, or high counts of air pollutants or pollen, can also bring on bronchitis. Even swallowing food that "goes down the wrong pipe" (known as aspiration) can cause this otherwise sterile area to become contaminated.

Chronic bronchitis is a persistent and often phlegm-producing cough that comes and goes or hangs around for long periods of time. This is most common in people who smoke, drink excessively, or are exposed habitually to harmful chemicals or pollutants.

AROMATHERAPY

A little dab will do. Essential oils are powerful agents against respiratory ailments such as bronchitis. Two of the most beneficial are eucalyptus and peppermint. Cedarwood, frankincense, lemon, myrrh, niaouli, and sandalwood work best for chronic bronchitis. Other essences are basil, bergamot, fennel, ginger, hyssop, juniper, lavender, marjoram, melissa, nutmeg, pine, rosemary, and tea tree. Take advantage of the healing power of these oils by putting a few drops on a handkerchief or tissue and inhaling the essence throughout the day. In addition, these essences can be diffused throughout your office or home to prevent illness in others. Electronic diffusers work best for this purpose.

BREATH WORK

Fill your chest with air. Deep-breathing exercises will help to fully expand the lungs, relax muscles, relieve anxiety, and even help you sleep.

To chest breathe, place your hands on your chest and concentrate on filling the upper chest as you slowly inhale. Slowly exhale.

For abdominal breathing, use the same technique while concentrating on filling the lower chest. Place your hands on your abdomen; you should feel it expand and fall.

Stretch to let air in. Stretching your rib cage and spine will open your breathing passages and allow air to flow more easily. Stand erect, slowly raising your arms above your head until you can clasp your hands. Inhale slowly to a count of three. Gradually lower your hands to your side, then to your lower back, until you can clasp your hands. Exhale to a count of four.

DIET

Garlic does you good. Garlic is well known for its antibacterial action. Get as much as you can. Roast whole cloves and liberally eat them as a spread on bread or crackers. Roasting takes the bite out of this breath killer and makes it very tasty. It's the best way to take it "straight." Garlic powder capsules, garlic oil macerate, and aged garlic extract are other ways to get your fill of garlic.

Keep the liquids flowing. Flushing your system with plenty of healthful liquids—water, herbal teas, and fruit and vegetables juices—will help move out the inflammation. Drink at least eight 8-ounce glasses a day. Stay away from caffeine-containing beverages such as coffee, black tea, and cola, which are dehydrating.

Lemon in a glass of warm water is also a good idea to purify and detoxify the body system. Add a slice or two of fresh ginger root to produce even more healthful benefits.

Say no to dairy. Abstain from dairy products, which can increase mucus production.

Take vitamin C. I recommend taking your vitamin C in the form of rose hips, because it alkalizes the body. There is ample research data documenting that vitamin C reduces the duration and severity of colds, improves lung capacity levels, and shields the lungs from damaging chemicals in the air. Take 500 to 1,000 milligrams per day. This amount is considered well within the safe range. If you experience diarrhea, decrease the amount you are taking. Three oranges is about 200 milligrams worth of vitamin C.

Feed the Stomach, Soothe the Lungs

This old-fashioned recipe is loaded with garlic and onions, the dynamic duo against disease. It helps treat, as well as prevent, respiratory ailments. Thyme and cayenne are other helpful healers. Stock up on it all winter long.

Old-Fashioned Garlic and Onion Soup

Sip this soup, warmed, throughout the day.

2 whole heads garlic, separated and peeled
4 large white or yellow onions, thinly sliced
4 tablespoons extra virgin olive oil
2 teaspoons dried thyme

6 cups vegetable broth

½ cup dry white wine

1 bay leaf

2 tablespoons raw honey

4 tablespoons dried basil

4 tablespoons dried parsley

¼ teaspoon cayenne pepper

Celtic Sea salt and freshly ground pepper to taste

Smash the garlic cloves with the side of a butcher knife or use a garlic press. In a large pot, sauté the garlic and onions in the olive oil until they are golden brown. Add the thyme, vegetable broth, wine, and bay leaf. Bring to a slow boil, reduce heat, cover, and simmer for 2½ hours.

Remove the bay leaf. Strain the liquid and return it to the pot. Add the honey, basil, parsley, cayenne, salt, and pepper.

INHALATION

Break it up. To loosen mucus and help clear out inflammation, try this inhalation three times a day. It contains eucalyptus, probably the most potent expectorant found in nature. Wrap a towel around your neck or wear a turtleneck or warm sweater to prevent a chill. Use this treatment three times a day.

✍ Eucalyptus Steam ✍

4 cups hot water

1 drop eucalyptus essential oil

1 drop lemon essential oil

1 drop sandalwood essential oil

Heat the water on the stove until it is very hot but not boiling (approximately 160 to 180 degrees) and pour it into a large, heavy metal, ceramic, or glass bowl. Add the essential oils.

Drape a towel over your head to form a tent and place your face about 8 inches above the water level. Be careful that the steam is not too hot. Breathe slowly and deeply with your eyes closed for 5 to 10 minutes. Pat your face and neck area dry with a towel.

For optimal benefits, follow with one of the chest rub recipes given below.

LIFESTYLE

Pamper yourself. If you have bronchitis, you won't feel much like doing anything. So don't. Get plenty of rest, dress warmly, and put an extra blanket on the bed at night. Herbal teas, hot-water bottles, and a good book can be your best friends when recuperating.

MASSAGE

Rub it in and rub it out. Certain essential oils made in the form of a rub can help diminish congestion. Because the oils are absorbed slowly into the skin, it is best to use these rubs two or three times throughout the day. I've developed two rubs: one for a moist cough and the other for a dry, nonproductive cough. The amounts should last for three treatments. They work best when applied to the chest and back. If you don't have a helper to work on your back, you will still benefit from the chest treatment.

❧ Moist Cough Chest Rub ❀

2 tablespoons vegetable oil
10 drops eucalyptus essential oil
5 drops hyssop essential oil
3 drops peppermint essential oil
2 drops cedarwood essential oil

❧ Dry Cough Chest Rub ❀

2 tablespoons vegetable oil
10 drops eucalyptus essential oil
5 drops hyssop essential oil

3 drops bergamot essential oil

2 drops sandalwood essential oil

Pour the vegetable oil into an amber glass bottle. Add the essential oils. Cap the bottle securely, and gently shake to mix. Label. Pour a small amount into your hands and warm by gently rubbing your palms together. To apply to the chest, stroke one side using the double stroke (hand over hand) method. Repeat several times and do the same on the other side. Repeat the method on your back.

Sound and Music Therapy

Good vibrations. Curing bronchitis isn't what The Beach Boys had in mind when they were singing about good vibrations, but vibrating sounds, known as toning, can have a healing effect on the lungs and sinuses. To make a healing vibration, take a fully expanded

Real-Life Cure

NATURE OUTSMARTS MEDICINE

Mary, a retired nurse, came to see me with a stubborn case of bronchitis that she had developed after a bout with the flu. Nothing she tried, including the medication her doctor prescribed, was helping her get better. She had the typical symptoms: a mild fever, fatigue, chest ache, and a persistent cough with occasional thick sputum. Mary was taking vitamin C as part of her routine health regimen, so the first thing I suggested was increasing her intake to 1 gram a day, spread out throughout the day. I also recommended the inhalations and massage rubs found in this section. I gave her my garlic and onion soup recipe, which she loved.

After three days her symptoms began to abate, so she stopped the inhalations. After one week, she was back to her former self—and her former health regimen. But the garlic and onion soup has become an added dietary habit. "I now eat it as a preventive," she reports. "It's a tasty way to stay healthy!"

When to Call the Doctor

Any illness involving the lungs has the risk of turning into pneumonia. Pneumonia means there is fluid and lymph in the lungs. This is potentially dangerous because fluid is taking up air space, therefore interfering with the delicate gas exchange that normally takes place in the lungs.

If breathing becomes shallow or if you detect abnormal breathing sounds, see a doctor immediately. Pneumonia is especially dangerous to the elderly, who commonly have depressed immune systems.

If you have a persistent cough that does not respond to treatment or your breathing is difficult or shallow, you should also be evaluated by a doctor.

Also, if your symptoms don't diminish after two or three days of self-treatment or if they get worse instead of better, see your doctor. You may need stronger treatment.

deep breath and make the sound "hum" while slowly exhaling. Repeat this at least three times and practice daily.

Bruises

SAY ADIEU TO BLACK AND BLUE

Color *over* the skin is fine to flaunt. But color *under* the skin is hardly fashionable.

A black-and-blue mark is the badge of a bruise (or contusion) caused by a bump, blow, or fall. The sudden contact causes capillaries just beneath the skin to break and bleed. When the blood clots, the skin displays its healing action through a rainbow of colors—blue, purple, then brown and yellow as blood slowly gets absorbed. Bruises can be painful and sore, depending on how extensive the trauma to underlying muscle and nerves. Given time, the typical bruise will heal on its own, but you can hasten the process by following the suggestions below.

AROMATHERAPY

Essential oils traditionally used for healing bruises are eucalyptus, fennel, geranium, hyssop, lavender, marjoram, and rosemary. Also, essential oils that are anti-inflammatory and increase circulation can be helpful. The anti-inflammatory oils include chamomile, clary sage, frankincense, geranium, lavender, myrrh, peppermint, rose, and sandalwood. These oils can be used topically in the form of massage oils, concentrated ointments, compresses, local baths (hand baths and footbaths), and full soaking baths.

HYDROTHERAPY

Start with cold. Basic first aid says to put an ice pack on an injury as soon as possible. This will help keep coloration to a minimum. Apply in 15-minute intervals for the first few hours after injury.

Then switch to hot. After 24 hours, heat, applied with a hot-water bottle, will help dilate blood vessels and improve circulation. Alternate heat with cold for optimum healing.

Freeze-frame further bruising. For a severe bruise, I suggest a cold compress made with essential oils. This formula will help heal the damaged tissue and hasten recovery. It can be used as soon as an injury occurs and later when the bruise develops, but it should not be used on broken skin that hasn't yet healed.

I've added witch hazel to the recipe below because of its astringent properties and ability to promote healing and tone the skin. You can substitute apple cider vinegar if witch hazel is not available. Neither should be used on broken skin.

Bad-Bruise Compress

The best aid for the baddest of bruises.

¼ cup water
¼ cup witch hazel or apple cider vinegar
2 drops lavender essential oil
2 drops hyssop essential oil
1 drop marjoram essential oil

Add the water and witch hazel to a small bowl. Add the essential oils and swish to disperse well. Soak a flannel cloth in the liquid, squeezing out as much moisture as possible, and place over the injured area. Cover with plastic wrap to help the essential oils absorb. Cover the wrap with a towel. Apply this compress for 30 minutes up to three times daily.

MASSAGE

Rub it away. For simple bruises with unbroken skin, this massage oil will help hasten healing time. It's been rated "excellent" by those who've used it. It can be used immediately following an injury and after coloration develops. Use gentle strokes at first. Massage gently into the area with outward circular motions and toward the heart. Once any soreness has subsided, firmer massage strokes can be applied to increase circulation to the area.

Bruise Oil

Accidents seem to happen while away from home. So, when my children were younger, I always kept this bruise oil in the first-aid kit at home and in the glove compartment of the car. It's especially handy when ice is not available. Now that my twin sons are teenagers, they carry a bottle of their own in their gym bag.

14 drops lavender essential oil

6 drops rosemary essential oil

5 drops hyssop essential oil

2 tablespoons arnica infusion oil or vegetable oil

400 international units vitamin E (1 or 2 capsules)

In an amber glass bottle, add the essential oils. Add the arnica infusion oil or vegetable oil to the essential oils. Break open the vitamin E capsule(s) and add it to the mixture. Cap securely and shake gently to mix. Label.

Put a few drops in your hands and rub your palms together to warm and massage gently into the wounded area for several minutes. Apply two or three times daily. For best results, follow with an ice pack for 10 to 15 minutes.

Real–Life Cure

OILS BRING SPEEDY RECOVERY

Veronica, a beautiful thirty-seven-year-old woman, had considerable bruising on her thighs and abdomen from liposuction surgery when she asked me if there was an aromatherapy solution to help the bruises go away. It had been four days since her surgery.

Her incisions were intact and dry at the time, with no signs of infection, so I told her to use Bruise Oil (see page 143). She faithfully applied the oils at least once a day, and sometimes twice a day on the weekends. She also applied the Bad-Bruise Compress (see page 143) for two weeks.

Ideally, it would have been more beneficial for Veronica to have started using essential oils *prior* to surgery to help diminish bleeding and swelling. However, she was pleased with the results: The bruises were long gone before the several weeks her doctor had said it would take. In fact, her surgeon was so pleasantly surprised by her quicker-than-usual recovery that he's been recommending essential oils to his surgery patients ever since.

Burnout

REFUEL SLOWLY

Do you go to work these days with that *couldn't care less, just show me the door* thinking going on in the back of your head? Okay, you may be developing a bad attitude about your job, but there is a logical reason why it is happening: burnout.

Burnout is a phenomenon that evolved from the 24/7 expectation of job commitment that started somewhere in the late seventies and eighties. It usually shows itself in mental and physical fatigue caused by a combination of factors including overwork, high levels of chronic stress, and lack of positive feedback. Perfectionism, the belief that you must do it all and do it perfectly, often underlies the exhaustion.

Clearly, a good stress reduction program was not in place or was not being practiced if you got to this point of extreme weariness. Realize that at this time you are prone to catching colds and infections, as the immune system, as well as the nervous system, has been overwhelmed.

AROMATHERAPY

Create balance through the senses. The helpful essential oils are those that affect the nervous system and aid in regulating and relaxing. Those used most often are basil, clary sage, eucalyptus, geranium, ginger, grapefruit, hyssop, jasmine, juniper, lavender, lemongrass, marjoram, neroli, nutmeg, patchouli, petitgrain, pine, rosemary, and ylang-ylang. Essential oil therapy includes inhalation, massage, and spa baths.

BREATH WORK

Catch your breath. Full, life-affirming deep breaths are highly recommended several times during the day, and especially during an aromatherapy inhalation session. These breathing exercises, described in detail on page 19, can be performed in your office, home, or anywhere.

Preferably, practice deep breathing in front of an open window or outside in the fresh air. Deep breathing oxygenates every cell and totally rejuvenates a tired, depleted state.

DIET

Get your eating habits in line. The misery that goes along with burnout often spurs bad eating habits, because food brings comfort. Avoid unhealthy foods in general, such as processed, fast foods that are devoid of nutrition and vital energy. Eat small, frequent healthy snacks during the day to prevent fatigue.

Eat from the sea. Potassium-rich and iodine-containing foods are often recommended for nervous disorders. Sea vegetables are a primary source of both. Make the Wholesome Sea Green Soup on page 389 for a delicious way to incorporate these healthful foods into your diet.

Add a dash of euphoria. Sprinkling nutmeg on your cappuccino, latte (decaffeinated, of course), or steamed milk will give you an extra pick me up and good feeling that you can't get from sugar or caffeine. Freshly ground nutmeg is the best and most potent.

HYDROTHERAPY

Lower the lights, please. There are many wonderfully relaxing and healthful benefits to the basic bath. However, a spa bath integrates soothing music, soft lighting, and pleasing scents to encourage renewal. This aromatic bath relieves nervous tension via the selected oils and specific healing water temperature. Designate a small block of time to take care of yourself, and don't forget the DO NOT DISTURB sign on the bathroom door.

Re-Fueling Spa Bath

4 tablespoons Celtic Sea or Dead Sea salt (or other carrier)
5 drops patchouli essential oil
3 drops clary sage essential oil
2 drops eucalyptus essential oil

Celtic and Dead Sea salts contain high concentrations of healthful minerals and trace elements that can be absorbed through the water, which make them perfect for depleted states. Also, they are completely natural, are alkalizing in nature, and carry the energy of the ocean. Add the essential oils to the salts and mix well. Pour the bath preparation into a full warm bath and stir with your hands. Soak for 20 to 30 minutes (or longer).

Wash negative thoughts from your mind. This therapeutic bath treatment is helpful when your racing mind is interfering with your ability to sleep. Darken the room, and light a few candles. Enjoy your time in perfect silence or play some soft serene music.

Serenity Blend

8 drops lavender essential oil
2 drops bergamot essential oil
2 drops mandarin essential oil
½ cup Epsom salt or Detoxifying Bath Salts (page 128)

Draw a very warm (92 to 100 degrees) to hot (100 to 104 degrees) bath. Mix the essential oils into the salt. Pour into the bath and swish to dissolve with your hands. Soak for as long as you wish. Sip on some chamomile herbal tea while you prepare for the best night's sleep you have had in a long time!

Turn around a bad day. If overwork and job pressures have depleted your energy stores, then this is the bath for you. It is effective for both mental and nervous exhaustion. The scent of this bath is one of contentment, lightheartedness, and optimism and prepares you for the weekend time off. If you are experiencing sensory overload, try taking your bath in total darkness (just keep a flashlight handy).

✢ TGIF Bath ✢

7 drops lavender essential oil
5 drops grapefruit essential oil
½ cup Celtic Sea salt

Draw a warm (92 to 100 degrees) to hot (100 to 104 degrees) bath. Mix the essential oils into the salt. Pour into the bath and stir. Soak for as long as you are comfortable. Wrap yourself in a thick cotton robe and rest for at least 15 minutes following the bath experience.

INHALATION

Just put on a happy face. For nervous tension, inhalation is very effective and can help transcend the tension you are experiencing. It is important to add the benefits of deep breathing to this treatment in order to increase the rewards of aromatherapy, oxygenation, and relaxation achieved from both.

The oils in the recipe on page 150 were selected for the following reasons: The lavender supports the exhausted nervous system and is uplifting; the basil and pine assist in general fatigue and nervousness and are brain stimulants that aid clarity of thought. The nutmeg is a special essence that is key for use in nervous fatigue states, is a powerful psycho-stimulant, and invigorates the mind. It basically can make you feel happy!

Real-Life Cure

RUNNING ON EMPTY

Bob, a successful forty-two-year-old business manager of a software company, talked to me about feeling "burdened and burned out." He had neglected his family, his personal needs, and much of the household responsibilities. He was working fifty to sixty hours per week. He traveled frequently and ate poorly, as he wasn't home most evenings in time for dinner.

Bob was a prime example of nervous and mental exhaustion, a man on the verge of burnout. In general, his health was good. His major complaint was fatigue and feeling "tightly wound up, like a rubber band." He was ready and willing to take the action necessary before it was too late.

First, he made priority lists and crossed out much of what he could delegate to others at work. He used my aromatherapy recommendations in the sauna at the exercise club, took baths at home (sometimes with his wife), and purchased a diffuser for his office. He did deep-breathing exercises regularly and started running again in the morning before work. He also started eating healthier and brought energizing snacks to work and on his business travels. Within a week Bob began feeling more in control of his life, more positive, and seemed to have more free time. Most important, he made the great divide between his work and personal life and finally found the time for both, without feeling guilty.

For other remedies, see Lethargy *and* Stress.

✍ Attitude–Altering Inhalant ✎

6 parts lavender essential oil
3 parts basil essential oil
2 parts pine essential oil
1 part nutmeg essential oil

Mix the essential oils in an amber glass bottle. Use a few drops in an aroma lamp or inhale from a tissue. Ideally, this blend is nice to use in a diffuser to disperse the essential oils into the room air two to three times per day.

Bursitis

✍

SEND PAIN PACKING

This condition, common to athletes and others who continuously overwork a joint, is an inflammation of the bursae, the serous sac or lubricant of a joint. The shoulder, knee, and elbow joints are the most commonly affected areas. Baseball pitchers, tennis players, and golfers are common targets, though anyone can come down with it. It's how tennis elbow, which is just bursitis of this joint, got its name.

Symptoms include sharp pain, restricted movement, skin that is hot and tender to the touch, and a swollen joint. But it's the sharp pain, even from the least amount of movement, that moves people to seek relief.

AROMATHERAPY

Muscle and joint aids. Essential oils helpful with bursitis are those that help any muscle and joint pain as well as those that help improve circulation. Many of them originated as herbs. They are chamomile (German and Roman), clary sage, cypress, eucalyptus, geranium, ginger, hyssop, juniper, lavender, lemongrass, marjoram, nutmeg, peppermint, pine, and rosemary. These helpful oils are used topically in the form of massage oils, concentrated ointments, compresses, and local baths (hand baths and footbaths), as well as in full soaking baths.

Herbs

Restore flexibility. Herbs are effective in rebalancing the body's chemistry and restoring flexibility through the removal of toxins (inorganic mineral deposits). Herbs that are most helpful in dissolving inorganic deposits are cranberry (powder and juice concentrate), citrus/lemon peel, kelp and other sea vegetables, and slippery elm.

To reduce inflammation that comes with decreased flexibility you will want to include a few of the following herbs: aloe vera, devil's claw, St. John's wort, yarrow, and yucca.

Hydrotherapy

Take the cold shoulder treatment. A cold compress made with essential oils followed by ice is the ideal treatment for alleviating joint swelling and pain. Use this compress as your initial treatment.

Cold Comfort Compress

1 cup cold water
3 drops cypress essential oil
2 drops chamomile essential oil
2 drops hyssop essential oil
1 drop juniper essential oil

In a metal or ceramic bowl, add the water. One at a time, add the essential oils, gently stirring after each addition to disperse the oils. Stir well. Soak a flannel cloth in the aromatic water and then wring out as much moisture as possible. Apply to the affected joint. Place a cold pack or ice pack over it to keep it cold. Cover with a towel. Leave this on for 20 to 30 minutes, changing the compress if it becomes warm or dry. Keep the joint (limb) elevated if possible. During acute and severe bursitis pain, the compress can be applied three times a day.

LIFESTYLE

Rest is best. There really is no way around the simple fact that resting the affected joint is crucial to alleviate bursitis discomfort and to encourage healing.

MASSAGE

This powerful and aromatic massage oil can be rubbed in prior to exercise to aid in the prevention of symptoms such as swelling and pain.

✍ Pain Prevention Oil ✍

10 drops rosemary essential oil
6 drops juniper essential oil
5 drops eucalyptus essential oil
4 drops chamomile essential oil (German chamomile recommended)
½ teaspoon carrot seed oil (optional)
1 tablespoon St. John's wort (hyperium) infusion oil
1 tablespoon vegetable oil

In an amber glass bottle, add the essential oils, carrot seed oil (if desired), St. John's wort (hypericum) oil, and vegetable oil. Cap securely and shake gently to mix well. Label.

Pour a few drops of the oil in your hands and gently rub your palms together to warm the oil. Gently massage into the affected area using small, circular motions until the oil is absorbed. Use up to three times a day.

Cellulite

❧

A FIRM SOLUTION

Cellulite: Now there's a set of dimples that is far from cute!

In some European countries, this scourge of womanhood is considered a medical condition. But here, in the United States, it's looked upon as a cosmetic problem brought on by aging and the accumulation of too much fat.

Cellulite is the name given to the unattractive dimpling and lumping of the skin, most often appearing on the outer thighs, hips, and buttocks. There are many theories as to the cause of cellulite. Some include swollen fat cells, fat cell malfunction, metabolic and circulatory disorders, hormonal imbalances, and fluid and toxin accumulation.

I personally believe the cause is a combination of poor circulation, poor elimination, poor diet, and general toxification. Sluggish fluids get trapped between fat cells, giving the trademark cottage-cheese appearance to the skin's surface. By poor elimination I mean that toxins and fluids are being stored in this tissue rather than purged from the system. Women with cellulite often experience constipation and inadequate fluid hydration. Bad diet is often the reason. Over the years, body tissue gets in a general state of toxicity. Our bodies simply cannot handle the daily doses of chemical-laden preservatives, additives, and colorants. The body has no easy way of eliminating many of these synthetic chemicals.

While opinons differ as to the cause of the problem, there is little controversy over the cure: It is difficult at best. Yet millions of dollars are spent each year on products, diets, appliances, supplements, and other gimmicks purporting some magical cure. But, I'm glad to report, cellulite is not inevitable. The best way to combat it is by preventing it. But I've also had success in helping women diminish the unsightly look of their thighs. It takes commitment and consistency on your part, but the end result is well worth it.

AROMATHERAPY

Essences that erase. Essences that combat cellulite are ones that help boost circulation, eliminate fluids, and detoxify. These include black pepper, cedarwood, cypress, fennel, geranium, grapefruit, juniper, lavender, lemon, lemongrass, mandarin, patchouli, rosemary, and tea tree.

In some commercial thigh creams, you will find salicylic acid as one of the active ingredients. This chemical constituent can be found naturally in birch and wintergreen essential oils. However, minute amounts are called for as they are considered dangerous in strong dilution. One half to 1 percent can be safely added to your lotion to stimulate local circulation.

Get your blood moving. The best way to attack poor circulation is a combination of aromatherapy, massage, and exfoliation. The cellulite scrub described below will tackle the toughest dimples—*if* you make it a faithful part of your body care. You can also opt for the ever-popular salt-glo treatment given here as well. The only thing you're missing is the Vichy shower and the $150 price tag!

⚮ Vanishing-Cellulite Scrub ⚮

Expect dramatic results when you use this scrub—along with the suggested lifestyle and dieting recommendations—within two to three months of use. I suggest using this scrub three times a week, alternating with dry skin brushing on the other days.

1 tablespoon sea salt (Celtic or Dead Sea salt works best)
10 drops mandarin or grapefruit essential oil
4 drops juniper essential oil
3 drops lemon essential oil
3 drops cypress essential oil
½ cup medium-ground cornmeal
½ cup coarse-ground oatmeal

Put the sea salt in a small bowl and add the essential oils. Mix to combine well. Add the cornmeal and oatmeal. Combine well. Store in a wide-mouth jar.

Use before or after your bath or shower. Simply wet the skin and apply a small handful to the affected areas by rubbing in a circular motion. Use light to medium pressure as this is very coarse. Rinse off and pat dry gently. Use three times per week.

ॐ Contouring Glo-Salts ॐ

*This all-over body contouring treatment to prevent cellulite and exfoliate dead skin cells
will produce a healthy glow in your skin—a sign of stimulated skin circulation.*

½ cup Dead Sea salt
½ cup Celtic Sea salt (coarse ground)
1 cup vegetable oil
2 drops eucalyptus essential oil
2 drops lemongrass essential oil
2 drops ginger essential oil
2 drops lemon essential oil
2 drops juniper essential oil

In a wide-mouth jar, add the sea salts. Pour the vegetable oil over the salts until they are barely covered. Add more if necessary. Add the essential oils to the mixture drop by drop. Mix well with a spoon or spatula. Cover and label.

To use, take a handful of the glo-salts and stand over a shower or tub area, since this gets a bit messy. Start at the feet and move upward toward the heart, using a circular motion. Avoid delicate skin areas such as the face.

Rinse off in a warm shower, and be careful to avoid slipping. Use these salts two to three times per week.

DIET

Make lemonade. Drink an 8-ounce glass of warm water with the juice of half or a whole lemon daily, preferably in the morning, to encourage detoxification and elimination. Lemon is also an effective diuretic and will stimulate the body to eliminate additional fluid.

Cut the fat with fiber. A diet low in saturated fat and high in fiber is imperative. Less fat eaten means less fat stored in the body. High fiber combats constipation and encourages elimination.

Eat plenty of vegetables, fruit, whole grains, and legumes. I recommend organics, as they are free of chemicals.

Asparagus is vegetable number one. Asparagus is a natural diuretic and especially beneficial for removal of fluids and impurities from the body. Eat as much as you can in your diet. As an alternative, you can take asparagus tablets.

Wash it out. The best way to flush toxins from the system is with water. Drink plenty of pure water to flush out the toxins, at least 8 to 10 glasses per day. Drink herbal tea and aloe vera juice (whole-leaf concentrate) to encourage the detoxification process.

Make friends with sea herbs. Dulse, kelp, and wakame are sea vegetables with extremely detoxifying properties. They are high in minerals and trace elements. Make the Wholesome Wholesome Sea Green Soup on page 389 for an easy and nutritious way to get to know these energizing and toxin-eliminating sea herbs.

Out with the bad. Eliminate water-retaining alcohol, coffee, and black tea. Also eliminate sugar and all highly refined and processed foods.

Make your oil flax. High-quality oil, such as flaxseed oil, will improve the cellular membranes, helping to eliminate toxins and excess fluid. You can add this oil to steamed vegetables and salads, but be sure not to cook with it. High temperature will destroy its benefits.

Hydrotherapy

Take the plunge. Epsom salt and sea salt assist the body in releasing toxins and excess fluids and make the best choices to use in your bath as carriers for essential oils. They can also be used alone. You can add the juice of one lemon into the bathwater for additional detoxifying benefits.

The recipe for Detoxifying Bath Salts on page 128 is also good for cellulite. Take two to three baths per week.

Skin stimulation for vitality. Scrubbing with a natural loofah sponge in the bathtub as you soak is another way to target the stubborn areas that need additional attention.

Bundle up. Wrap yourself in a warm bathrobe or bath towel to encourage perspiration immediately following the bath. The body continues to react and respond to the essential oils for up to an hour after a bath is taken.

Cool down to tone up. Follow your daily shower by turning the water to cold for a few seconds to close the pores, aid in circulation, and help firm tissues. This is an optional but effective tool in promoting excellent circulation and body toning. Start out slow and work up to a more dramatic temperature change.

Lifestyle

Move it to lose it. Movement increases blood flow. Walking at a brisk pace, swinging the arms from side to side, is a great form of exercise you can enjoy outside in the fresh air. Dancing, yoga, hiking, and even sex are considered forms of exercise.

Exercise does not have to be (and shouldn't be) painful, boring, difficult, expensive, or inconvenient. Take stretch breaks during your working schedule to avoid long periods of sitting or standing while at the office.

Massage

Defy the thigh. The essential oils in this lotion recipe are natural diuretics and will encourage the kidneys to produce more urine, therefore excreting additional body fluids. The essential oils were chosen for their ability to increase and stimulate circulation and for their firming ability. Use this lotion during the day rather than before you go to bed, as you may need to empty your bladder more frequently.

This recipe must be prepared with a natural-base lotion. If the lotion contains any mineral oil by-products, the skin will not be able to readily absorb the essential oils. Mineral oil has a large molecular structure and blocks moisture (and essential oils) from getting in.

✍ Firming Lotion ✍

This is not just another thigh cream!

6 ounces unscented base lotion

1 ounce distilled witch hazel lotion

30 drops lemon essential oil

20 drops cypress essential oil

15 drops lavender essential oil

10 drops juniper essential oil

5 drops black pepper essential oil

Purchase an 8-ounce bottle of your favorite natural unscented base lotion. Empty a quarter of the lotion, or use it up first. The extra room is needed to completely blend the lotion. Otherwise you can mix it in a jar or bowl and use a funnel to get it back into the bottle.

Tip: Try a Dry Massage

To boost circulation and slough off dry skin, dry skin brush with a good-quality, natural bristle brush prior to your cellulite bath treatment. A form of stimulating massage, dry brushing prepares the skin to more readily absorb essential oils. Always dry brush and massage toward the direction of the heart, focusing on problem areas such as the back of the arms, hips, and thighs.

In a small cup or dish, add the distilled witch hazel lotion. Add the essential oils and stir to mix well. Pour the mixture into the base lotion. Cap securely and shake very well. Label.

To apply, put a small amount on your hand and massage cellulite areas with circular, upward, firm strokes toward the heart. Massage until it is completely absorbed. It is best to put this on in the morning after showering.

Real-Life Cure

SHE'S NOW THIGH-HIGH

Sharon, forty-two, was so embarrassed by the appearance of her thighs that she came to me looking for a solution. After hearing her story, I was amazed that cellulite was her major complaint!

She told me she had low energy, irregular bowel habits, and a history of sinus problems. She was mildly overweight and only relatively active. I advised her to alter her diet—low fat, no caffeine, high fiber, natural foods—and exercise regularly. I also told her to take the baths and use the lotions outlined in this section. She even drank detox tea and lemon juice daily. She eliminated all soft drinks and drank only pure water along with the tea and lemon juice.

Within a month's time Sharon called with excitement in her voice to say that her husband had noticed the difference! She became less ashamed of and shy about her thighs and began wearing shorts more often. All in all, she started loving her body again, which, I'm convinced, changed how she presented herself to others.

TEAS AND TONICS

Sip an herbal drainer. Here is a detoxification tea I recommend to anyone complaining about cellulite. The herbs used are all natural diuretics.

Toning Tea

This tea can be made in larger portions and kept in the refrigerator.

> 4 parts peppermint
> 1 part red clover tops
> 1 part ground fennel seed

1 part dried parsley

1 part dandelion herb or root

Lemon juice or stevia as sweetener (optional)

In a jar, add the herbs listed and shake to mix. Label contents. To make the tea, use 1 teaspoon of the tea mixture per cup of water. Simmer for 5 to 10 minutes. Strain. Flavor with lemon juice or stevia, if desired. Drink 1 to 3 cups per day, hot or cold.

Chicken Pox

🖎

STOP THE ITCHING

Chicken pox is kind of a rite of passage for the elementary years. The virus is so contagious that even indirect contact with an infected child likely means that your child will come down with it, too.

Symptoms include general malaise, fever for 24 hours or less, and a rash of small red spots on the face and trunk that turns into blisters that break open and crust over to form scabs. But, to the child, it's the itching more than anything else that drives them to distraction—and what should concern you the most. Scratching the scabs can lead to infection and scarring.

The common age at which most children contract chicken pox is between two and eight years of age. The incubation time is 14 to 21 days after exposure to the virus. But the communicability period is from the onset of

Nothing to Fear

Chicken pox is a common childhood disease that typically comes around but once in a lifetime. However, those who have had chicken pox as a child can get shingles, which is caused by the same virus in adults. Because the illness is often more persistent in adults than in children, it is best not to fight it when your child is exposed.

fever—usually 1 day before lesions appear—until the last vesicle has dried and scabbed over completely, about 5 to 7 days.

AROMATHERAPY

Spray the itch away. Due to their astringent nature, the essential oils used in this recipe help relieve symptoms. The witch hazel is also astringent and will aid in drying the blisters as well. Aloe vera is anti-inflammatory and will help heal and prevent scarring. Honey is used primarily as a carrier for the essential oils, since they will not emulsify in the liquids on their own. It is also an antibacterial and anti-inflammatory agent.

Carrot seed oil is an essential oil and is often used in 10 percent dilutions (or less) to aid in skin healing, prevent scarring, and serve as an antioxidant. It is optional in this recipe; however, if you are concerned with scarring, I strongly suggest you include it.

Note: Remember to do a skin patch test on your child to check for skin sensitivity before applying this (or any new essential oil) to a large area. See page 10 for directions on how to do a skin patch test.

✺ Spray Away for Chicken Pox ✺

1 tablespoon honey
40 drops lavender essential oil
15 drops lemon essential oil
15 drops bergamot essential oil
5 drops peppermint essential oil
1 teaspoon carrot seed oil (optional)
½ cup aloe vera gel (or concentrated spray)
½ cup distilled witch hazel

In a measuring cup, add the honey, essential oils, carrot seed oil (if desired), and aloe vera gel. Stir to mix completely. Add the witch hazel, stirring again to mix. Pour into a spray bottle or mister with a fine spray nozzle. Label. Spray onto affected body areas, avoiding the eye area. For use on the face, spray a small amount onto a cotton ball and dab on affected areas. Use as needed several times a day.

Give calamine an extra kick. In the recipe on page 161, you can substitute the traditional anti-itching cream, calamine lotion, for the aloe and witch hazel. To make, add the essential oils to 8 ounces of calamine lotion. Shake well to combine the oils completely in the lotion. Keep away from eye and mouth areas.

Diet

Drink like a bunny. Drink plenty of liquids. Encourage drinking diluted herbal teas and juices (especially carrot juice) and plenty of water. Make the Old-Fashioned Garlic and Onion Soup on page 137 to aid healing and prevent infection.

Real-Life Cure

THE ALL-IN-THE-FAMILY CURE

There are many case histories I could share with you, but I think my own family's story highlights just about every possibility you could experience with your own children.

When my youngest boys were in first grade, one of them came home with a minor fever and a note from school. There was a chicken pox outbreak in the school and surrounding areas. Kristopher was the first of the twins to develop it. To no surprise, his brother Ryan came down with it 1½ weeks later. But we were really surprised when our eldest son, who was fifteen, got it—for the second time. All in all, I was housebound with children for close to 6 weeks!

I can personally vouch for the recipes given here. They were a godsend for my kids. They healed quickly, had very little scarring, and at most the itching was mild or moderate.

My fifteen-year-old, Jeremy, experienced a horrendous amount of pox all over his body, including his eyes, throat, and ears. He had a mild case of chicken

continued . . .

pox when he was in preschool, so we thought he was done. When adults or teenagers get chicken pox, the symptoms and rash can be much more pronounced. The spray seemed to be the most helpful and the easiest to use. Jeremy opted for a tepid shower in lieu of the aromatic bath and misted with the chicken pox spray afterward.

All healed well with little scarring.

HYDROTHERAPY

Take an old-fashioned bath. Most young children love baths and can be entertained—and distracted from itching—for quite a while with water toys. This aromatic bath is very effective at providing cooling relief from itching. It contains baking soda, a classic home remedy for easing the itching caused by chicken pox. The essential oils used here are skin friendly and safe. They guard against infection and inflammation and help calm the nervous system. The best water temperature for itching conditions is warm to tepid, approximately 80 to 100 degrees.

❧ Anti-Itch Bath Batch ❧

1 cup baking soda
2 drops lavender essential oil
1 drop chamomile essential oil
   (German chamomile recommended)
1 drop tea tree essential oil

In a shallow bowl, add the baking soda and essential oils. Mix well with a spoon. Fill a bath with tepid water, adding the baking soda mixture when nearly full. Stir the bath with your hand to dissolve the mixture. Allow the child to soak for up to 30 minutes, depending on comfort level. Do not allow the child to chill.

LIFESTYLE

Pass time wisely. Parents should have a dual purpose in treating chicken pox: ensuring a speedy recovery and keeping your child from infecting others. That means you can expect to keep your child at home for at least 1½ to 2 weeks. In the meantime, here's what to keep in mind:

- Keep your child's fingernails clipped as short as possible in order to avoid scratching and breaking open the blister that can lead to infection.
- Keep the child isolated from other children until all lesions have crusted and completely scabbed over.
- Sleep heals, so make sure your child gets plenty of rest.
- Spray the air with Pure-for-Sure Spray on page 392 to keep the indoor air clean. Use pure eucalyptus essential oil for disinfecting clothing and towels by adding a few drops to the wash cycle while doing laundry.
- Make sure to wash your hands well after treating your child so as not to spread the virus to others.

Childbirth

✍

A TOTAL EXPERIENCE

I wish I could turn back the clock and use what I know now when I had my children. It would have been a much more pleasurable and relaxing experience, I'm sure. Soft lighting, gentle music in the background, and soothing scents would have filled the room, relaxing me and welcoming my babies to the world.

Today, it's a different world. More than ever, couples are requesting personalized childbirths, including home births, birthing rooms in hospitals, and independent birthing centers. Methods of birthing include the Bradley method, Lamaze method, and water birth, among others—things unheard of in our mothers' time. And I'm glad to see many women requesting supportive therapies, such as aromatherapy, for their childbirth experiences.

Aromatherapy is the perfect way to enhance the childbirth experience. Not only does it help control pain but also relaxes the body, disinfects the air, and welcomes the newborn in a very special, aromatic way.

AROMATHERAPY

Lavender's the leader. Lavender essential oil is key to your overall labor experience because it is well known for relieving pain and decreasing the need for analgesic drugs. It's used in all the blends suggested here. Other essential oils frequently used in labor are clary sage, jasmine, lavender, nutmeg, and rose. Those that encourage relaxation and reduce anxiety include bergamot, chamomile, frankincense, jasmine, lemon, mandarin, neroli, orange, rose, and spikenard.

> ## Tip: Ease Labor–Caused Nausea
>
> Nausea during labor is a common but very unpleasant experience. To minimize the feeling, place a drop of peppermint essential oil on a tissue and put it under the mother's nose so she can inhale it.

If you want to use essential oils in your childbirth, discuss it in advance with your caregiver and get any necessary approvals in advance. Time of delivery is not the time to make special requests.

HYDROTHERAPY

Pamper tender tissue. Emptying the bladder after childbirth is not always a pleasant experience. Toilet tissue is harsh on delicate tissue. This aromatic warm water spray wash, however, feels comforting and can be used immediately following delivery. Keep it in a plastic bottle in the bathroom for convenience.

If you have any itching, try bergamot essential oil instead of the patchouli. If there is any tearing or sutures, substitute tea tree for the patchouli. You may want to use the lavender essential oil all by itself as another option. It doesn't have to be complicated to work well.

Mother's Safety and Comfort Come First

Several of the essential oils used for labor and childbirth are ones on the cautionary list for pregnancy. These include clary sage, jasmine, nutmeg, and rose. But they should be considered safe when used properly and with the guidance of a qualified practitioner.

Also, be aware that hormonal changes during pregnancy can change a woman's appeal to certain scents. What was appealing before could be appalling now. There is nothing unusual about this. More often than not, however, aromatherapy is very well received by mother, father, and birthing staff. It helps relax everyone and bring focus to the event at hand. But first and foremost is the mother-to-be's comfort.

✍ Postdelivery Periwash ✍

1 drop lavender essential oil
1 drop patchouli essential oil
2 tablespoons witch hazel (optional)
7 ounces warm distilled water

In a clean plastic bottle, add the essential oils and, if desired, the witch hazel. Cap securely and shake well. Add the warm water and shake again. Shake well before each use, as the essential oils float to the top quickly. Alternatively, you can mix the essential oils in a little honey to emulsify them, making them water soluble. After voiding, clean the perineum by rinsing with this aromatic solution to be fresh and clean.

Try these alternatives. Other essential oils useful in healing the perineum are bergamot, chamomile, and myrrh. Herbs traditionally used for healing are calendula, comfrey, pilewort, and St. John's wort.

Refresh her face. A facial mist consisting of hydrosols can be purchased to spray on the mother's face and upper chest during delivery. Hydrosols are the floral waters left over from the distillation of essential oils. Most are skin friendly and safe to use as a facial mist. They are very light and cooling for a tired and warm mother in stressful times. Look for hydrosols of citrus, neroli, or rose for options.

Soothe the after-pain. Warm sitz baths using essential oils can help increase healing and decrease swelling after birth. Most hospitals have sitz baths on their postpartum floors. At home you can use the bathtub by filling it partially. A low level of water is used to cover the perineum area only.

If there is considerable swelling, use a cool water (70 to 80 degrees) bath or cold packs. Otherwise, a warm water (92 to 100 degrees) bath is soothing and relaxing. Witch hazel lotion can be included in the sitz bath treatment for its astringent quality but is optional. The honey is used as a carrier for the oils and for its anti-inflammatory and antibacterial properties.

～ After-Birth Bath ～

2 drops lavender essential oil
1 drop patchouli essential oil
1 drop tea tree essential oil
1 tablespoon raw honey
¼ cup witch hazel lotion (optional)

In a small bowl, add the essential oils and honey. Stir to blend. Fill a tub with just a few inches of warm water. Add the witch hazel, if desired, to the honey blend. Stir the water with your hands to disperse the oils completely. Sit in the water with knees up and slightly apart for 15 to 20 minutes. This can be done twice a day.

INHALATION

Diffuse pain, stay centered. This inhalation blend helps decrease the need for pain medication, promotes relaxation, relieves anxiety, and helps the mother (and birth team) stay focused and centered during the labor process.

The lavender essential oil is also a mild antiseptic, which is helpful in purifying the room air. If a stronger disinfecting blend is needed, as perhaps in a hospital setting, then the Pure-for-Sure Spray found on page 392 may be a good option as it contains essences with more effective antibacterial properties.

⟨⟩ Labor-of-Love Spray ⟨⟩

8 parts lavender essential oil
1 part frankincense essential oil

Mix the essential oils together in a bottle. Fill an automated electric diffuser according to manufacturer's directions. Place in a safe location in the room, away from close proximity to the activity. This spray can be diffused for 15 to 20 minutes at a time every few hours as desired.

MASSAGE

Soothe contractions. Add some pleasure to the labor process through this soothing massage. A combination of lavender, clary sage, and chamomile essential oils will help relax inner tensions and control pain. This massage oil can be applied between contractions to the lower abdomen, lower back, and sacrum (the triangular-shaped bone at the base of the spine). Massaging this area of the back with counterpressure, applying pressure against or toward the area experiencing pressure, with the palm of the hand provides additional relief. The oil also can be massaged into the mother's feet.

❧ Labor-of-Love Oil ❧

A blend to soothe away pain.

8 drops lavender essential oil

3 drops clary sage essential oil

1 drop chamomile essential oil

2 tablespoons sweet almond oil or vegetable oil

2 tablespoons St. John's wort infusion oil or arnica infusion oil

In an amber glass bottle, add the essential oils one by one. Add the sweet almond or vegetable oil and the infusion oil. Cap the bottle securely and shake well to thoroughly combine. Label.

To use, pour a small amount in your hands and warm by gently rubbing the palms together. Apply using gentle, circular motions.

SOUND AND MUSIC THERAPY

Bring music to her ears. Prior to birth, the mother-to-be should pick out some soothing music to play in the background while she's in labor. It will help relieve anxiety and help distract her from the pain. There are many varieties of soothing music available today at music stores, and a few popular pieces are listed here. Most harp music and enhanced ocean sounds are popular options. Some selections are:

Goldman—*Dolphin Dreams*

Murooka—*Lullaby from the Womb*

Brahms—*Lullaby*

Braga—*Angel's Serenade*

Wagner—*Evening Star*

Koto Flute

Real–Life Cure

A LABOR TO REMEMBER

Wendy, a thirty-one-year-old first-time mother, wanted to deliver her baby at home. We started planning for the event several months in advance.

Wendy experimented with different essential oils and found what she wanted—lavender and frankincense. She decided she wanted it used in a spray diffuser to help her relax, control her pain, and keep her focused and grounded. Massage oils were prepared ahead of time that included lavender and clary sage to aid the labor process. They were massaged into her lower back with counter-pressure when she experienced back labor and discomfort and also used on her lower abdomen to increase and strengthen contractions when needed.

One of her favorite aromatherapy treatments was a simple neroli facial mist, which she used often over her face and chest for relaxation. "It lifted my emotions and felt so refreshing," she reported afterward. It was very pleasant for the birth team members, too! There were also flowers, soft lighting, and music.

Wendy had a birthing tub available, which she used through dilatation to help her relax. After a seventeen hour labor, she gave birth to a healthy baby girl. She described the experience as "wonderful" and can't wait to have another baby. For everyone involved—the mother, father, and support team—the experience was magically memorable.

Circulation Problems

GO FOR THE FLOW

Poor circulation is a broad term linked to an even broader variety of health conditions: low blood pressure, varicose veins, angina, and arterial disease, just to name a few. For certain, it's something you can do without.

The potential dangers and complications due to poor and inadequate circulation are many. They range from ulcerations, congested lymph glands, abnormal blood clotting, and coldness to more serious blood clots, heart attack, and stroke.

When the "plumbing" isn't working optimally, the entire body is affected. When nutrients and oxygenated blood do not make it to their destination on time, the tissue cells begin to suffer poor nutrition and work less efficiently. Over time, veins become distended (varicose veins), blood pressure is compromised (low blood pressure), smaller blood vessels in the extremities get less oxygen-rich blood (numbness, coldness), and the greatest muscle of all—the heart—can suffer damage in the form of angina pectoris or heart attack.

A pretty grim picture, isn't it? Yet it is one of the major areas where we can make a difference in our health! And aromatherapy plays a central role. But let's be realistic. You can't expect aromatherapy, or any other complementary medicine, to completely remedy this problem. A steady routine followed slowly but consistently and in concert with your doctor will benefit the circulatory system and help get it back in working order.

AROMATHERAPY

The therapeutic value of essential oils in assisting poor circulation is more than simply supportive. There are oils that help stimulate circulation, especially if the problem is localized to a certain part of the body, like the arms and legs. General toning of the circulatory system is important, and essential oils can be applied here as well. Aromatherapy is extremely effective in releasing and preventing stress, which only aggravates the situation and can lead to high blood pressure and heart disease.

Improve blood flow. Essential oils that are invigorating, oxygenating, and stimulating to circulation are bergamot, cypress, eucalyptus, geranium, ginger, grapefruit, lavender, lemon, lemongrass, neroli, nutmeg, peppermint, pine, rose, rosemary, and spruce. If hypertension and stress are major factors in your poor circulation, then the essential oils that relax and calm the nervous system will be particularly helpful. These are basil, cedarwood, chamomile, clary sage, frankincense, geranium, jasmine, juniper, lavender, lemon, lemongrass, lime, marjoram, melissa, myrtle, orange, palmarosa, patchouli, petitgrain, pine, sandalwood, vetivert, and ylang-ylang. These essential oils can be utilized by inhalation methods, in baths, lotions, and for massage.

BREATH WORK

Do it right! Breathing, the most important function of the body, has a direct effect on our circulatory system. It is the primary source of energy. In 1732, when blood pressure was first measured by Stephen Hales, he found that the blood pressure fell and rose with every breath.

There is, however, an effective and an ineffective way to breathe. Many people with circulation problems are chest breathers, meaning they draw their air by using the chest muscles. They take shallow, short breaths. This actually puts them in a state of mild hyperventilation, causing them to discharge too much carbon dioxide from the blood. This forces the heart and circulatory system to work harder, thereby stressing this system.

The proper way to breathe is through the abdomen. It fully expands the lungs and oxygenates the blood most effectively. Abdominal breathing takes practice. At first you will need to make a conscious effort to breathe this way, but with practice it will become more natural.

Here's how to do it: Place your hands on your abdomen, just under your rib cage, near your diaphragm. Concentrate on filling the lower lungs with your breath and observe the abdomen (not your chest) rise and fall with each slow and deep breath. You will feel and see your hands move, confirming that you are doing the exercise correctly. Breathing with your diaphragm promotes full lung expansion and therefore fully oxygenates the body, producing calmness.

DIET

Don't go too sweet or too salty. Mounting evidence suggests the importance of food choices on our circulatory health. Adopting a diet that emphasizes fruits, vegetables, and whole grains and limits animal products will have many benefits, such as a lower risk of heart disease, obesity, and poor circulation.

Decrease refined sugar and dairy products and avoid table salt, all of which have been implicated in circulatory problems. Celtic Sea salt is much better for you than the iodized chemically and electrically altered commercial version, because it is completely natural and contains vital minerals. It can be found in natural health food stores. (See "Much More Than a Grain of Salt" on page 262 in Fluid Retention.

Love those onions! Eat plenty of onions and garlic for their circulation-promoting benefits. Try my Old-Fashioned Garlic and Onion Soup recipe on page 137.

Get your vitamins. Eat foods high in the antistress B vitamins, the antioxidants like vitamins C and E, and the minerals zinc and selenium. They assist circulation and strengthen blood vessel walls and thus may help to prevent future problems.

HERBS

Take your choice. Some of the common and traditionally used herbs for circulatory problems are garlic, ginkgo, gotu kola, hawthorn, horse chestnut, and prickly ash bark, typically purchased in loose tea form, capsules, or tincture. Follow directions on the manufacturer's label for proper dosing.

HYDROTHERAPY

Boost blood flow. A therapeutic bath made with detoxifying bath salts is just what the natural folk doctor ordered. The ingredients in this bath not only help pump up the circulatory system but nourish the skin as well.

The water temperature should be warm but not too hot, as this can raise your blood pressure. For best results, use a dry-skin brush before stepping into the tub to increase circulation to the skin's surface or use a loofah sponge in the bath and scrub in circular motion toward the heart. After soaking a while, try elevating your feet above the heart level by resting them on the edge of the tub. Dry briskly with a towel to further stimulate and slough dead skin cells that have become loosened during the soak. Taking three aromatic baths per week will do wonders to tone and stimulate your body.

Get-in-Circulation Bath

You'll love what this does to your skin, too!

1 cup Celtic Sea salt
4 drops cypress essential oil

3 drops grapefruit essential oil

1 drop nutmeg essential oil

In a small bowl, add the sea salt. Add the essential oils and mix well with a spoon. Fill the bathtub with warm water (92 to 100 degrees). Pour in the salt mixture, and, using your hands, stir to dissolve into the bath. Soak for 20 to 30 minutes. Sip room temperature water or herbal tea while soaking.

INHALATION

The sweet smell of success. Take advantage of the air you breathe all day long. By placing several drops of this blend in an aroma lamp, potpourri burner, humidifier, or electric diffuser, you can be breathing in your aromatherapy treatment without a second thought.

The diffuser is the most effective way to experience aromatherapy, especially for circulation, nervous system, and respiratory benefits. To make sure you get regular exposure to these essential oils and to make it easy, hook up a timer to the diffuser and place it in the main part of your living or work space.

This particular blend includes circulation stimulators and toners, nervous system relaxing oils, and emotional uplifting essences. Spray it around your living space on a regular basis—three to four times per day. It will purify the air as well as support your circulatory and nervous systems.

⌀ Blood-Flowing Blend ⌀

This has a bright, clean, natural scent I think you will enjoy.

3 parts cypress essential oil

3 parts lemon essential oil

2 parts bergamot essential oil

1 part ginger essential oil

1 part geranium essential oil

In an amber glass bottle, add the essential oils using an eyedropper or teaspoon. Cap and shake well. Label. Add the desired amount to your electric diffuser, according to the manufacturer's instructions.

LIFESTYLE

Practice healthy habits. The following lifestyle habits have all been found to help increase circulation:

- Get heart-pumping exercise at least three times a week. Brisk walking works.
- If you smoke, stop. Nothing is worse for your circulation than cigarette smoking.
- Use alcohol moderately. Occasionally drinking red wine can have antioxidant benefits.
- Maintain an ideal weight.
- When outside during cold-weather conditions, dress warm and keep hands and feet well protected.

MASSAGE

Back to basics. A back massage blend using stimulating aromatherapy oils will invigorate poor circulation. Massaging over the chakra area governing circulation will prove most helpful. This area, which is above the heart, is called the heart chakra and is also known as the heart plexus.

Massage gently in a clockwise circular motion with the blend given below. In general, a clockwise motion favors release of tension and strengthens the body. In contrast, the counterclockwise motion will stir up energy. It is the former circular direction that is most widely used.

❧ Poor-Circulation Massage Oil ❧

12 drops cypress essential oil
6 drops rosemary essential oil

4 drops lemon essential oil

3 drops nutmeg essential oil

2 tablespoons vegetable oil

In a clean amber glass bottle, add the essential oils one by one, using an eye-dropper. Add the vegetable oil. Cap securely and shake gently to mix. Label. To use, warm the oil by placing the aromatherapy oil bottle into a hot water bath or rubbing a few drops between your palms. Apply to the back area with firm, upward stroke movements, always working toward the heart, assisting circulation. Also apply to the heart chakra with a circular motion.

Try a Little Ankle Therapy

According to Creative Healing, a hands-on approach to healing founded by Joseph B. Stephenson in 1956, blood flow can be enhanced with ankle massage. This massage involves circular movement and downward pressure over what Stephenson called the "ankle filter area."

Place your forefinger in the cavity at the ankle, located on the outside of the foot, slightly in front of the ankle bone (the prominent ball-shaped bone). Press down and gently move your finger in a circular motion. As blood flow increases, your foot will begin to feel warm. Massage for 1 minute or longer.

Colds

∞

STOP SYMPTOMS COLD

When it comes to cold germs, there's nowhere to hide. We are in contact with germs all the time, everyday and everywhere we go. When our immune system is lowered, our defense mechanisms are weakened, and we "catch" a cold.

It is not the damp, cold weather, as our great-grandmothers might have presumed, but our immune system that predetermines whether or not we get sick. The viral or bacterial organisms only infect the body if our natural defenses are down.

Early signs of a cold include a scratchy throat, nasal congestion, slight fever, mild headache, and a general feeling of being unwell. Colds typically reach their peak within two to three days' time. Early treatment and prevention are the best approach to cold symptoms.

AROMATHERAPY

Antiseptic essences. The essential oils most helpful with colds are those that have antiseptic (germ killing) properties, stimulate the immune system, and have the ability to help dry up mucus flow. They are basil, bay, black pepper, cajeput, cedarwood, eucalyptus, ginger, helichrysm, hyssop, lavender, lemon, marjoram, melissa, niaouli, oregano, peppermint, pine, ravensara, rosemary, tea tree, and thyme.

Take a peppermint drop. Peppermint is best known as a digestive aid, but it's also the best essential oil for alleviating the complaints of colds and flu. Because of its antispasmodic and analgesic properties, it can work wonders on the respiratory system.

Put a peppermint drop on the back of your hand and take a lick. Or mix 3 drops with a small amount of honey and add it to 1 cup of warm water or tea to drink several times a day. This is not recommended for small children, however.

The Hard Cold Facts

As many as 40 percent of the common colds are caused by one of the more than one hundred varieties of the rhinoviral—*rhino* means nose—strains. These organisms enter the body through the mouth or nose. Influenza, the flu virus, accounts for only about 10 percent of common colds.

The average person gets three colds every winter. That's more than 700 million cold and flu cases annually in the United States alone.

Give it the cold treatment. Essential oils are common fighters of the common cold. I consider this recipe the perfect germ killer. Use it, as indicated, in the remedies that follow.

Conquer-a-Cold Combo

Use as your first line of defense for combating colds.

4 drops hyssop essential oil
3 drops rosemary essential oil
3 drops peppermint essential oil
3 drops eucalyptus essential oil
3 drops lemon essential oil

In a small amber bottle, add the essential oils one by one, using an eyedropper. Cap securely and shake well. Label. Use this oil combination topically as a massage oil or compress, or in a bath. See Appendix B for dilution ratios.

The Zinc Cure

Zinc lozenges are well known for shortening the course of a cold or flu. I've taken it one step better by zapping the zinc with an antiseptic and antiviral essential oil. Simply take one natural zinc lozenge and place one drop of ravensara or thyme (linalool) essential oil on it. Put it in your mouth and suck on it slowly. You can take one lozenge every 3 to 4 hours.

Look for brands of zinc that do not contain sugar and that are large and flat so the drop of essential oil can be readily absorbed on it.

DIET

Get your C. Vitamin C has long been acknowledged as a cold stopper. But it is often recommended in large doses and only works at the onset of a cold. Megadoses of vitamin C can produce unpleasant side effects—diarrhea being the most common. This is why I recommend getting your vitamin C from fruit juices such as orange, grapefruit, and cranberry. They feel really good going down, too.

Getting plenty of liquids. Liquids literally help wash away cold symptoms. In addition to the above juices, drink plenty of water and make herbal teas from the list found below.

Avoid the dairy aisle. Dairy products promote mucus production. They'll only make you feel worse.

Eat something spicy. On the contrary, spicy foods make mucus flow. Go for foods made with cayenne pepper, garlic, ginger, horseradish, and onions, which are also antibacterial.

HERBS

Pick your favorite fighting herb. Herbal medicine has much to offer in treating the common cold. Herbal teas, capsules, and tinctures help build the immune system, stimulate the thymus gland, and fight cold germs.

The Medicinal Power of Mushrooms

Mushrooms have been used in Asian cultures for thousands of years as both food and medicine. Here are some of the world's most prized medicinal mushrooms, possessing a long history of proven effectiveness in directly stimulating the immune system and fighting colds.

Caterpillar Fungus or Deer Mushroom (*Cordyceps sinensis*)
Maitake (*Grifola frondosus*)
Old Man's Beard (*Hericum erinaceus*)
Reishi (*Ganoderma lucidum*)
Shiitake (*Lentinula edodes*)
Turkey Tail (*Trametes versicolor*)
Velvet Foot (*Flamulina velutipes*)
Whitewood Ear or White Fungus (*Tremella fuciformis*)

Traditional herbs used to treat colds are astragalus, boneset, calendula, echinacea, elderberry, eyebright, garlic, ginger root, goldenseal, licorice root, olive leaf, peppermint, sage, and yarrow.

For long-term prevention, build up the immune system with ashwaganda root and Siberian ginseng root. They help increase your resilience and act as adaptogens, which support you in times of stress.

Do the Thymus Thump

To stimulate the thymus gland, a major player in stimulating the immune system, gently but firmly, with a fisted hand, "thump" on your thymus gland, which is located behind your breastbone in the center of your chest. This aids in activating the immune response and production of T-cells, which help fight cold and flu germs and other immune system insults.

HYDROTHERAPY

Soak and stoke up your temperature. Viruses and bacteria are very sensitive to body temperature. This spa treatment will encourage you to sweat and raise your body temperature. This is advantageous, as the body's natural defense against germs is to do this very same thing.

For a full-body spa soak, mix 10 drops of Conquer-a-Cold Combo (page 178) in 1 cup of baking soda and pour into a hot bath. Soak for at least 20 to 30 minutes. Dry yourself completely and wrap up in a cotton terry bathrobe or blanket. Rest for half an hour or more. The warmth of the robe will help keep heat in and keep the essential oils working longer.

INHALATION

Steam inhalation. Steam heat is very effective at breaking up a stuffy nose and getting mucus to flow. Adding essential oils to the steam maximizes the effect.

Bring a pot of water to a simmer on the stove. Do not let it boil. Transfer to a counter or pour into a large ceramic bowl. Add 3 or 4 drops of Conquer-a-Cold Combo to the water.

Hold your head approximately 8 inches from the water level and put a towel over your head in the form of a tent. Breathe deeply for 5 minutes or longer. Do two or three treatments a day, especially the first day of symptoms, for best results.

MASSAGE

Rub your chest. For a natural alternative to synthetic, petroleum-based chest medicine, make your own by adding 12 drops of Conquer-a-Cold Combo to 1 tablespoon of vegetable oil. Massage into chest and back areas. Include the neck if the lymph nodes are swollen.

Drain those nodes. Swollen glands are a common side effect of a cold. This massage rub will help drain the lymphatic system and bring the swelling down.

∞ Cold Rub ∞

A massage oil for cold symptoms and swollen glands.

4 drops eucalyptus essential oil
4 drops geranium essential oil
4 drops rosemary essential oil
1 tablespoon vegetable oil

In an amber glass bottle, add the essential oils using an eyedropper. Add the vegetable oil. Cap securely and shake to mix well. Apply and massage the cold rub in downward strokes, beginning on the neck and shoulders, moving down and outward toward the sides of the back. This encourages mucus drainage from the head and chest.

When the massage is complete, inhale the remaining oil on your hands. Then wash them thoroughly. Wrap your neck in a scarf or towel or put on a turtleneck sweater or jersey. Apply this oil in the morning, once during the afternoon, and again before retiring at night.

You may opt to make a larger amount for repeated usage. Simply multiply the recipe by four, or more.

SOUND AND MUSIC THERAPY

Hum for me. There are specific healing sounds, referred to as toning, that vibrate particular areas of the body to create balance, clear stagnation, and renew energy. For ailments of the lungs, sinus, and head region, practice making the sounds "hum" and "ma."

Take a deep breath, fully inhaling and filling the lungs. As you start to exhale, begin to tone the sound of "hum." Repeat three times. Repeat using the tone "ma." Practice these healing tones daily for optimal results.

When to Call the Doctor

While most cold and flu symptoms can be dealt with on your own, contact your health-care practitioner if you have any of the following symptoms:

- Fever exceeds 102 degrees
- Severe nausea, vomiting, and can't keep fluids down
- Moderate or severe headache
- Difficulty breathing
- Mucus has turned thick yellow or green
- Moderate to severe earache
- Symptoms persist for a week or more

Colitis

⁄∅

THE STRESS CONNECTION

Here's a disease that goes by different names: colitis, spastic colon, and inflammatory bowel syndrome (IBS). Those who have it call it something else: misery.

Whatever you call it, this disease of the colon is typically associated with inflammation and intermittent spasms. The cause is not always clear, but it seems to be related to the nervous system and diet.

Symptoms alternate between those related to constipation and diarrhea. At times the stools will be "pebblelike," dry, and hard and then the next day may be very loose, or mucouslike. Bloating of the abdomen, mild cramping or strong spasms, flatulence, depression, and an overall diminished feeling of vitality are common. High stress levels, imbalances within the immune system, food allergies, and genetic factors have been implicated as possible contributors to the disease.

Though colitis is difficult to treat, here are some remedies that offer some comfort to an otherwise miserable disease.

AROMATHERAPY

Oils that are kind to the colon. Essential oils used for colitis are calming to the nervous system. They are basil, bergamot, chamomile, geranium, lavender, lemongrass, niaouli, peppermint, pine, rosemary, and tea tree. Those with colitis should also take essential oils that promote relaxation and fight stress (see the section on Stress). These oils are most effective used in a bath, diffuser, or a massage oil blend.

The Peppermint Twist

It's not just for mouthwash anymore.

When people go through a medical examination of the rectum and colon, known as an endoscopy, doctors have found that adding the essential oil of peppermint to the preparation used in the procedure helps relax patients and prevent colon spasms.

In Germany and now in the United States, you can find peppermint enteric-coated pearles or capsules for internal use for ailments of the digestive tract.

DIET

Eat more fish. Omega-3 fatty acids found in abundant amounts in fish and flaxseed oil help reduce intestinal inflammation. Also, juices from chlorophyll-rich green leafy vegetables are also beneficial.

Stay out of Thai restaurants, and other places that serve highly spiced foods. Spicy foods irritate the colon and can cause a colitis attack or make a current condition worse. However, there are some spices that have actually been proven to be beneficial to the colon: anise seed, cinnamon, garlic, and thyme.

Hard to stomach. Those with colitis should also avoid dairy products, caffeine, nuts, and seeds.

HERBS

Balance the bowel. Several herbs have been found to help normalize the bowel, gently cleanse the system, and reduce inflammation and spasms. However, they should be used in moderation and are not for long-term use. Butternut bark, cascara sagrada, fennel seed, flaxseed, licorice root, and rhubarb root are colon cleansers. Antispasmodic herbs include chamomile, fenugreek seed, Irish moss, lobelia, marshmallow root, peppermint, slippery elm bark, thyme, and valerian root. Anti-inflammatory botanicals are alfalfa, aloe vera, calendula, chamomile, comfrey root, echinacea root, gentian root, licorice root, St. John's wort, skullcap, and turmeric.

MASSAGE

Get a tummy rub. Gentle massage, deep breathing, and relaxation are key components to your treatment plan. The following recipe is for mild cases of colitis, especially if the condition is exacerbated by stress. The essential oils chosen are relaxing, antispasmodic, slightly antidepressant, and anti-inflammatory.

✒ Colitis Chill–Out Lotion ∽

*This lotion was named by a patient of mine who
discovered stress brought on her colitis outbreaks.*

30 drops lavender essential oil
10 drops ylang-ylang essential oil
5 drops bergamot essential oil
3 drops chamomile essential oil
4 ounces unscented body lotion or vegetable oil

In an amber jar or bottle, add the essential oils. Cap securely and shake well to
mix. Add the body lotion or vegetable oil. Shake again to mix thoroughly. To use, put
a little lotion in your hands and apply to the lower half of the abdomen using gentle,
circular clockwise motion. Use daily. When finished, inhale essences from your
cupped hands.

TEAS AND TONICS

Drink up! The lemon balm, and chamomile herbs in this herbal tea blend are antispasmodic, while the calendula is added for its healing benefits. This tea happens to be very
soothing, slightly cooling, and makes a great refreshing ice tea for the summer months.

✒ Cool, Calm, and Collected Tea ∽

You don't have to have colitis to enjoy it!

1 part lemon balm dried herb
1 part catnip dried herb
1 part calendula flower tops
1 part chamomile flowers
Honey or stevia to taste

In a bowl, combine dried herbs and flowers and mix well. Store in a clean glass jar and label. Use 1 teaspoon per cup of hot water. Steep for 5 minutes, then strain. Drink as often as desired.

Call in the heavy healer. This odd tea must steep overnight, but it's well worth the time if you're suffering with colitis. The secret ingredient is flax, which provides an omega-3 oil, calms the digestive tract, and gently heals.

✺ Restorative Flax Tea ✜

12 ounces boiling water

1 tablespoon organic flaxseeds

Pour the boiling water over the flaxseeds and steep overnight. Drain and drink. The liquid may be reheated and served warm.

When to Call the Doctor

Any sudden change in bowel habits, blood in the stool, or pain with movement of the bowels warrants an examination by your doctor since it could be more than colitis. One of the most ignored symptoms of colon cancer is a change of bowel habits, especially if noted for more than a week or two. Not everyone who experiences any of the above warning signs has cancer, but it is a good idea to rule out the possibility. Ignorance is sometimes much more harmful than the disease itself. Early detection and treatment determine your success in most health problems.

Real–Life Cure

COLITIS RELIEVED WITH ESSENTIAL OILS

Rachel, forty-three, has a history of colitis going back to her teenage years. She came to see me during a week of acute symptoms. She was experiencing episodes of colitis-related symptoms six to eight times per year: typically, a change in stools, alternating constipation and diarrhea with some abdominal bloating, and cramping several hours following meals.

She said she frequently felt depressed and gradually was withdrawing from her social life during times of distress related to the colitis. She refused to see a physician for medication, as she is opposed to taking drugs unless absolutely necessary. She had already recognized foods that seemed to aggravate her condition, such as corn, large amounts of raw vegetables, fatty foods (especially fried foods), and coffee. But ignoring them wasn't doing her much good.

I asked Rachel about stress, but she insisted that her colitis couldn't be related to anything very stressful in her life; she didn't think her life was very stressful! I suspected, however, that she was not fully aware of her stress levels and ability to cope with change. She refused any type of stress evaluation, but she was willing to try an aromatherapy lotion and bath regime. I made further recommendations in her diet, which included decreasing other stimulant beverages like cola, chocolate drinks, and tea blends that contained black tea leaves. She was unaware that these had almost as much caffeine as coffee.

She used the massage lotion recipe provided earlier in this section, which she called her "Chill-Out" lotion, and drank Cool, Calm, and Collected Tea occasionally. I also gave her an inhalation recipe for depression, which she used whenever she was feeling blue. (You can find the recipe on page 218.) During the next six months she had only two episodes of colitis. She attributes her improvement to the essential oils.

Conjunctivitis

Not Just Kid's Stuff

Can you be "in the pink" and feeling irritated at the same time? Yes—if you have pinkeye.

Pinkeye, or conjunctivitis, is an inflammation of the transparent tissue covering the white (sclera) of the eye and the underlid. While known as a common, contagious childhood infection, it's common in adults, too.

The cause can be either bacterial or viral, and each is highly contagious. Hint: If the tearing matter is clear and watery, chances are it is of a viral origin. The bacterial-type infection produces a yellowish- or green-colored discharge. Often, upon awakening in the morning, you may find a crusty discharge on or around the eye.

Conjunctivitis typically does not cause visual changes. It is associated with allergies or exposure to environmental irritants such as smoke or chlorine in swimming pools.

All of the following treatments are safe for children as well as adults.

AROMATHERAPY

Mellow the yellow. Hydrosols or floral waters are recommended rather than essential oils. They are gentle and safe to use for delicate areas such as the eyes. Chamomile, rose, myrtle, and lavender floral waters are excellent choices for an eye compress. Personally I like chamomile the best because it is so mild and extremely soothing.

HERBS

Eyebright is eye right. Certain herbs are good for inflammation and irritations of the delicate and sensitive eye areas. Eyebright (euphrasia) is particularly known for its benefit to the eyes, as reflected by the name. Other herbs traditionally used in the treatment of eye disorders such as conjunctivitis are elderflower, ginseng, goldenseal, and quince. Preparations can be made or purchased as eyewashes, tinctures, or herbal capsules to take by mouth.

HYDROTHERAPY

Wash out carefully. With inflamed tissue, such as conjunctivitis, always use cool or tepid water temperatures (70 to 92 degrees) to encourage a decrease in the swelling and to aid the itching that often accompanies this ailment. Be sure to thoroughly wash the eye cup as well as your hands with soap and water. Do not re-use towels, as this infection can spread to other members of the family or to the other eye.

❧ Gentle Eyewash ❧

¼ teaspoon Celtic Sea salt
1 cup boiled tepid water or distilled bottled water

In a cup or small bowl, dissolve the salt in the water and stir well. Fill an eyewash cup or a shot glass with the saltwater solution. Standing at the sink, bend over the eye cup and fit it as snugly as you can over the eye area to prevent any leakage. Tilt your head back and blink several times, washing the eyeball and eyelids with the liquid. Bring your head back to the forward and down position and empty the eye cup contents into the sink. Refill and wash several times. Pat eye area gently. For best results, follow with the compress recipe below.

Cool the eye. The eyes must stay closed during this treatment to avoid irritation from the herbs. The herbal and aromatic properties of the compress will be absorbed through the eyelids.

This treatment makes a great follow-up to an eyewash. Since a cool temperature is recommended, you can make this ahead of time and let it cool in the refrigerator before using it.

❧ Bright-Eye Compress ❧

2 cups water or distilled bottled water
2 teaspoons chamomile, eyebright herb, or calendula petals

1 teaspoon distilled witch hazel (optional)
Several 2-inch-round cosmetic cotton pads/wipes (or cotton balls)

Heat the water to a boil. Add the herbs and let them steep, covered, for 5 to 10 minutes. Strain through a paper coffee filter or several layers of cheesecloth. Pour into a clean glass jar. Add the witch hazel if desired. Close the jar and shake well. Refrigerate to cool.

When ready to use, shake contents well and pour over cotton pads. Wring out the pads and lie down in a relaxing place. Apply the moist compress to the affected eye for 5 to 10 minutes. Do this two or three times a day. Remember to keep eyes closed during application! Do not use this application on small children who are unable to follow directions.

Constipation

✍

STIMULATION FOR STUBBORN BOWELS

It's a common problem but one that's seldom talked about.

Constipation is the absence of a bowel movement over a period of time—for most people, about 24 hours. In general, it involves some difficulty in passing stools, which are often hard and dry. Sometimes there can be pain in the lower abdomen. Constipation is easy to treat, but over a period of time a chronic condition can lead to hemorrhoids.

Some of the causes of sluggish bowels and constipation are nervous tension, a diet consistently low in fiber, dehydration, and a sedentary lifestyle. In recent years, constipation has been increasingly related to overuse of laxatives; this can promote "lazy" bowels because the body loses the ability to regulate the passage of stools. Even herbal laxatives can have a negative effect if used too frequently. Laxatives should only be used on an occasional basis. If you find yourself reaching for a laxative more than once a month, consider dietary and lifestyle changes to support your body-regulating function.

BREATH WORK

Breathe deeply. Deep breathing has a very beneficial effect on the large intestines via the lungs. According to Oriental medicine, the lungs and large intestine have a strong relationship. By taking deep breaths, you automatically relax the abdomen. While applying massage oil to your abdomen, do several slow, deep breaths to increase the benefits.

DIET

Make friends with fiber. Fiber is your best insurance to keep bowels in good working order, but it must be introduced into your diet slowly. Taking in too much too quickly can result in excess gas.

The best fiber for your diet is bran. For example, sprinkle ½ teaspoon or more on whole-grain cereal each morning. Or try this muffin, a great tasting way to get things moving.

Guaranteed-to-Work Bran Muffins

A muffin a day . . .

1 cup bran
½ cup oat bran
1½ cups whole-wheat flour
1 teaspoon baking soda
½ cup chopped prune pieces
2 egg whites or 4 tablespoons ground flaxseed
1 banana
½ cup molasses
2 tablespoons safflower oil
¾ cup nonfat, soy, or almond milk
12 walnut halves (optional)

Preheat the oven to 400 degrees. In a bowl, combine the bran, oat bran, flour, and baking soda. Add the prune pieces. In a food processor or blender, mix together the egg whites, banana, molasses, oil, and milk. Add the wet mixture to the dry ingredients. Fold together until moist (don't overstir).

Spray muffin tins with oil or use paper cups. Fill muffin tins ¾ full and top with a walnut half if desired. Bake for 15 to 18 minutes. Do not overbake, or they will turn out dry. Makes one dozen. Enjoy one every day.

These muffins freeze well, so you can make a batch or two and store them seven per bag for a one week supply.

Keep your whistle wet. Dehydration is the most common cause of constipation. Without adequate hydration, bowel movements get hard and too hard to move. Excretions collect water on their exit route, making for easy elimination. That's why you need to drink a minimum of 8 glasses of water every day.

LIFESTYLE

Develop a routine. As odd as this may sound, it works. By developing a routine of sitting in the bathroom first thing every morning (with your cup of hot herbal tea), you can encourage and actually train your bowels to move. Remember not to strain.

Exercise helps all areas of the body to perform better, especially the large intestines. A look into your lifestyle and habits may enlighten you as to whether stress plays a part in your problem.

MASSAGE

Move in the right direction. Massage encourages peristalsis, the wavelike contractions of the intestinal wall that supports the movement of material through the bowels. Massage in general helps eliminate stress and aid in relaxing the body, thus making bowel movements a lot easier. The following massage oil is designed to stimulate sluggish bowels.

❧ Moving-On Oil ❧

7 drops rosemary essential oil

5 drops fennel essential oil

2 tablespoons vegetable oil

In a small amber glass bottle, mix the essential oils with the vegetable oil. Cap securely and shake to mix. Label. Pour a small amount of the oil in your hand and massage the lower abdomen and sacrum area (lower back over spine) on a daily basis. Massage in a clockwise direction to encourage the correct flow.

TEAS AND TONICS

Since dehydration is the most common cause of constipation, a laxative tea provides both extra liquid and gentle stimulation. Some herbs that are helpful in alleviating constipation are fennel, ginger, licorice, marshmallow root, psyllium husk, rhubarb root, and slippery elm.

Real-Life Cure

A BRAN FAN IS BORN

Donna, an elderly woman experiencing occasional bouts of constipation, asked for my advice while visiting her family near my home during the summer. After evaluation, it appeared to be a simple case of constipation due to lack of exercise, the stress of traveling, and a change in her typical eating pattern.

She was curious to give herbs and aromatherapy a try since this was entirely new to her. She was one of the most conscientious clients I have ever worked with! She did everything that was recommended and called with questions and feedback. She made dietary changes, which called for increasing fiber and liquids. Donna looked forward to her bran muffin every day, and she enjoyed her "special potion," as she called her aromatherapy blend.

✍ Herbal Laxative Tea ✍

⅛ slice fresh ginger root
½ teaspoon ground fennel seed
½ teaspoon ground licorice root
1 cup boiling water
Honey or stevia to taste (optional)

Place the herbs in a mug. Pour the boiling water over the herbs and allow to steep for 5 to 10 minutes. Strain. Sweeten with honey if desired. Drink this tea for occasional constipation as needed. Best taken at bedtime.

Cough
✍

RUB THE RIGHT WAY

We cough every day. We cough to clear our throats. We cough to expel irritants we breathe into our lungs. We cough to get someone's attention. But there are days when we just cough and cough and cough and cough.

This kind of coughing is often associated with a cold or flu, an infection such as bronchitis, or postnasal drip. Postnasal drip causes a tickle in the back of the throat, and coughing is the body's reflex attempt to clear it.

Coughs can be moist or dry in nature, depending upon how much mucus is present and whether or not the cough is related to a cold or to an irritant exposure. There are different cures for different coughs. For moist coughs, the expectorant and mucolytic essential oils will be best to use. For dry coughs, antispasmolytic and antitussive essential oils will be called for. Antitussive, anticough agents are especially good at night if a cough prevents sound sleep.

AROMATHERAPY

Fragrant cough-cutters. Essential oils that assist with allaying coughing attacks are cypress, eucalyptus, frankincense, hyssop, juniper, lavender, myrrh, peppermint, rosemary, and sandalwood. They are best used in rubs, baths, and inhalations.

HERBS

Natural Cough Cures

CUSTOMIZING HERBAL REMEDIES ACCORDING TO YOUR COUGH

Antiviral: elderberry syrup, elder flower tea, astragalus extract, and olive leaf extract

Cough suppressant: anise seed tea and cherry bark tea

Expectorant: mullein and horehound tea, garlic syrup or soup (page 137)

Immune support: echinacea and green tea

Spasmodic coughs: lobelia leaf and lemon thyme tea

HYDROTHERAPY

An aromatic bath soak will help with all types of coughs, colds, or flu. The warm water temperature, therapeutic essential oils, and taking time out for yourself all add up to a faster recovery and improved health and well-being. The essential oils do not mix with water, so a carrier or bath base is needed. If you have dry skin (or it's midwinter), try the heavy cream as the bath base because it will add moisture and protect your skin; and if you want to try something new and chic, blend your oils in natural honey.

Takin'-Care-of-Me Bath

5 drops lavender essential oil
3 drops geranium essential oil
2 drops hyssop essential oil
¼ cup honey or cream

Fill the bathtub with comfortably hot water. Mix the essential oils in with the honey or cream. Add to the bathwater and stir with your hand to disperse. Soak for 15 to 20 minutes. Inhale deeply; this is an inhalation as well. Wrap up in a warm blanket or robe immediately upon getting out of the bath. Rest for 30 minutes under blankets. Follow with a chest rub before retiring.

INHALATION

Get all steamed up. The time-tested, old-fashioned steam inhalation is still the unrivaled treatment for coughs linked to colds and other respiratory conditions. The steam carries the essential oil molecules into the upper respiratory tract where they work directly on bacteria, viruses, and mucus. The oils have antispasmodic properties as well, which aid in the alleviation of coughing spasms.

Steam Heat for Coughs

4 cups water
1 drop cedarwood essential oil
1 drop eucalyptus essential oil
1 drop hyssop essential oil

Heat the water on the stove until it comes to a simmer. Do not boil. Pour the water into a ceramic bowl. Add the essential oils. Hold your head 8 inches over the bowl, close your eyes, and put a towel over your head to form a tent.

Inhale slowly and deeply, keeping your eyes closed. Steam for 5 to 10 minutes.

Cover your neck and upper chest with a warm towel, blanket, or scarf to keep the warmth in and the oils working. Repeat two or three times a day.

LIFESTYLE

A few suggestions to help keeps coughs at bay:

- Avoid dairy products. They can increase mucus production.
- Drink plenty of fluids. This not only keeps your mouth moist but also thins mucous secretions.
- Avoid environmental irritants.
- If you have postnasal drip, sleep with a couple of pillows to elevate your head.
- Keep a cool-water humidifier in your bedroom, and don't forget to put several drops of eucalyptus essential oil in the appliance for an all-night treatment. To increase oxygen content, you can add ½ cup of hydrogen peroxide.

MASSAGE

Rub it in. I've selected different rubs here for dry and moist coughs. Rosemary is the special agent for the moist cough, due to its expectorant properties. Lemon and pine are added to the dry cough remedy because they are diuretic and antibacterial.

✑ Moist Cough Rub ✑

12 drops eucalyptus essential oil
8 drops hyssop essential oil
4 drops rosemary essential oil
2 tablespoons vegetable oil

✿ Dry Cough Rub ✿

12 drops eucalyptus essential oil
6 drops hyssop essential oil
3 drops pine essential oil
3 drops lemon essential oil
2 tablespoons vegetable oil

In an amber glass bottle, add the essential oils, drop by drop, with an eyedropper. Add the vegetable oil. Cap and shake to mix. Label.

To use, warm the oil by placing some in your hands and rubbing them together. Massage upper chest and lower neck area on both front and back. When finished, inhale the essences from your hands before washing them well. Use twice a day.

Cuts

✿

EASY FIRST-AID ACTION

Oooo—ouch! How can something so tiny like a paper cut hurt so much?

Slices, slivers, and scrapes to the skin can bring a tear to the eye, but for the most part they will disappear almost as quickly as they appeared. Often, a strong immune system, excellent skin integrity, and a thorough cleaning with soap and water or an antiseptic vinegar are the only cures warranted. If, however, you feel your minor cut or wound needs some more attention, here is what to do.

AROMATHERAPY

First to the rescue. First-aid essential oils, called vulneraries or cicatrizants, possess antibacterial, anti-inflammatory properties that aid healing and prevent infection. Among them are bergamot, cajeput, chamomile (German and Roman), clary sage, eucalyptus, fennel, fir, frankincense, galbanum, geranium, helichrysm, hyssop, jasmine, juniper, lavender, lemon, lemongrass, myrrh, neroli, niaouli, patchouli, pine, rosemary, sandalwood, tea tree, and thyme.

Yes, rub vinegar into the wound. Vinegar and honey have been used since ancient times as a treatment for minor cuts, scrapes, and burns. I use honey as the carrier for the essential oils in this recipe in order for them to combine well with the vinegar and water.

The vinegar is an important ingredient because it is antiseptic and discourages fungal growth. It also helps reduce itching, which often occurs during the healing process. This recipe makes 8 ounces and is an excellent first-aid treatment. It stores well.

ᴏ First-Aid Antiseptic Vinegar ᴏ

This is the ultimate wound cleaner and should be a staple in your medicine chest.

6 drops lavender essential oil
2 drops tea tree essential oil
1 drop chamomile essential oil
1 drop lemon essential oil
1 teaspoon honey
½ cup distilled warm water
½ cup apple cider vinegar

You will need an 8-ounce amber glass or high-density plastic bottle. Mix the essential oils with the honey. In a glass measuring cup or bowl, combine the aromatic honey with the water and vinegar. Stir well and pour into the bottle. Shake well to mix. Label the contents with directions for use. To use, simply soak a cotton ball with the solution and clean the wound.

SALVES

A honey of a heal. Honey and other bee products are perfect healing agents for superficial wounds and minor burns (including sunburn). Other bee products include bee pollen, beeswax, propolis, and royal jelly. This honey balm recipe is highly curative and easy to prepare. Any honey can be used, but I prefer raw honey because it contains live enzymes and active ingredients such as the propolis and pollen.

✧ Healing Honey Balm ✧

For minor cuts, scrapes, and burns.

2 tablespoons pure, raw honey
12 drops tea tree essential oil
8 drops lavender essential oil
2 drops helichrysm essential oil
2 drops niaouli essential oil

In a small bowl, measure out the honey and essential oils. Mix thoroughly using a small spoon. Pour into a clean 1-ounce glass jar and label. To use, spread a thin film of the balm over the injury. Bandage if necessary. Dress three times per day and observe for signs of infection.

Go for the best. When more than a good cleaning is warranted, use this healing ointment to prevent the wound from drying and getting infected. It contains the best essential oils in existence for first-aid treatment and promotes tissue growth from the inside out. This ointment uses Heavy-Duty Ointment on page 240 for the base.

✍ Antiseptic Ointment ❧

This skin-friendly blend kills germs and speeds healing.

40 drops lavender essential oil
20 drops tea tree essential oil
10 drops chamomile essential oil
10 drops lemon essential oil
3 drops citrus seed extract (optional)
Heavy-Duty Ointment

Prepare the Heavy-Duty Ointment according to the directions given on page 240. In a clean storage jar, add each of the essential oils and, if desired, the citrus seed extract, using an eyedropper. Add the Heavy-Duty Ointment. Cap securely and shake to mix thoroughly.

To use, apply a small amount of this ointment to the cleaned wound. Cover with bandaging if necessary or leave open to air.

The Specialized Nature of Honey

When it comes to marketing their trade, bees offer lots of choices. Besides how the honey is sold or processed (comb, extracted, strained, raw, or wild), there are different types of honey, depending upon which plants the honey bees frequented to gather pollen.

They include alfalfa, barberry, buckwheat, cleome, cotton, currant, eucalyptus, goldenrod, hawthorn, heather, locust, orange blossom, sage, sycamore, thyme, and white or sweet clover and can be found or purchased for the want.

Although all are delicious and can be used for medicinal purposes, I recommend using the alfalfa, eucalyptus, orange blossom, sage, and thyme honey for skin therapy because of their additional antiseptic benefits.

When to Call the Doctor

Any sign of infection calls for a trip to the doctor or emergency room. These include swelling, increased redness, and/or pain and discharge, especially with a foul odor. If you see red streaks forming toward the heart, it is a sign of blood poisoning and requires immediate attention. See your health-care practitioner immediately.

Keep Safe: Keep Up with Your Booster

Tetanus, or lockjaw, is a life-threatening disease caused by anaerobic bacteria (*clostridium tetani*), which is found in soil and animal fecal matter and can be introduced into the body by any break in the skin. The major symptom is stiffening of the muscles, including the jaw, and requires immediate medical attention.

Since any wound, especially one occurring in the outdoors from rusty nails and old wood, carrys the potential for lockjaw. Medical professionals recommend a preventive tetanus, or booster, shot every 10 years.

Cystitis

⁄

BLADDER MADE BETTER

There is no rest for the restroom weary.

Cystitis is one of those problems that beckons you to empty your bladder at all hours—and especially at night. To make matters worse, the bathroom call is more of a sensation than a need. What passes is often merely a trickle. And, no matter what the amount, it causes a burning pain.

Cystitis occurs when the bladder becomes inflamed due to bacterial infection or local irritation (e.g., following sex). Of the 1 million Americans who contract it annually, 90 percent are women.

AROMATHERAPY

Soothe with the softness of sandalwood. Essential oils that contain antibacterial and anti-inflammatory properties are the aromatics chosen for this ailment; however, they must also be gentle enough to be used on delicate tissues such as the perineum. Sandalwood essential oil is both a gentle astringent and disinfectant and is included in most of my blends for urinary tract ailments.

> ## Tip: Public Restroom Faux Pas
>
> Squatting to avoid contact with public toilets may help prevent you from coming into contact with nasty germs, but it actually increases your risk of cystitis. The posture does not allow for complete emptying of the bladder, which complicates the ailment.

Other essential oils known to be useful in bladder inflammation and infections are bergamot, cedarwood, chamomile, cypress, eucalyptus, fennel, frankincense, hyssop, juniper, lavender, marjoram, niaouli, pine, rosemary, and sandalwood.

No to peppermint. Peppermint is often classified with the oils above because it is best known as an anti-inflammatory agent, but it is not recommended for cystitis because it can irritate sensitive tissue in this area.

DIET

Flush your system. Recommendations include drinking plenty of water, at least 8 glasses per day. Extra fluids, like fresh lemon water and herbal teas, will encourage dilution of local bacteria and aid in flushing them from the system. Get more rest and avoid stimulants like caffeine, alcohol, and black tea. Avoid sweets or sweetened juices (unsweetened cranberry juice is okay), because sugar actually encourages the bacteria to multiply.

Take a slug of vinegar. A tablespoon of natural apple cider vinegar diluted in water is an excellent remedy for balancing the pH of the urinary tract.

HERBS

Reach for natural assistance. Thankfully, nature has provided us with many effective herbs for overcoming and preventing bladder infections. Some of the primary herbs useful in this ailment are chickweed, cranberry, dandelion leaf, fennel seed, goldenseal root, horsetail, oat straw, parsley, pau de arco, pipsissewa, and uva ursi.

A few specific herbs known for their soothing and antispasmodic properties are Irish moss, marshmallow root, and thyme. Among the antibacterial botanicals are burdock root, chaparral, echinacea root, goldenseal root, myrrh gum, and pau de arco.

Herbs can be purchased and used in the form of herbal teas and tinctures as well as in capsule form.

HYDROTHERAPY

Sitz it out. The most appropriate therapeutic cure for a bladder infection is the sitz bath, which literally means "to sit." It is a local bath treatment that delivers the healing agents directly to the area in need. It is a very effective and soothing remedy. A bath in a regular tub with a few inches of water or a large basin in which you can sit comfortably will suffice.

✺ Sitz Bath for Cystitis ✺

3 drops sandalwood essential oil
2 drops tea tree essential oil
1 drop chamomile essential oil
1 to 2 tablespoons honey
2 tablespoons apple cider vinegar

Fill a large basin with warm to tepid water or use the bathtub and fill to hip level. If there is severe burning and local irritation, use tepid water to relieve these symptoms. Otherwise, use warm water.

In a small dish, combine the essential oils and honey. Mix well to blend. Add the vinegar to the bathwater and then the aromatic honey blend. Soak by sitting in the bath (with knees bent out of the water) for at least 15 to 20 minutes. Sip on herbal tea while in the tub if you wish.

Wash, not wipe. After voiding, many find bathroom tissue too abrasive. A pleasant option for cleaning this area is an aromatic periwash made of distilled water, cider vinegar, and a few drops of essential oil. Use after every trip to the bathroom (which is often!).

A plastic squirt bottle is handy to use as a peri bottle or use a plastic water bottle with the pull-out drinking spout.

Aromatic Periwash

2 tablespoons apple cider vinegar
1 drop lavender essential oil
1 drop sandalwood essential oil
7 ounces distilled warm water

In a clean plastic bottle, add the vinegar and essential oils. Cap and shake well. Add the water and shake again to mix. Shake each time before use, as the essential oils separate from the water. Rinse with this immediately after voiding. Pat dry with a clean, soft cotton towel.

MASSAGE

Therapeutic massage. According to Chinese medicine, the sacral area (the base of the spine) is a major chakra (focal point) for the genitourinary system. The infusion oils listed in this recipe are optional, as well as the carrot seed oil; however, they have anti-inflammatory and healing properties and add to the efficacy of this blend.

Massage Blend for Cystitis

10 drops lavender essential oil

6 drops sandalwood essential oil

5 drops cedarwood essential oil

4 drops bergamot essential oil

¼ teaspoon carrot seed oil (optional)

1 tablespoon vegetable oil

1 tablespoon mullein or calendula infusion oil (optional)

In an amber glass bottle, add the essential oils and, if desired, the carrot seed oil. Pour in the vegetable oil and, if desired, the infusion oil. Cap securely and shake gently to combine well. Label. Apply a small amount to the lower abdomen, above

Make Your Own Infusion Oil

To make your own infusion oils at home, follow these simple instructions. A variety of herbs and flowers can be gathered or purchased to make several different infused oils for an assortment of uses. The most common are arnica (*Arnica Montana*), calendula (*Calendula officinalis*), and St. John's wort (*Hypericum perforatum*). However, in more exotic locations you will find monoi-, gardenia-, centella-, and jasmine-infused oils to include in your beauty and skin spa preparations. You may use fresh or dried flower heads. However, if you choose to make your infusion with fresh flowers, be sure all the moisture has been removed.

Fill a slow cooker or Crock-Pot with the clean, dry flower tops. Pour in enough virgin olive oil to cover them completely, and heat the mixture very slowly on the lowest setting for 24 hours. Alternatively, you can place them in a large glass jar in the sun for a few days up to one month. The later, longer period of time is recommended for St. John's wort infusion oil. Strain well into squeaky-clean amber glass bottles and label. Add several vitamin E capsules or oil to prolong the infusion's shelf life. Keep refrigerated.

the bladder area, in addition to the lower back. Apply this treatment oil twice per day, once in the morning and then just before retiring.

Dandruff

❧

REIGN IN THE SHOWER

Feeling flaky lately? Spotting a bit of "snow" on the shoulders is a common occurrence, especially during dry, cold seasons when the skin has a tendency to get dry.

For some people, however, dandruff, medically termed *seborrheic dermatitis,* is a chronic condition. In addition to dry skin, it can be caused by poor circulation, fungal infection, or overuse of high alkaline shampoo or hair products.

Whatever the cause, there is no need to pack away the navy and black wardrobe. Try these easy solutions.

AROMATHERAPY

Reach for the birch. Many commercial dandruff treatments contain salicylate constituents, which are closely related to aspirin or salicylic acid. Certain herbs and essential oils naturally contain this constituent and can be used in aromatherapy applications such as scalp treatment oils and rinses. Of these, the essential oil I recommend for individual use is the birch essential oil. It is best used as part of a blend, incorporating other beneficial essences. When used by itself, you should dilute it to 0.2 percent essential oil or less.

Make use of scalp-friendly oils. Essential oils that are useful for dandruff conditions are basil, birch, cedarwood, clary sage, cypress, eucalyptus, lavender, lemon, lime, patchouli, rosemary, and tea tree. They can be mixed with borage, carrot seed, evening primrose, jojoba, and sweet almond as carrier oils.

Baby your scalp. Baby shampoo makes this formula extra easy on the scalp. And it really works!

✧ Dandruff Shampoo ✧

40 drops lavender essential oil
20 drops rosemary essential oil
10 drops birch essential oil
10 drops cedarwood essential oil
8 ounces baby shampoo

In a small bowl, mix together the essential oils. Add the essential oils to the shampoo. Cap securely and shake well to mix. Label.

To use, massage a small amount into wet hair. Massage into your scalp for 3 to 5 minutes. Rinse several times, ending with a cold-water application. The latter is an optional step but helps close pores and stimulate scalp circulation. Follow with the Vintage Victorian Hair Rinse given below.

Note: Though this is made with baby shampoo, it should not be used by young children. Keep labeled and out of the hands of children.

Herbs

Try the Victorian vinegar cure. During the Victorian era, herbal vinegars were popular for hair and skin care. They were easy to make from herbs found in the garden and countryside.

Along the way, these herbal and floral vinegars lost popularity as store-bought and perfumed preparations became widely available. But when it comes to dandruff control, these herbal hair rinses that contain vinegar are still some of the most beneficial after-shampoo rinses you can use. Vinegar, diluted in herbal infusions or floral waters, helps to normalize the scalp's delicate pH balance and aids in toning the scalp. It also successfully removes oil and shampoo residue from the hair. Witch hazel lotion can also be used in this way.

Traditional herbs used in scalp conditions such as dandruff are aloe vera, borage, lavender, myrtle, nettles, rosemary, sage, and witch hazel. Any of these can be made into herbal infusions and vinegars for hair rinses.

Make Your Own Herbal or Floral Vinegar

Herbal and floral vinegars are easy to make. Obtain a good apple cider vinegar (preferably organic) and pour 1 quart into a wide-mouth glass jar. Add one to two handfuls of fresh-picked flowers and herbs. Set the mixture in the sun for a few weeks, shaking daily. If you are in a hurry, gently heat the vinegar and add to the herbs, allowing to steep for several days. Strain and bottle. Label contents. This can be added to baths, hair rinses, and diluted even further for use as a facial toner. For dandruff, use basil, lavender, and rosemary.

～ Vintage Victorian Hair Rinse ～

*Mix up this recipe and store it in a plastic bottle with a squeeze top,
by recycling one of your old shampoo or conditioner bottles.*

8 ounces floral water or herbal infusion
2 tablespoons cider vinegar or herbal vinegar

Lavender floral water can be used, or you can make your own herbal infusion. Simply take fresh or dried flowers and herbs (from the list in the box on page 206) and pour hot water over them, about 2 to 3 tablespoons per cup, to make a strong infusion. Nettles and rosemary herb make a nice tea to add to this recipe.

Massage

Treat your scalp. Use the scalp treatment preparation given below for tough cases of dandruff or for an occasional special scalp treatment. It is made with nutritive, but fairly light, oils as well as known anti-dandruff essences. It is preferable to warm the aromatic oil first, prior to massaging into the scalp, to increase absorption and promote circulation to that area. For best results, leave it in overnight and shampoo in the morning. Follow with the Vintage Victorian Hair Rinse.

Scalp Treatment Oil

Apply at night after brushing your hair and scalp completely.

2 tablespoons jojoba oil
½ teaspoon carrot seed oil
10 drops lavender essential oil
5 drops rosemary essential oil
3 drops cedarwood essential oil
2 drops birch essential oil (optional)

In a small amber bottle, mix the jojoba and carrot seed oils. Add the essential oils and shake gently to mix well. Label. To use, put several drops on your fingertips and massage into your scalp and the roots of your hair.

Tip: Brush and Brush Some More

I'm not going to recommend one hundred strokes a day, though that would certainly be good for your scalp and hair. But to control dandruff, you need to brush your hair vigorously before shampooing. This not only will help loosen dead skin cells but also will increase circulation in the scalp.

Moreover, the type of brush *does* matters. Use only a natural bristle brush. Plastic and other synthetic brushes will not massage your scalp adequately and can cause damage to your hair.

Dental Plaque

A PLANNED ATTACK

Most people brush their teeth regularly, but do they brush their teeth properly? According to dentists, the answer is a loud *NO*. The average person brushes for an average of 51 seconds, while dentists say we should brush for 2 to 3 minutes.

So what is the penalty for this egregious lack of attention to our teeth? Plaque or, specifically, plaque buildup, the seed that leads to dental decay and gum problems.

When teeth are not cleaned properly, a filmy layer forms on the surface, creating a nesting ground for bacteria. As bacteria, calcium phosphate, and old food deposits accumulate, they harden into plaque. Once plaque develops, it is unlikely you will be able to clean your teeth without the help of a dental professional. Therefore, the goal is to prevent plaque by brushing long enough, regularly, and with a healthy tooth-cleaning product.

AROMATHERAPY

Check for these oils. Essential oils of clove, coriander, eucalyptus, fennel, geranium, ginger, lavender, lemon, myrrh, peppermint, spearmint, star anise, and tea tree are used for their natural flavoring, as well as the antiseptic, astringent, and healing benefits they provide in natural toothpastes and mouth rinses. Look for them on the labels when buying natural toothpaste or mouth-rinse products.

Make your own. I've been using homemade tooth powder since I was a kid, and I'm proud to say that I have few dental problems. Here's the powder my family favors.

❧ Teeth-White Tooth Powder ❧

4 parts baking soda
1 part Celtic Sea salt, finely ground

1 part rubbed sage herb (optional)

5 drops fennel or tea tree essential oil

Lemon juice or water

Combine the baking soda, sea salt, and, if desired, sage in a dish or mortar and pestle if you have one. Carefully check that the sage is finely ground or "rubbed," discarding any large or stick pieces. Add the essential oil and mix well with the pestle. Store in an airtight wide-mouth jar, covered dish, or bottle.

To use, moisten your toothbrush with lemon juice or water and sprinkle the powder onto the brush. Brush gently for a few minutes and rinse thoroughly. Follow with Kiss-Me Mouthwash, which can be found on page 112.

My Father's Sage Advice

My father had me brushing my teeth with baking soda and lemon juice as soon as I could hold a toothbrush. As I got older and more adventuresome, he suggested an added ingredient: sage.

Finely ground, rubbed sage has many positive effects on the teeth and on the delicate mucous membranes. Next time you're in the garden, pick a fresh sage leaf and rub it over your teeth for an instant polish. Then chew the leaf to freshen your breath.

HERBS

Healthy alternatives. Herbs effective for maintaining healthy teeth and gums are echinacea, goldenseal, krameria, myrrh, neem, peelu, propolis, and witch hazel. Other natural ingredients sometimes found in natural, healthier toothpastes are baking soda, chalk, hydrogen peroxide, sea salt, and silica. Other natural flavoring to look for in natural tooth-cleaning products are cherry, elderberry, hibiscus, licorice, and orange.

One Brush Is Not Enough

It takes about 36 hours for a toothbrush to dry completely. If you use the same brush daily, germs can easily live on the moist surface. You have options to avoid contamination and bacterial growth: Keep three different toothbrushes and rotate them daily. Or do what I do and keep your brush soaking in a baking soda solution.

To make a solution, add 1 teaspoon of baking soda to ½ cup of water. To flavor the solution and increase antibacterial properties, you can add 1 drop of tea tree oil or lemon oil.

For more information and remedies, see Bad Breath *and* Bleeding Gums.

Depression

ELATION THERAPY

We all get the blues now and then, that powerless "who cares" feeling that can leave us bored, anxious, listless, and ready to snap at anyone who looks at us the wrong way. On the other end of the spectrum is depression, a life-absorbing condition with emotional pain too hard to comprehend except by those who've actually "been there."

The word *depression* means to "push down." No one is immune to it. It strikes adults, teenagers, and even children and is especially common among those in the helping professions, such as nurses. It hits those in poor health and those in grief over the loss of a loved one.

Symptoms of depression range from mild to severe. Causes of depression are still debated and theorized in medical circles, but it's widely believed to be linked to a chemical imbalance in the brain. There's also evidence that genes are a factor in our vulnerability to depression. It is most common in women, which leads many to believe that hormones and body-image perceptions are a root cause.

It should go without saying that serious (clinical) depression cannot be solved alone. Professional intervention is needed. One beneficial treatment is cognitive behavior therapy, which looks at changing the belief system and unhealthy behaviors of a person having difficulty functioning. Professionally monitored support groups and therapy are also helpful.

In my mind, however, too many doctors resort to prescribing drugs too quickly. Serotonergic drugs, known as serotonin reuptake inhibitors, are widely prescribed to both children and adults for a variety of diagnoses; however, depression and anxiety-related disorders top the list. These medications are designed to block serotonin in the brain, thereby increasing brain levels of this neurochemical. It is now becoming obvious that raising serotonin levels by lowering the metabolism of serotonin can produce serious, long-term problems. For example, one popular drug in this group has approximately 44,000 adverse reports filed with the FDA. Out of this appalling statistic, 2,500 of them were deaths associated with suicide or violence.

As I said, clinical cases of depression are beyond this book's application to heal. But if you're feeling blue or mildly depressed or even feel that a lift in your mood is needed, try these pleasant, spirit-lifting treatments.

AROMATHERAPY

Smell the fragrances of life. Notice that many of the essential oils used for depression are from flowers and fruit. These essences tend to be light and ethereal in nature, with an uplifting effect on the mind and emotions. Essential oils used for depression are basil, bergamot, cedarwood, clary sage, frankincense, geranium, grapefruit, jasmine, laurel, lavender, lemon, melissa, myrrh, neroli, orange, rose, sandalwood, spruce, and ylang-ylang.

Essential oil therapy that supports serotorin production via raphe nucleus stimulation are primarily the sedative oils, which include: laverder, neroli, Roman chamomile, and sweet marjoran.

Essential oils that can have a positive influence on feelings of anger that are associated with depression can be useful as well and include chamomile, rose, rosemary, and ylang-ylang. If the depression is associated with a loss, then essential oils helpful for grief and bereavement, such as frankincense, hyssop, lavender, marjoram, neroli, and rose, should be

Better Than Drugs

Serotonin is a naturally occurring neurotransmitter (produced by receptors in the brain and intestinal tract) that is responsible for elevating mood, improving memory, controlling anxiety, increasing libido, and boosting metabolism.

There's no need to resort to drugs to increase serotonin levels in the brain. Studies have found that doing exhilarating or feel-good activities can help increase serotonin levels naturally. I suggest the following:

- Exercise vigorously for 10 to 15 minutes.
- Get a massage.
- Take a roller-coaster ride.
- Think happy thoughts.
- Watch a funny movie.
- Go to a party and talk with people.
- Listen to comedy (radio, cassette tape in car).
- Meditate or pray.
- Practice yoga.
- Practice deep, relaxed breathing for 10 to 15 minutes.
- Eat foods high in carbohydrates.
- Use serotonin-enhancing aromas.

included. Any of these oils, or a combination, can be enjoyed by simply inhaling their aromas for several minutes, when used in a diffuser, by massaging with them, or in an aromatic bath.

BREATH WORK

Among the enormous benefits to performing Healing Breath is that it retunes and stimulates your brain and readjusts your bioelectrical field. Getting plenty of oxygen through

Rose Petal Perk Me Up

Every summer I make up a large batch of rose vinegar to add to my baths. It has a lovely, rich red color and is a fresh change from the typical bath oils and salts.

To prepare, simply pick an ample amount of nonsprayed, fragrant red and pink rose petals. Place freshly picked flowers into a large gallon-sized glass jar and pack loosely. Gently heat raw apple cider vinegar on the stove and pour over the flowers in the jar until they are completely covered. Put the lid on and store for several weeks. Strain and bottle. I place mine in a pretty wine decanter near the bathtub. You can add a few fresh or dried rose petals into the bath for extra luxury! This Victorian-inspired bath vinegar lasts for a year or more and can offer great relief for the mid-winter blues.

long, deep breathing will provide you with renewed energy and a brighter outlook on life. This refreshed outlook kindles your "prana," or vital life force, which is essential for a balanced, blissful existence.

The Healing Breath

Relax yourself, focusing your attention on your breath. Breathe in a slow, calm manner as you follow these steps:

1. Sit in a relaxed position in a chair or on the floor with your legs folded in front of you.
2. Raise your arms over your head and gently twist your torso from side to side to stretch your rib cage and spine.
3. Bring your arms down and place your hands comfortably in your lap.
4. Inhale through your nose for a count of three.
5. Exhale for a count of four, completely emptying your lungs.

HYDROTHERAPY

Soak in some mental energy. Sometimes a little personal pampering is all you need to chase away the blues. This bath helps lift the mood because it contains many of the essential oils that are proven helpers against depression.

Draw a warm bath and soak for as long as you are comfortable. Taking time for yourself is part of the cure. Combine with the inhalation blend below to double the effectiveness.

✺ Bye–Bye Blues Bath ✺

Add music, candles, and a warm cup of herbal tea.

3 drops lavender essential oil
3 drops ylang-ylang essential oil
2 drops basil essential oil
2 drops geranium essential oil
1 drop grapefruit essential oil
¼ cup honey
Fresh rose petals or geranium leaves (optional)

Mix the essential oils in the honey. Fill the bathtub with warm water and then add the aromatic honey mixture. Toss in the flower petals if desired. Stir well using your hands. Soak for at least 30 minutes.

INHALATION

Heaven on earth. This formula emanates a heavenly scent. It's entirely made of essential oils that fight depression. Clients tell me that it works miracles.

Selected ingredients: Clary sage is euphoric and an antidepressant. Ylang-ylang is useful in states of anger and is an anti-depressant. Geranium is regulating and balancing, while basil is helpful in clearing the mind, is an anti-depressant, and is useful for mental fatigue. Sandalwood eases nervous tension and improves concentration.

This blend is meant to be used in a diffuser. It can also be used in an aroma lamp, potpourri burner, or a few drops on a tissue.

⁄⊘ Mind/Mood Blend ⊘⟋

This is my personal favorite!

4 parts clary sage essential oil
4 parts ylang-ylang essential oil
3 parts geranium essential oil
2 parts basil essential oil
1 part sandalwood essential oil

In an amber glass bottle, add the essential oils. Cap securely and shake gently to mix. Label. To use, add 4 to 6 drops to a diffuser or lamp several times a day. If using an electric diffuser, allow to run for 15 minutes.

Take it with you. Place a few drops of the Mind/Mood Blend in a perfume pendant and wear it around your neck. It's a perfect and fashionable way to feel good throughout the day.

LIFESTYLE

Don't isolate yourself. Being in the company of others might be the last thing you feel like doing, but it's actually the best thing you can do. Aloneness only allows you to brood and think about your problems. Surround yourself with happy people.

Don't fret. Plan your day to fill your time. Set each day's tasks by prioritizing, and be realistic in your goal setting.

Treat yourself with flowers. Be kind and give yourself a special treat, such as fresh flowers. My favorite aromatic bouquets include fragrant roses, stargazer lilies, lily of the valley, hyacinth, and gardenias. Avoid using food as a reward, because it often backfires.

Help others. Deflect your feelings by helping those less fortunate than you. Volunteer work in a charity is a wonderful way to feel good about yourself.

Affirm yourself. Create more positive energy in your life by reprogramming your thoughts. Consciously focus on empowering statements instead of negative self-talk. For example: "I am loved"; "I am blessed"; "I feel safe."

MASSAGE

Go undercover. An aromatherapy full-body massage is a wonderful and pleasant way to pamper yourself when you are feeling down. It is affirming and nurturing, in addition to being very satisfying, as touch is a basic need.

Massage and aromatherapy go hand in hand in treating nervous-system ailments such as depression. For a special treat, take a diluted blend of the oil given below when you go to your massage therapist.

Go for the heart chakra. According to Ayurveda, massaging the heart chakra area, located halfway between the sternum and the throat, can help transform and balance this energy center. Ayurvedic healing believes that it is here where pain, sorrow, and emotional trauma are stored. Releasing these energies heals by increasing your sense of well-being and vital life energy flow. I recommend doing it with this massage oil formula and your personalized affirmations.

❧ Elation Formulation ❧

> 8 drops lavender essential oil
> 8 drops ylang-ylang essential oil
> 2 drops basil essential oil
> 2 drops geranium essential oil
> 2 drops bergamot essential oil
> 2 tablespoons sweet almond oil or vegetable oil
> 1 teaspoon wheat germ oil

In an amber glass bottle, add the essential oils. Add the sweet almond oil and wheat germ oil. Shake gently to mix well. Label.

To use, apply a small amount onto the back of the hands and chest area (heart chakra). Massage using slow, clockwise, rhythmic, circular strokes. Inhale the essences from your hands after application to the skin. During the day, inhale from the back of the hands. The oils will be absorbed through the skin. Apply two or three times daily.

SOUND AND MUSIC THERAPY

Mellow out with melodies. Music that treats depression and fear and alleviates boredom is nothing new. Harmonics have been used since the beginning of civilization to comfort the human soul and carry our emotions to brighter inner landscapes. Here are a few of my favorites. Explore, venture out, and find your own special music that will lift you up when you are feeling otherwise.

Beethoven—*Piano Concerto No. 5*
Mozart—*Symphony No. 35*
Handel—*Water Music*
Handel—*Choruses from Messiah*
Liszt—*Hungarian Rhapsodies*
Respighi—*Ancient Dances and Airs; Pines of Rome*
When You Wish Upon a Star (Disney Songs)

TEAS AND TONICS

Sip something good. A good cup of herbal tea is the ultimate feel-good tonic. This special tea incorporates herbs that are helpful in combating depression by nourishing and supporting the nervous system.

⟋ Feel-Good Herbal Tea ⟍

3 parts lemon balm herb
1 part lavender flowers

1 part rose petals

1 part spearmint leaf

1 part St. John's wort

1 part marjoram

Vanilla Honey (see recipe on page 221),

    stevia, or lemon to taste (optional)

Mix the herbs and flowers in a bowl. Store in a glass jar and label. To prepare, use 1 to 2 teaspoons of herbal tea per cup. Pour hot water over the herbs and allow them to steep for 5 to 10 minutes. Strain and flavor with Vanilla Honey, stevia, or lemon if desired. Drink up to 3 cups per day.

❧ Vanilla Honey ❧

1½ cups raw honey

1 to 2 4-inch pieces vanilla bean

Gently heat honey over low setting, taking care not to boil. Pour honey into a clean glass jar. Add 1 to 2 pieces of vanilla bean. Let it age for a week or two, if you're able to stay away from it that long! This aromatic honey is delicious in herbal tea, blended with whipping cream, and even used as a face mask.

YOGA AND MOVEMENT

Release those endorphins. Ever see anyone returning from the gym in a really bad mood? Not very often, I bet, if ever. That's because heart-pumping exercise has been found to release feel-good chemicals called endorphins into the brain. It's what gives runners their so-called "high." Exercise also boosts circulation, trims the body, and strengthens the immune system.

If you can't get to the gym (or, better yet, in addition to the gym), take daily walks, preferably in the park or along the seashore, to connect with nature and appreciate the beauty it offers. Fresh air and deep breathing exercises are both good in aiding relaxation and promoting good oxygenation of the entire body.

Real–Life Cure

AROMATHERAPY FOR DEPRESSION

Karen, a fifty-five-year-old psychotherapist, had been taking antidepressants for years when she came to see me for an alternative solution to her bouts of depression. She had to take the drugs for several months, she told me, before she "came out of it."

To complicate matters, Karen had experienced several losses in her life over the prior six months and was experiencing anxiety. It also didn't help that Karen was in a profession in which she dealt with the problems of others all day.

We worked together to implement an aromatherapy plan that would benefit her lifestyle and emotional needs. She changed her eating habits to a healthy diet and started taking daily walks outside on her lunch break. More important, she began using essential oils in her bath, in massage preparations, and in a diffuser that she used in her office between appointments and in her bedroom at home. She also used a blend of oils for a hand and chest massage.

Working with Karen turned out to be a positive experience for both of us. Her quick recovery prompted me to incorporate the anger and sadness oils into the depression blends. She was drug-free and completely over her depressed feelings within about two weeks.

When to Call the Doctor

If you or someone you know experiences four or more of the following symptoms for more than two weeks and none of the remedies mentioned here has helped, it may be time to see a professional trained in psychotherapy or medicine.

continued . . .

- Persistent sadness or feelings of emptiness
- Hopelessness
- Guilt
- Loss of interest in normal activities
- Change in appetite
- Fatigue or decreased energy
- Suicidal thoughts or thoughts of death
- Irritability
- Difficulty in concentration and/or remembering

Stretch your body, ease your mind. On the opposite end of the spectrum is yoga, a technique of gentle movement and stretching that is as good for your mental outlook as it is for your body.

Dermatitis

SMOOTHING OUT THE BUMPS

A red itchy rash that abruptly erupts on your skin is a telltale sign that something has rubbed you the wrong way.

Referred to as contact dermatitis, the most common causes are exposure to poison plants, such as ivy, oak, and sumac; industrial chemicals, textiles and metals, solvents, detergents, and dyes; cosmetics; and even some medicines.

The most suspect cosmetic ingredients include synthetic fragrance, preservatives, propylene glycol, formaldehyde, sunscreens, and deodorants.

Be Wary of These Additives

Of the thousands of newly released synthetic chemicals introduced into the commercial market yearly, here are but a few of the common, yet questionably unsafe, cosmetic ingredients you may find in your skin-care products at home. Many of them are derived from petroleum.

- *Mineral oil:* Linked to cancer, skin and eye irritation, and clogged pores
- *DEA (diethanolamine):* May cause cancer in laboratory animals. FDA presently investigating this ingredient, which can be found in forms of cocamide DEA and lauramide DEA
- *Proplyene glycol:* Skin and eye irritant
- *Talc:* Linked to ovarian and lung cancers
- *Sodium lauryl sulfate:* Skin and eye irritant; linked to some cases of canker sores

Tip: Homeopathic Helper

Rescue Remedy is a brand name homeopathic remedy that can provide welcome relief for dermatitis. It's best used right after initial contact with the allergen. It should calm the inflammation process quite readily and aid the healing process. Look for it in cream or tincture form.

The liquid form can be combined in the Cooling Relief Compress on page 226, mixed in a bath or mixed in with a homeopathic cream and applied three times per day.

AROMATHERAPY

Contact these. Essential oils that help relieve itching are bergamot, cedarwood, chamomile (especially German chamomile), jasmine, lemon, and peppermint (use 1 percent dilution or less). Anti-inflammatory essential oils are useful in dermatitis, as this is an inflammatory process involving the dermal layer of the skin. The essential oils effective in decreasing swelling are carrot seed, chamomile, clary sage, frankincense, geranium, lavender, lemon, myrrh, patchouli, peppermint (1 percent or less), rose, and sandalwood. Rose has proven able to decrease histamine production, which is important in allergy-related conditions. Other essential oils useful for dermatitis include benzoin, hyssop, juniper, and neroli.

HERBS

Added relief. Anti-inflammatory herbs are calendula, chamomile, comfrey, elderflower, lavender, lemon juice, oats, parsley, St. John's wort, and yarrow flowers. These can be made into strong infusions and applied by compress or spray.

Ointments and creams made with calendula, comfrey, and plantain are also very effective. Aloe vera gel mixed with one of the essential oils listed above can be extremely useful to the healing process and can alleviate redness and itching.

HYDROTHERAPY

To wash or not to wash. Immediate washing of the area is necessary when a rash appears from direct contact with skin irritants. However, in the case of poison ivy or oak, do not use soap, as this will spread the irritant to other areas of the skin. Rinse with cold water to flush the substance from the skin and then apply hot water for a few seconds.

Feel your oats. An old-fashioned home remedy for treating rashes and simple skin inflammations is to soak in bathwater infused with oats. Steep a muslin bath bag in a bathtub filled with hot water. Allow the bathwater to cool to a safe temperature.

Alternatively, quick cooking oats can be used. Soak the oats in three times as much water over-night. Strain and then pour into the bathwater. Some natural, unscented soaps are made with oat flour for this type of ailment as well.

> ## Tip: Chill to Perfection
>
> Keep your aloe vera gel in the refrigerator. By storing it in a cold place you will prolong its shelf life, preserve its potency, and provide cool relief to such problems as dermatitis, sunburn, and accidental thermal burns.

First aid first. At the first sign of a rash, especially poison ivy or oak, rub it with aloe vera juice or gel or rinse it with floral waters of chamomile or lavender. Following this initial first aid, cool compresses, baths, or oils can be used as a more intensive form of treatment.

Compress the itch. This compress is for general use for red and inflamed skin rashes. Depending on the size of the area that is affected, a washcloth, small flannel cloth, or large toweling can be used. If a large area is covered with the rash, the baths may be more appropriate.

Vinegar and witch hazel are astringents that are effective for itching skin. One half cup of either can be used in the compress water or a combination of both as shown here.

This treatment aids swelling and itching in the form of a cool aromatic compress.

Cooling Relief Compress

Tames itching and swelling.

¼ cup apple cider vinegar

¼ cup witch hazel lotion

1 to 2 cups cold water

2 teaspoons baking soda

4 drops lavender essential oil

2 drops chamomile essential oil

2 drops bergamot essential oil

In a bowl or basin (or sink if a larger area needs to be covered), add the vinegar, witch hazel, and water. To the baking soda, add the essential oils and mix well. The

When to Call the Doctor

If you get a rash that rapidly spreads and involves raised bumps that become pimplelike in appearance, you could have chicken pox or measles. If any rashlike areas develop into ulcers (with or without pain) in the mouth, genitals, palms of the hands, or soles of the feet, you should also see a doctor.

baking soda is used as the carrier for the oils and to help with itching. Add to the water and mix well by stirring. Soak the cloth and wring most of the water from it. Apply to the rash-afflicted area. Lay an ice pack over this and wrap with a towel. Leave on for 20 minutes. Change the compress once it becomes body temperature or begins to dry. Apply the compresses three times per day as needed.

For more remedies and information, see Allergies *and* Sensitive Skin.

Diaper Rash

Wipe It Out

Baby's bottom is red and sore. Baby is crying, and Mom and Dad feel guilty. Well, they shouldn't. Baby simply has a case of diaper rash, which is very common. The comforting solutions I offer will have baby cooing in no time.

Aromatherapy

Essential oil therapies along with soothing herbal infusion oils are a perfect combination for treating the delicate skin of little ones. However, due to their potency, essential oils must be used with caution and with the proper instruction for a safe and effective outcome. See page 17 for cautions about children's dosages.

Say "never again." This oil blend will prevent diaper rash and treat mild cases. Use it sparingly to protect baby's delicate skin. The calendula infusion oil is very healing and protective and is highly recommended for this recipe. If you cannot find it in your natural health store, you can substitute jojoba, safflower oil, or sweet almond.

✌ Baby–Bottom Oil ✌

10 drops lavender essential oil
1 drop chamomile essential oil
4 tablespoons calendula infusion oil

In a 2-ounce amber glass bottle, add the essential oils. Add the calendula oil. Shake well to mix. Label with directions for use. Apply in small amounts on dry skin when changing diapers, up to three times per day.

LIFESTYLE

Stay dry. Keeping baby in wet diapers too long is the major cause of diaper rash. For prevention, here's what to do:

- Wash baby's buttocks and perineum thoroughly and dry well before applying a new diaper. Allow baby to air dry for a few minutes in the sunlight when possible.
- Change diapers as soon as they become soiled or wet.
- Avoid powders, which can cake to the skin, and mineral oil, which can clog pores and prevent adequate drying of the skin.

Baby Bottom—Cleaning Solution

A mixture of white distilled vinegar and water—one part vinegar to four parts water—is a great solution to cleaning a baby after a soiled diaper is removed. It neutralizes the concentrated urine and ammonia present on the buttocks and helps balance the skin's pH. It also discourages yeast, a common cause of rash.

When taking baby out and about, soak cotton cosmetic pads or towelettes in this solution and store in a resealable plastic bag.

- Avoid plastic pants and disposable diapers; they discourage air circulation and retain body heat and moisture. Use all-cotton diapers most of the time, and disposable diapers when traveling and for convenience only occasionally.
- Wash cloth diapers with vinegar or borax; this will neutralize the ammonia that is produced from urine.

Diarrhea

The Counterattack

Diarrhea is often nature's way of expelling something harmful from your body—fast.

Common causes include eating something that disagreed with you, food poisoning, water contamination, viral infection, inflammation (as in colitis and diverticulitis), and nervous conditions such as fear and anxiety.

While diarrhea can be good because it gets rid of the unwanted, it is not normal. It can range from mild to severe and can be accompanied by abdominal cramping and bloating. Extreme or prolonged diarrhea can result in dehydration, bleeding, malnutrition, and overall weakness.

Diarrhea caused by a viral infection or food poisoning should be allowed to run its course, usually about twelve hours. Sometimes this is all that is needed to get rid of the offending organism. It is just your body's natural response to try to expel as much of the harmful organisms or poison as possible. However, if you want to slow the flow, try these remedies.

Aromatherapy

Essential oils that have been used traditionally to slow diarrhea are chamomile, cypress, eucalyptus, geranium, ginger, juniper, lavender, myrrh, nutmeg, peppermint, rosemary, and sandalwood. Oils that aid in calming the spasms and irritability of the bowels include geranium, juniper, lemon, and rosemary. For chronic diarrhea, try neroli and sandalwood essential oils; they are especially useful for long-standing conditions of nervous origin.

DIET

Easy does it. Diarrhea overworks and overstimulates the bowels, so it's a good idea to eat bland foods and drink plenty of liquids during and after a siege. Avoid sweets, high roughage foods such as fruits and vegetables, stimulants such as caffeinated drinks, and highly spiced foods.

Squeeze a lemon. The juice of a fresh lemon is antiseptic and antibacterial. Add the juice of a lemon to an 8-ounce glass of purified water as often as possible.

Milk plus one is better. Warm milk spiked with a pinch of freshly ground nutmeg can help calm diarrhea and a nervous, hyperactive digestive tract.

Call for lassi. A traditional Indian drink called lassi primarily consists of yogurt and water. It is made sweet with honey or sugar, or sour with salt.

Salt helps the body hold on to fluids; therefore, this salty version is beneficial if you have diarrhea. Use natural yogurt or kefir that contains live cultures of acidophilus and lactobacillus (probiotics) to help restore the "good" flora being lost through the bowels with diarrhea.

Actually, our family makes many versions of this drink to enjoy as a refreshing beverage during the summer months. I flavor it with rosewater, ginger, honey or stevia, and fresh mint leaves and whip it in the blender with crushed ice.

✆ Healing Frappé ✆

Good enough to drink any time.

½ cup natural plain yogurt or kefir
(organic, with active cultures)
½ cup cold water or ice

1 teaspoon finely grated fresh ginger root
¼ teaspoon Celtic Sea salt
Pinch of nutmeg
Pinch of cinnamon

Combine all the ingredients in a blender and blend on high. Drink as needed.

MASSAGE

Get a belly rub. Massaging the lower abdomen and lower back area with the palm of your (or someone else's) hand can help relax the colon. Using the essential oils is essential.

Belly Rub Remedy

8 drops lavender essential oil
2 drops ginger essential oil
1 drop chamomile essential oil
1 drop peppermint essential oil
2 tablespoons vegetable oil

Measure essential oils into an amber glass bottle. Add the vegetable oil and shake gently to mix. Label contents with directions for use. To use, apply in a slow, rhythmic, counter-clockwise motion over the lower abdomen and lower back. Inhale the essences from your hands with several slow, deep breaths following the massage. Lie still and relax for 15 to 20 minutes. Apply twice per day.

Note: Be careful not to massage too deeply or too fast, as this can further stimulate the bowels.

When to Call the Doctor

If diarrhea persists for more than 24 hours, there is danger of dehydration, especially if it is accompanied by vomiting. This can happen quickly, especially in small children and the elderly. See a doctor immediately.

Dry Nose

⁊

SNIFFING FOR RELIEF

A dry nose is more than an uncomfortable nuisance. It can set the stage for other problems, such as nasal sores, nosebleeds, and infection. Dry nose is most common in winter climates where houses are closed up tight, the central heat is cranking, and the outside air is dry and cold for months on end. It's a sign that you are dry, too. You can also end up with a dry, achy nose during or after an illness, such as a cold or flu.

AROMATHERAPY

Don't get sore. If your nose gets irritated to the point that it starts forming sores and scabs, reach for the heavy artillery: tea tree essential oil. Tea tree oil has antibacterial and antifungal qualities and is a good choice for preventing infection. Try this recipe, which also contains calendula infusion oil, known to be healing as well as moisturizing. If you can't find calendula infusion oil, you can use all sesame oil (2 tablespoons).

⁊ Healing Nasal Oil ⁊

1 tablespoon natural sesame oil
1 tablespoon calendula infusion oil
1 capsule vitamin E (400 IU)
1 to 2 drops tea tree essential oil

Mix the sesame oil and calendula oil in a small dish or wide-mouth amber glass bottle. Cut off the end of the vitamin E capsule and squeeze the gel into the oil. Add the tea tree essential oil and mix thoroughly. Label contents with directions for use. Warm the bottle by placing it in hot water prior to use.

To use dip your small finger into the aromatic oil. Close one nostril with your index finger and sniff the oil from your finger through the other nostril. Repeat on the other side. Use several times a day as needed.

Diet

Drink up. A dry nose is a sign of dehydration, so increase your fluid intake. Pure water, herbal teas, and diluted fruit and vegetable juices are best. Get the equivalent of eight 8-ounce glasses of fluid a day.

Avoid caffeine. Coffee, black tea, cola drinks, and other beverages containing caffeine are natural dehydrators and will only contribute to the problem. Same goes for alcohol. If you must imbibe such liquids, figure on drinking two to three extra glasses of water for every glass of the above you consume.

Inhalation

Open sesame. According to the holistic practice of Ayurvedic medicine, sesame oil helps balance the nervous system and moisturize the skin. Sniffing sesame oil is especially useful if you are a *Vata* body type (*dosha*). Vata characteristics and bio-energies are dry, cold, mobile, light, penetrating, clear, and rough. This ancient healing art also believes that a total body massage with sesame oil is very grounding, healthful, and balancing. Here's a healing recipe I find helpful for all sore, dry noses, no matter what your *dosha*.

Moisturizing Nasal Oil

1 tablespoon natural sesame oil, warmed or at room temperature

Put the sesame oil in a shallow dish or saucer. If warming the oil, put it in a ramekin and place it in a hot-water bath. In the morning upon waking, and several times a day as needed, dip your little finger in the oil and insert it into one nostril. Close the other nostril and sniff or inhale. Repeat on the other side. The further you can insert your little finger into your nose, the better. You'll want to do this in the privacy of your bathroom or a restroom for obvious reasons!

Spike your steam. Steam inhalations can do wonders for making a dry nose flow. Use only warm or mildly hot water, not exceeding 160 to 170 degrees. You should be able to touch the water without burning. If the water is too hot, it can actually cause more drying or aggravate the delicate lining of the nasal passages.

Add 1 to 2 drops of tea tree oil (to help promote healing) to the steam inhalation treatment described on page 180.

LIFESTYLE

A warm, buttoned-up house or office can be nice and cozy, but it can also turn a dry nose into a chronic problem. Here's how to make your environment more nasal friendly.

Crack a window. Make that several windows. This allows for air exchange.

Go for the layered look. Heating systems are huge contributors to dry, stale indoor air. Keep the indoor temperature set to at least 68 degrees, or as low as you can stand it. If you layer your clothing, you'll never know the difference.

Dry, Hot, and Bothered

Cold weather dwellers aren't the only ones who stick their noses into sore, dry danger. Those who live and breathe the hot dry air of America's desert southwest are just as prone. Unlike hot climates with a lot of humidity, dry air can be deceptively dangerous.

Drink water and other nondehydrating liquids continuously throughout the day, plus follow the other tips in this lifestyle section. Replacing lost minerals and electrolytes is also important; as we sweat we evaporate not only water but also crucial minerals such as sodium and potassium. A pinch of Celtic Sea salt helps prevent dehydration and mineral depletion.

Get your house potted. On really cold, dry days, simmer pans of hot water on the stove, radiator, or wood-burning stove. It will add moisture to the air. Better yet, make long simmering soups and stews, which have the added benefit of a wonderful aroma.

Use a humidifier. Cold water humidifiers are best. To keep it constant, put it on a timer to go on and off automatically throughout the day. Make sure to clean it regularly (read the directions carefully), or you could create a host of other problems such as mildew. Optional: You can add eucalyptus essential oil to the reservoir per manufacturer's directions on certain models.

Create a green feeling. Houseplants are natural air filters and will help absorb the stale air that can congest pure air flow. So scatter plants around the house, preferably the green plants such as Areca palm, Boston fern, golden pathos, peace lily, and spider plants.

Say misty for me. Room mists help add moisture and purify the air. But don't use store-bought ones. They often contain chemicals that can aggravate the problem. Instead, make your own simply by adding 10 to 20 drops of your favorite essential oil to 6 ounces of water in a mister.

Take a long walk. The best way to escape stale indoor air is to get outdoors a few times a day. Breathe in deeply every several paces, and you'll literally feel the fresh air give your health a lift.

Dry Skin
∿

NOURISH AND REPLENISH

Need a good example of environmental stress? Well, take a look at your skin.

Chances are it's in some stage of dryness. Maybe it's just a little scaly and flaky when you rub your arms or elbows. Or it could be chapped, cracked, or even fissured.

Real-Life Cure

A FRESH-AIR CONVERT

Tina was a very physically active forty-year-old when she developed a chronic sore nose after she took a full-time job in a sealed-window office building. Deeply distressed, she ended up in my office after she developed painful sores in her nose.

I prescribed the Healing Nasal Oil, which gave her immediate relief. (You can find the recipe on page 232.)She later added tea tree essential oil, which helped heal the sores. She's now a fresh-air convert: She uses homemade room mists at home and the office and always keeps her windows at home open a crack, no matter what the temperature. Plus, she says, "I never go a day without drinking my eight glasses of water. My problem is gone and I feel great!"

Dry skin is particularly a problem in winter climes where the air is dry (and the central heat is on indoors) or if you work in a dehydrated environment, such as an air-conditioned office building, hospital, or airplane.

Dry skin can also be inherited. If you have fair skin and blond or red hair you are more likely to experience dry-skin conditions than those with dark characteristics.

AROMATHERAPY

Start early. Adapting an aromatherapy program early when symptoms of dryness are first recognized makes this condition relatively easy to remedy. Chronic and severe cases of dryness, which include eczema or dermatitis, however, may take a bit longer because the skin has to heal before it can be replenished.

Skin-loving oils. Essential oils provide moisture, healing, and nourishment to the dermal layers of the skin because the skin has the ability to absorb these small molecules through the superficial blood vessels and hair follicles. Essential oils known to help dry skin conditions are carrot seed, cedarwood, chamomile, frankincense, geranium, jasmine, lavender, myrrh, neroli, patchouli, rose, sandalwood, and ylang-ylang. These oils can be blended into personal skin-care products such as lotions, oils, and creams.

Throw Out the Towel

Here's a technique for keeping moisture in after a bath or shower: Instead of drying your skin with a towel, use your hands to rub off excess water from your body. Start at the shoulders and move to the arms and chest, working downward to the legs.

You won't be completely dry, but that is the point. Apply your favorite aromatherapy body oil over your entire body while it is still moist. Let yourself dry the rest of the way naturally. The oil blend will seal the moisture in as needed.

Mask the problem. A facial mask is a special treatment for replenishing the skin with moisture and for soothing minor skin irritations. Its aim is to nourish and calm the skin's surface.

Good for dry skin types and combination skin, there are endless possibilities as to what can be added to this type of facial mask—floral and herbal waters, seaweed extracts, oils, yogurt, honey, mashed avocado, or papaya are among the most popular.

This recipe is easy to prepare, very moisturizing, and has a good consistency. I suggest that you select your own essential oils for dry skin from the list given above. You'll need a total of 5 drops. This mask can be done several times per week.

❧ Moisture–Balancing Facial Mask ❧

1 teaspoon natural plain yogurt (with active cultures)

2 teaspoons raw honey

1 vitamin E capsule (400 IUs)

1 teaspoon oat flour or finely ground oatmeal

5 drops essential oil (total)

Combine the yogurt and honey. Cut off the end of the vitamin E capsule and squeeze the contents into this mixture and stir well. Add the oat flour and blend into a smooth paste. Adjust the flour as necessary. When it looks right, add the essential oils and mix. Apply to the face and neck areas with your fingertips, using small circular motions. Avoid the eye area. Lie down and relax. After 15 to 20 minutes, remove with warm water. Apply three to four times a week.

Opulent oils. This is a wonderful aromatherapy recipe for those who are prone to dry facial skin. I love its aroma. Make sure to apply a floral water or facial mist before using. You can make this facial oil into body oil by following the General Treatment Blending Chart on page 501.

✍ Opulent Face Oil ✍

1 teaspoon jojoba oil
1 teaspoon calendula infusion oil
¼ teaspoon carrot seed oil
1 teaspoon sesame oil
6 drops sandalwood essential oil
4 drops neroli essential oil
2 drops geranium essential oil
400 IUs vitamin E (optional)

In a 1-ounce amber glass bottle, add the jojoba, calendula, carrot, and sesame oils. Add the essential oils and, if desired, the vitamin E. Shake well to mix completely. Label. To use, gently pour 4 to 6 drops on your fingertips. Apply in upward strokes on moistened skin.

HYDROTHERAPY

Milk baths. Moisturizing warm baths are another way to slough off dead skin cells gently and effectively. This milk-based recipe is especially good for dry skin that comes from cold winter temperatures.

∿ Milkmaid's Bath ∿

6 drops carrot seed essential oil
1 drop chamomile essential oil
5 drops lavender essential oil
½ cup heavy cream, buttermilk, or goat's milk
   (or you can substitute ¼ cup powdered milk to make a paste)

Mix the essential oils with the cream or milk in a small bowl. After the bath is filled, add the milk to the bath and stir with your hands. Soak for 30 minutes. Follow with a moisturizing body oil. This bath can be enjoyed several times a week as desired.

Don't forget to spray. A floral water (hydrosol) spray is important to use before applying a facial oil to the skin because the oil helps keep the moisture close to the pores. Most floral waters are excellent for dry skin; however chamomile, lavender, neroli (orange blossom), and rose floral waters are among the best.

Lifestyle

Avoid excess drainage. Some of the things we do to help nourish our skin have an opposite effect on dry skin. Here are some don'ts for dry skin conditions:

- Do not use clay facial masks, as they remove some of the protective facial "film" from your skin.
- Avoid using products containing alcohol or other harsh chemicals. Petroleum by-products such as Vaseline, mineral oil, and baby oil should be avoided, since they create a barrier that does not allow moisture or essential oils to get through.
- Avoid extreme heat, such as hot baths, saunas, and Jacuzzis. Also, chlorinated swimming pools seem to worsen dry skin, whereas swimming in the ocean will help.

MASSAGE

Stimulate the skin. The major factor in many dry-skin conditions is that the sebaceous glands are producing insufficient amounts of sebum, the skin's natural moisturizer. To stimulate sebum production and circulation, follow the dry skin brushing technique described on page 40. This technique improves circulation to the skin, cleans pores, and triggers the sebaceous glands to manufacture more sebum. However, you will want to proceed gently and use light pressure so you don't cause undue irritation.

Feel your oats. Finely ground oatmeal–type scrubs are great for gently exfoliating the skin. Oats provide moisture in addition to safely sloughing off dead skin cells. The recipe for Farm-Fresh Facial Scrub on page 58 is perfect to use for dry skin. This scrub can be done up to three times per week, depending on how your skin feels.

SALVES

Extra help for dry skin. This Heavy-Duty Ointment can be made with various oils or fats and beeswax to form a coating over weakened or soft areas of skin that need extra protection to heal. You can make the ointment soft or firm, depending on the ratio of oils to beeswax that you use. This preparation is one of the highest concentrations of essential oils used, about an 8 percent dilution. However, as a general rule, ointments are designed to be used sparingly and in acute situations. This ointment or balm can be made when extra help is needed for dry skin areas such as on elbows, cuticles, and heels. It is a widely used base for many preparations, including wound-care and replenishing salves for menopausal dryness.

✧ Heavy-Duty Ointment ✧

¼ cup extra virgin olive oil or calendula infusion oil (see recipe for infusion oils on page 206)

1 tablespoon natural beeswax (if you desire a softer ointment, use less beeswax)

800 IUs vitamin E (capsules)

80 to 100 drops essential oil (total)

Combine the first three ingredients in the top of a double boiler and melt together. Once melted, remove from heat and allow to cool. If adding essential oils, wait until the oils have cooled somewhat so they don't evaporate away quickly. Stir them in completely and pour into a sterile or very clean, colored glass jar. Cap tightly and label contents. You can hasten the cooling by putting the jar in the refrigerator. Use a tongue depressor or small spatula to take out what you need with each use, so as not to contaminate the contents.

Dull Hair

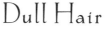

MAGICAL MANE INGREDIENTS

Dull, lifeless, brittle, dry. If this describes your hair, you have a chronic case of bad hair blues.

Dull, lifeless hair is usually of our own creation. Chemical hair treatments, extreme sun exposure, chlorinated swimming pools, hot tubs, a bad diet, overshampooing, or even using the wrong shampoo or conditioner can change the texture of hair. Some medications are also to blame.

There is no reason, however, to hide your hair under a hat. There are plenty of ways to avoid waking up to a bad-hair day.

AROMATHERAPY

Custom-make your own shampoo. Specific essential oils can bring back luster to your hair simply by adding them to natural or neutral shampoos and conditioners. Certain oils, however, respond best to certain types of hair. To make your own, simply add 80 drops of essential oil to 8 ounces of shampoo or conditioner using these guidelines:

Dry hair: Use cedarwood, lavender, or sandalwood.
Oily hair: Use lemongrass, rosemary, or ylang-ylang.
Normal hair: Use clary sage, geranium, or lavender.

HERBS

Hide behind herbs. Herbs diluted and made into vinegars can add highlights and shine to the hair. They can even cover gray hair. My friend Ellen has used strong infusions of rosemary to cover her gray for the last several years. It works so nicely, I never knew she had any gray hair until she told me! There's an herb for every color, though the formulas for brunette and dark hair work best.

Dark hair: Use rosemary and sage herbs.
Light hair: Use chamomile herb and fresh lemon juice.
Red and auburn hair: Use calendula and madder root.
Gray hair: Use rosemary and sage herbs.

Any of the herbs listed above can be made into herbal vinegars and diluted to make excellent hair rinses. For instructions on brewing your own herbal vinegars, see page 209.

Add a booster herb. In general, herbs that stimulate circulation are an added benefit and include butcher's broom, cayenne, chamomile, ginger root, Ginkgo biloba, rosemary, and turmeric. To make hair thicker and healthier overall, incorporate the silica rich herbs such as burdock root, dulse, echinacea root, goldenseal, horsetail herb, and oatstraw. These may be taken in the form of teas, tincture, or capsules in addition to preparing hair treatment rinses.

Lavender-Scented Locks

Add shine and luster to your locks by adding a few drops of lavender or rosemary essential oil to your hairbrush before brushing. It will also give your hair a wonderful scent. You may find yourself brushing your hair every evening (like in the old movies) as this is an aromatic way to end a long day and naturally perfumes your hair for bedtime. The lavender essential oil will even help you sleep!

LIFESTYLE

Be a boarhead. I doubt anyone actually follows the old wive's tale that claims brushing your hair one hundred strokes a night will keep it healthy forever. Brushing, no matter how many strokes, is good for the hair—if you use the correct hairbrush!

Most hairbrushes are made of synthetics, such as plastic and nylon, and can damage the hair by stretching and stripping it. These materials can be too stiff against the scalp as well. Natural boar and vegetable-based bristles are still the best, as they give your hair a healthy glow and do not pull or stretch the hair shaft. Natural bristles can help clean your hair by removing excess oil and dirt. Boar bristles can also be safer to use for scalp exfoliation and stimulation.

Buy the right brush. In addition to finding a good natural bristle brush, the correct hairbrush designed for your hair type is necessary to get shiny and lustrous hair. The following styles of hairbrushes can be found in specialty stores or beauty supply stores:

Long hair and blow-dry style: Use a half-round brush.
Strong, thick, short hair: Use a club brush.
Delicate and thinning hair: Use a soft club brush.
Long straight hair: Use an oval brush.
Short, fine hair: Use a professional hairbrush.

Earache

HERE'S SOUND ADVICE

Now hear this. The ear is a potential site for a lot of trouble. We put things in it we shouldn't—like bobby pins and Q-tips. We subject it to high altitudes in airplanes and sky-high elevators. We take it naked into the cold, drench it in chlorinated water, and blast it with boom boxes, thigh-high speakers, and personal cell phones.

It's no wonder that there are so many ear problems going around! The problem that's familiar to us all is the common garden-variety earache or ear infection, the kind we get from a cold or flu and the kind that makes babies and toddlers wail through the night. This is the type of ear pain I'm covering here.

AROMATHERAPY

Turn to warm, soothing oils. Chamomile and lavender essential oils are gentle enough for use in the ear and possess anti-inflammatory and analgesic properties. Other essential oils that have been successful in alleviating ear pain are basil, cajeput, hyssop, rose, and tea tree. You will want to mix these essences with a vegetable or herbal infusion oil before applying inside the ear.

✺ Aromatic Ear Oil ✺

½ teaspoon mullein infusion oil*
½ teaspoon garlic infusion oil*
1 drop lavender essential oil
1 drop chamomile essential oil

Combine the mullein and garlic oils in an amber glass bottle. Add the essential oils and mix well. Gently warm the bottle of oil in a hot-water bath. Apply 2 to 3 drops of aromatic ear oil into the ear canal with an eyedropper. Plug your ear with a cotton ball to protect clothes or bedding and to keep the ear warm and protected.

*Note: These are specialty herbal oils that can be purchased at most natural health stores. If these oils are not available, substitute extra virgin olive oil or sesame oil.

HERBS

Helpful botanicals. Mullein flowers, with strong antibacterial properties, have been widely used for treating the nerve-type pain associated with earaches. Garlic oil is used for its natural antibiotic effects as well. St. John's wort infusion oil is very effective for all nerve-related pain, including the discomfort of earaches.

Other effective herbs for earaches are catnip, chamomile, echinacea, rosemary, skullcap, and valerian root. Ginger root is helpful if there is nasal congestion present.

SOUND AND MUSIC THERAPY

Say **Nnnnnnn.** The specific sound that can be made, or toned, to vibrationally heal the ears is the sound "N." Take a deep breath and perform the sound on the exhalation. Repeat three times daily for best results. For a small child experiencing ear pain, although not as effective, you can hold or rock the child with his or her head (bad ear) on your chest while you make the vibratory sounds.

Folk Remedies for "Sick Ear"

In traditional folk medicine, a small muslin bag or sock filled with sea salt, flaxseeds, or buckwheat was heated and placed over the affected ear to draw moisture from the ear canal. Similarly, mothers would instinctively rock their babies with their "sick ear" against their bosoms. A hot-water bottle works well, too!

Is It an Allergy?

If your child has chronic ear infections, it's possible it could be caused by a food allergy.

Many children's earaches and infections stem from an allergic reaction to dairy or wheat products. Cow's milk and sugar intolerances are also common in children.

Breast-feeding reduces the risk of ear infections in infants because breast milk is rich in lactoferrin and other immune-stimulating compounds.

Eczema

🜋

SOOTHING SMOOTHING RESULTS

Patchy knees and elbows are often exhibit number one.

If the verdict on your skin problem turns out to be eczema, there's no need to fear a life sentence of red, sore, itchy, thick red patches all over your body. There is plenty you can do to tame the problem.

Most often the inflammation shows up on the hands, wrists, ears, face, and creases of the knees and elbows. Eczema is associated with asthma and is partially an allergic-type reaction of the body. It has been linked to food allergies, genetics, low stomach acid, a dysfunctional immune system, and stress.

AROMATHERAPY

Attack the symptoms. The primary goals of aromatherapy treatment are to decrease the sometimes intense itching that accompanies eczema, to increase local circulation to the affected site, and to promote new, healthy skin tissue. Anti-inflammatory agents are useful, in addition to essential oils that ease dry skin conditions.

Essential oils useful for eczema are bergamot, carrot seed, cedarwood, chamomile, geranium, hyssop, juniper, lavender, myrrh, patchouli, rose, and rosemary. Bergamot and juniper are especially useful if the eczema is the weeping (wet) type, as they provide additional drying properties.

Carrier oils and special additive oils that will increase healing are calendula, evening primrose, jojoba, rosehip seed, and vitamin E.

Go for the concentrated treatment. This massage oil concentrate is extremely effective for dry eczema with redness, itching, and swelling present. In most acute cases, healing occurs within four to five days when the oil is applied three times daily and followed with a compress treatment. The rose oil is a key component of this recipe as it is known to decrease histamine production, which is associated with allergy-related skin ailments. Carrot seed and rosehip seed are extremely beneficial in healing and nourishing inflamed skin.

✍ Healing Skin–Oil Concentrate ✍

1 tablespoon calendula infusion oil
1 tablespoon safflower oil
¼ teaspoon carrot seed oil
¼ teaspoon rosehip seed oil
12 drops lavender essential oil
6 drops bergamot essential oil
3 drops chamomile essential oil
3 drops rose essential oil
1 400-IU vitamin E capsule

In an amber glass bottle, combine the calendula and safflower oils. Add the carrot seed and rosehip oils. Mix well. Add the essential oils. Cut open the vitamin E capsule and squeeze into the mixture. Cap securely and shake. Label.

Apply in small amounts to affected areas. Massage into the skin until absorbed. Apply three times daily.

DIET

Check out your diet. Since flare-ups are associated with certain foods in some people, examine your diet to find out if any food or food group is affecting you. Common suspects include wheat, dairy, and corn. If you suspect a certain food, stay away from it for several weeks and observe how your skin reacts. Reintroduce the food into your diet. If your skin reacts, you have your culprit.

Eat these oils. A daily dose of flaxseed oil and raw nuts and seeds have been found to help improve dry skin conditions such as eczema.

Get plenty of fluids. Drink plenty of pure water and herbal tea to keep your skin well hydrated and your entire system detoxified.

Herbs

Healing formulas. Effective herbs for skin nourishment and healing are those with a high alkaline and mineral content. They include aloe vera, burdock root, calendula, chamomile, dandelion root, marshmallow root, and yellow dock root. Herbs that stimulate circulation are also helpful. They include hawthorn leaf, lobelia, rosemary, St. John's wort, and turmeric. These can be taken in combination or individually in capsule, tea, or tincture form according to the manufacturer's recommendations for internal use.

Alternatively, strong herbal infusions can be prepared and poured into the bath to provide healing benefits.

Hydrotherapy

Cool down the heat. Cool compresses can help ease intense itching, swelling, and inflammation. It's best to apply them after treating your skin with a healing oil.

This recipe contains chamomile and lemon essential oils, which are well known for their antipruriginous (itch-relieving) properties.

⦾ Anti-Itch Compress ⦾

8 ounces cool water
2 drops geranium essential oil
2 drops lemon essential oil
1 drop chamomile essential oil

In a glass or ceramic bowl, pour the cool water. Add the essential oils and stir with a spoon or your hands to disperse well. Soak a small towel or flannel cloth large enough to cover the affected area. Wring out the cloth and apply it to the skin.

Cover with an additional towel or lay an ice pack over this. When the compress becomes warm or dry, replace with a fresh compress. Do this treatment for 20 minutes up to three times daily.

Bathe in baking soda. Adding a cup of baking soda to your daily bath is another way to calm the itching. For an aromatic bath with baking soda and bath salts, see page 127. Always use a mild soap to prevent irritating the skin even more.

See also Dry Skin.

Eye Strain

VISION SAVERS

Seeing is believing.

If you suffer from eye strain due to exposure to such things as computer screens, big screen TVs, poor lighting, sun glare, night driving, or bad eyewear, here's what you can do to get rid of itchy, watery, tired eyes.

While you're following these recommendations to ease the ache, do a little searching to get to the root of the cause. Correcting the problem is the only way to prevent future problems.

HERBS

Eyebright is eye right. The herbs eyebright and bilberry have been used for ages for general eye weakness and eye strain. Herbs containing beta-carotene are especially useful for eye problems and include barley grass, bee pollen, bilberry, eyebright, parsley leaf, peppermint, and spirulina. Herbal eyewashes can also be made from the herbs. Chamomile, green tea, and rosemary, along with the eyebright, are favorites for this method.

Rest with an Eye Pillow

Ever hear of an eye pillow? It's a rectangular-shaped puff filled with lentils, rice, oats, or other grains that lays snugly across your eyes and offers relief from eye strain, tension, and mental fatigue.

Eye pillows have a nice, gentle pressure or weight to them and often smell nice. I keep my own homemade one on my nightstand and would not be without it. The pillow should fit sideways across your face, covering your eyes and a little beyond to each side. An average size is about 3½ by 8½ inches. I use a soft fabric like satin or silk to make mine and fill with flaxseeds and lavender flowers. Here's my recipe.

✍ Eye Pillow ✍

1 cup flaxseeds
1 cup dried lavender flowers
3 to 5 drops lavender essential oil

Mix the flaxseeds and lavender flowers together in a bowl. Sprinkle the lavender essential oil in the mixture and blend well with a spoon or spatula. Put into an eye pillow and sew the opening. Lie down and rest the pillow on your closed eyes.

HYDROTHERAPY

Compress those tired eyes. A cool compress over the eyes will be of great help in relieving eye strain after a long day. Use the eye compress recipe on page 189. Lie quietly for 10 minutes or longer with the eye compresses over your eyes.

Bag 'em. Take two chamomile tea bags soaked in hot water and cool in the refrigerator. Lie quietly and put the bags on your closed eyelids for 10 minutes.

Soak away the cause. Because eye strain usually has an emotional or physical stress component, you will also benefit from antistress blends for your bath. I recommend the TGIF aromatic bath recipe for sensory overload found on page 148.

Be prepared. Commercial eye packs made of gel-filled plastic can be purchased and stored in the refrigerator.

Practice Smart Eye Nutrition

Good nutrition has been linked to the prevention of a number of eye conditions.

Flavonoids: May lower your risk of age-related macular degeneration. Incorporating the spice turmeric into your cooking and drinking green tea are among the flavonoid-rich herbs to include.

Omega-3 fatty acids: May prevent eye problems related to inflammation and high blood fats. Fish such as mackerel, Pacific salmon, and albacore tuna as well as flaxseeds are rich sources.

Zinc: Research shows that visual loss is reduced with zinc supplementation. Organic eggs, whole grains, nuts, and yogurt are good food sources.

LIFESTYLE

Be kind, unwind. Being kind to your eyes is the long-term answer to this common ailment. This means you have to give them time to relax.

- Wear sunglasses and a hat on bright days to protect your eyes.
- Install full-spectrum lighting in your work space. The ideal lighting arrangement for reading or detailed work is bright lighting at shoulder level, placed behind you and off to one side.
- Use an antiglare computer screen frame to cut down on glare and light reflection.

- And let's not forget to take breaks! Get up and walk around periodically. Allow your eyes to rest and adjust.
- Under less optimal conditions, look up every so often to focus on a corner of a room or distant object to rest your eyes.

Yoga and Movement

Use a simple ancient secret. Palming is an old yoga practice that relieves eye strain and promotes relaxation of this area. Simply rub your palms together vigorously until they feel warm. Cup your hands over your eyes gently without causing any pressure. The heat and darkness created by doing this soothes and relaxes the eyes.

Fever

⟋

Fanning the Fire

The temperature is rising. And what you feel isn't good.

A rise in normal body temperature—above 98.6 degrees—means you have a fever. Besides the reading on your thermometer, clues of a fever include the shivers, hot sweats, and, depending upon the extent of the temperature rise, delirium.

A fever in and of itself is actually a good thing. It is the body's natural response to stave off germs that are trying to infect the body. Interfering with the body's attempt to protect itself is necessary, however, when the fever gets too high or causes discomfort. I would give the fever a chance to do what it is meant to do for at least three to four hours before initiating the first-aid recommendations.

Aromatherapy

Febrifuge fragrances. Essential oils capable of lowering fevers typically are those that can produce a sweat. They include basil, bergamot, chamomile, eucalyptus, ginger, hyssop, juniper, lavender, lemon, lemongrass, peppermint, rosemary, and tea tree. These are most often used in compresses or baths.

DIET

Drink up. No one with a fever feels like eating, but it is essential that liquids keep flowing. This means drinking as much pure water as possible. Fruit juices containing vitamin C, such as orange and carrot, are also great choices.

Soup is souper. A light broth-type soup is a way to get extra nutrition in the body. Try my Old-Fashioned Onion and Garlic Soup on page 137. It's a favorite at my house.

Keeping the Household Well

To help keep others from being sick, I recommend misting the air with antibacterial and antiseptic essential oils. This can be done by dispensing the oils with a diffuser in your main living area every few hours or using a room mist spray. Scents I like the best for this purpose are eucalyptus, lavender, lemon, and pine.

HYDROTHERAPY

De-escalate a fever fast. A cold compress is the simplest thing to do to bring down a fever. The compress should be placed over the forehead area, because the head is a major source of heat loss in the body.

Common Causes of Fevers

- Infection (viruses, bacteria, fungi, protozoa)
- Muscle activity (vigorous physical activity)
- Tissue death (injury, heart attack, pulmonary embolism)
- Dehydration (heat, sweating, decreased fluid intake)
- Foreign protein in blood (venomous bites, internal absorption)
- Increased thyroid activity
- Cancer (lymphomas)

To speed the healing process, I recommend a compress made with essential oils. This is especially designed for kids.

✺ Cool Compress for Kids ✺

1 cup ice-cold water
3 drops lavender essential oil
1 drop eucalyptus
  (*E. radiata* or *E. smithii*) essential oil

In a bowl, pour the ice cold water. Add the essential oils and swish to disperse in the water. Soak a washcloth and then wring it out to release most of the moisture so it is not dripping wet. Apply to the forehead. After it dries or warms to body temperature, reapply a fresh compress. Check the body temperature every 30 minutes.

Caution: Do not use this on children younger than three years old without advice from your health-care practitioner.

Take a whole-body sponge. Folk medicine and grandmothers have been recommending this technique for centuries: sponge down the body with tepid or cool water. Colder temperatures are too extreme for whole-body treatment. The feverish person should be lying on a bath towel. It is not necessary to remove all clothing; just the upper chest, back, and legs need to be exposed.

Try my sponging remedy using essential oils.

✺ Aromatic Sponge ✺

1 quart tepid water
2 drops chamomile essential oil

Fill a bowl with the water. Add the chamomile oil and swish the water to disperse as much as possible. Soak the sponge (or cloth) in the water. Gently squeeze out the sponge, leaving it wet enough to cool the body. Have the person lie face up on a towel. Starting from the neck and working your way down, sponge the body. Re-soak the sponge as needed. Have the person turn over and do the same on the back. Do not allow the person to chill, as this will cause the body to heat.

Take a cool bath. Hydrotherapy principles state that cool water temperatures, between 70 and 80 degrees, are optimal for fever conditions. If the water is too cold, the body's response is to shiver, which creates heat and counteracts the goal of the treatment bath. Be sure to confirm the water temperature by using a thermometer.

Soak in the bath for a few minutes at a time. Pat dry, rest, and retake temperature. Repeat if necessary.

Tip: Aspirin Warning

Do not give aspirin for fever conditions in young children and teenagers, as this has been linked to Reye's syndrome, which can lead to liver and brain damage. Also, pregnant women should not use aspirin in their last trimester.

When to Call the Doctor

Fevers can be dangerous in children and the elderly. Call your physician immediately if:

- A baby (under 3 months old) has a fever of 102 degrees or higher
- A child or elderly person has a fever above 103 degrees
- A child is inconsolable and irritable
- A child or elderly person is very lethargic
- Someone is confused, delirious, or unconscious
- Someone complains of severe pain, intense headache, or stiff neck
- Someone has difficulty breathing

Flatulence

✺

GAS GUZZLERS

Is gas cramping your style? We all experience gas—every day, in fact—but it only becomes a problem when it starts interfering with your life.

Flatulence occurs when small air or gas pockets get trapped in the stomach and small intestines. The fastest way to escape is the shortest exit possible—the colon. All perfectly natural. However, sometimes gas can cause severe pain.

To avoid or contain the problem, here's what to do.

AROMATHERAPY

Smell, don't swallow. Essential oils that come to the aid of gas are those that help relax muscles (antispasmodics and those that aid digestion). The most recognized for these qualities are anise, basil, bergamot, chamomile, coriander, fennel, ginger, hyssop, juniper, lavender, marjoram, melissa, myrrh, peppermint, and rosemary.

These oils can be used in diluted form as massage oils for the abdominal area, as inhalants on a tissue, from an aroma lamp, or simply from the bottle or hands. They should not be taken by mouth unless prescribed by a physician, because they are extremely concentrated.

The peppermint treat. An exception to the rule is peppermint. Peppermint is one of the few essential oils I recommend taking by mouth for digestive problems and only so by a single drop on a sugar cube or teaspoon of honey, which acts as the medicinal carrier. Peppermint is considered a GRAS (Generally Regarded As Safe) oil and is listed in the United States pharmacopoeia as such. It is incorporated extensively in food and flavoring in the pure form as well as its synthetic components.

Peppermint helps to equalize the pressure in the stomach caused by gas and has an antifoaming action to help prevent further gas formation. It continues to be highly regarded as a primary remedy for relief of gas today, as it has been for many ages prior.

❧ Antigas Lozenge ❧

1 sugar cube (or 1 teaspoon of honey)
1 drop peppermint essential oil

Put a single drop of essential oil of peppermint on the sugar cube. Slowly suck on it to release the essence into the stomach.

DIET

Some less extreme symptoms related to abdominal cramping and gas are bloating, burping, and flatulence. Gas formation in the stomach can be caused by eating or drinking too fast and literally swallowing air. However, more frequently the cause is a sluggish digestive system, which causes undigested food to sit in the stomach where fermentation takes place.

Get your combos right. Proper food combining can be especially important to some people since certain foods (protein) take hours to digest while others (fruit) take only 20 to 30 minutes. So if these two types of food are eaten at the same meal, the fruit will stay in the stomach longer than it should, while the proteins are being digested. There are a number of books written on this topic of food combining, also known as "natural hygiene." Much of the work in this area is based on studies of the digestive system and its inherent natural rhythms and cycles done by nutritionists and physicians William Hay and Herbert Shelton.

Beans you can be around. Avoid refined foods with chemical additives, as these are clearly the major source of digestive problems. Proper cooking of beans and legumes— that is, slowly—will decrease gas formation. Adding cumin or a piece of kombu (sea vegetable) to the beans will also help.

Too much is too much. Too much red meat and too little soluble fiber can also cause more digestive problems, so be aware of this and increase your consumption of slightly steamed or fresh vegetables with your meals.

Check your meds. The interaction of specific medications or drugs taken on an empty stomach can produce digestive upset and possibly cramping. Check your medicines. If you don't have to take them on an empty stomach, then don't.

Herbs

Gripe about it. Among traditional European remedies for intestinal problems such as gas is a syrupy liquid called "gripe water. " It contains anise, caraway, dill, and fennel as the active ingredients. A mere tablespoon can put an end to gas pains. Gripe water can be found in natural health stores. Tea for Tiny Tummies contains these ingredients in tea form (see page 259). Other herbs traditionally used for gas problems include catnip, chamomile, hyssop, marjoram, sage, savory, tarragon, and thyme. Spices known to help in this area are cinnamon, clove, coriander, ginger, and nutmeg.

Lifestyle

Take a look at your life. Look into your daily life routines and find ways to relax and incorporate pleasurable ways to dampen the damaging effects of stress on your health, emotions, and spirit. I have personally experienced and observed the paramount results of using essential oils for relief of all stress-related problems.

Also, you should:

- Eat in a relaxed, slow manner. Avoid situations where you may eat too fast and under stress.
- Avoid wearing tight clothing, especially around the waist and abdominal area; this can impede both digestion and elimination.

Massage

Uncramp with style. This pleasant massage blend helps to alleviate cramping in the abdominal area caused by gas and spasms. Warming the oil prior to its application encourages absorption and the muscles to relax. Use a light and gentle, clockwise, circular massage stroke with the palm of the hands to further stimulate the gas to disperse down the gastrointestinal tract.

✍ Antispasm Massage Blend ✍

1 drop chamomile essential oil
1 drop coriander, fennel essential oil, ginger, or lavender
1 teaspoon vegetable oil

Mix a total of 2 drops (1 drop chamomile plus 1 drop of other chosen oil) with the vegetable oil. Massage gently over your abdominal area (and solar plexus) with

Tea for Tiny Tummies

If you have children (ages 3 and up) prone to tummy aches caused by gas problems, you may want to make some of this ahead and keep it in the cupboard. That's what I did for my son Kris when he was a toddler. It is also great for overindulgent adults.

This sweetly aromatic herbal tea can be taken at the onset of gas cramping or 15 minutes before meals to prevent cramping and relax the stomach.

✍ Tea for Tiny Tummies ✍

⅓ teaspoon cardamom spice
⅓ teaspoon ground fennel seed
⅓ teaspoon ground caraway seed
⅛-inch slice fresh ginger root
1 cup water

Place the herbs in a mug and mix well. Heat water to boiling and pour over the herb and spice mixture. Let it steep for 10 minutes. Strain and sip while still warm.

the palm of your hand in a clockwise direction. Afterward, inhale essential oils from your hands with slow, deep, full breaths.

Put a hot-water bottle or heating pad over the abdomen for additional relief and to help relax muscle spasms. Sometimes lying at a 30-degree angle with your head slightly elevated will help as well.

Yoga and Movement

Break the wind. The double wind-relieving movement in yoga, or the roll back exercise, helps release any gases from the intestines and gently massages the abdominal organs. It is a simple rocking practice and is described fully on page 109.

Real-Life Cure

A PAINFUL SCHOOLDAY

My children are so rarely ill that it sounds strange when I share this story, but it demonstrates the severity of gas pain in some individuals and its link to the emotions.

Kris, one of my twin sons, went to the nurse's office at school with extreme abdominal pain when he was eight years old. His temperature was normal, and he had not eaten anything likely to cause cramping. I was called to come and pick him up as soon as possible, since he was so uncomfortable. When I got to school, Kris was doubled over in pain and could not walk upright. It looked serious. When we returned home he lay on the couch with a hot-water bottle while I confirmed his temperature.

I gently massaged him with the oil blend (given on page 259), while he sucked on a sugar cube that I had spiked with a drop of peppermint essential oil. Within 15 minutes Kris felt considerably better. After drinking sips of Tea for Tiny Tummies (see page 259) he felt 90 percent better. In less than half an hour, he had bounced back and appeared perfectly normal!

At the time, I was very much aware of how the nervous system interacts closely with the digestive system, especially in children. We got to spend a quiet afternoon together, but I've always wondered what role Kris's emotions played in his problem that day.

Fluid Retention

SWELL SOLUTIONS

See the difference. *Feel* the difference.

Swollen hands, feet, and ankles are hard to ignore. They make walking uncomfortable and getting into shoes impossible. Rings don't slip on, and, worse, you can't get them off.

Swollen limbs are a sign of fluid retention. This can be the result of overindulgence in anything that works the body hard, like gardening or, foolishly, like walking a mile in three-inch heels. But it's also a common side effect of conditions associated with circulation such as arthritis, varicose veins, constipation, high blood pressure, and general fluid retention (edema, when the body holds on to fluid). Also, in the last trimester of pregnancy there may be extremity swelling, typically of the hands and feet, due to the additional weight bearing on the pelvic veins.

AROMATHERAPY

The great escape route. Essential oils help eliminate excess fluid by way of the kidneys or the skin. The lungs and digestive system are also ways the body uses up water and bodily fluids, but they are secondary escape routes.

The essential oils that work on the kidneys are natural diuretics; they encourage an increase in urine production, which must flow through the bladder and kidneys. Diaphoretic essential oils are those that aid the production of sweat and therefore help the body to secrete bodily fluids via the skin, specifically the sweat glands.

The essential oils considered useful in both of these exit pathways are cedarwood, chamomile, cypress, eucalyptus, fennel, frankincense, geranium, grapefruit, hyssop, juniper, lavender, lemon, lemongrass, mandarin, orange, patchouli, rosemary, and ylang-ylang. You can use these oils alone or in combination in many therapies including compresses, massage, footbaths, and full spa soaks.

D I E T

Ban the water savers. Changes in your food fare include avoiding high sodium-containing foods, especially canned and processed foods.

- Substitute real Celtic Sea salt for table salt, as it provides natural minerals, is hand harvested, and is rich in trace elements and electrolytes.
- Eat a healthy, high-fiber diet to avoid constipation and varicose veins.

Much More Than a Grain of Salt

The bad reputation of table salt is well deserved. Refined salt, sea salt, and macrobiotic salts are approximately 97.5 to 98 percent pure sodium and chlorine (NaCl). They are completely unnatural, refined, and, in my mind, chemically and biologically dangerous.

The salt industry is huge. Hundreds of tons of salt are produced each year, but only about 4 percent of purified salt ends up at your grocery store, restaurant, and food-processing plant. Pure sodium chloride is a necessary ingredient in the processing of many chemicals. As a matter of fact, salt is made for chemicals, not people. Refined salt is stripped of all natural nutrients essential to good health. Refined salt contributes to multiple health problems, including fluid retention, due to the following additives:

- Excessive concentration of iodine (twenty times the natural amount)
- Dextrose (sugar), added as a stabilizer to protect the iodine from oxidizing
- Sodium carbonate, a bleaching agent
- Anticaking agents

The only ecologically harvested salt that I consider whole and bio-energetically conducive to health when taken internally is Celtic Sea salt. It is an organic, complete, and natural form of sea minerals containing the highest percentage of all the essential trace and macro elements needed to restore human health and energy. Natural sea salt is light gray in color, moist to the touch, and will have a cubic crystal shape.

- Drink fresh-squeezed lemon juice in water, as this is a natural diuretic.
- Eat more onions and garlic, which are also diuretic agents.
- Chew the Sweet-Breath Seed Mix given on page 114. These seeds are diuretic, too!

HERBS

The chosen few. Herbal remedies for water retention include chickweed, cornsilk, dandelion leaf, and horsetail. They are best used in herbal teas or footbaths. They can also be taken in capsule or tincture form by mouth according to the product label instructions.

HYDROTHERAPY

Take a sensible soak. For generalized swelling and fluid retention, a full aromatic bath is your best bet. The bath is best at a warm temperature—about 98 to 101 degrees—not hot. The goal is to encourage circulation and promote sweating. If the temperature is too cool, the body will not respond as quickly.

A full bath is an excellent way to take in essential oils, since a large area of your body's skin surface is absorbing the active ingredients. Following the bath, wrap yourself in a warm bath towel or cotton bathrobe to encourage further sweating. Sipping cool water or herbal tea while in a warm bath can stimulate the kidneys, too! Keep warm and rest by lying down for at least 20 to 30 minutes following the aromatic bath.

You can make up your own blend by using any of the essential oils listed here, singly or in combination. Use 6 to 10 drops of essential oil per spa bath.

> ### Tip: Marble Bath Is Marvelous
>
> Sore feet? Before you put your battered toes into your next footbath, empty a bag of marbles into the bottom of your tub and give yourself an acupressure treatment while you soak by rolling your feet back and forth along the marbles. Then ask your mate for a foot massage. A test of true love!

Going local. A hand bath or footbath is a very soothing, cooling, and effective relief for swelling that is localized to the limbs. A cold to tepid water temperature (70 to 92 degrees) is advantageous to decrease local inflammation and swelling. This treatment uses cold water because it involves a smaller body area that can easily tolerate the cooler temperature. This footbath is designed for ankle and foot swelling.

⚬ The Shrinking Footbath ⚬

This can be used for swollen hands, too!

2 to 4 tablespoons Celtic Sea salt
  or Detoxifying Bath Salts (page 128)
2 drops lemon essential oil
1 drop cypress essential oil
1 drop juniper essential oil

Combine the salt and essential oils. Add to a full basin of water. Swish the water well to combine. Sit in a comfortable place and allow your feet to soak for at least 15 minutes. Pat your feet dry and elevate them at least 6 to 8 inches above heart level by lying down for another 15 minutes or more. This further encourages blood to return to the heart and decreases local fluid accumulation.

While lying down and elevating your feet, take a series of deep breaths to help promote relaxation and good blood circulation.

Hot weather helpers. Cold packs, cold compresses, and ice will also ease and diminish swelling of the hands and feet, especially during hot weather.

LIFESTYLE

Take supportive measures. A few simple strategies will help prevent swelling and fluid accumulation due to poor or inadequate circulation.
- Avoid tight-fitting clothing; yes, the pressure around your body can make you swell.
- Wear shoes that *fit*.
- Wear support hose or knee-highs.
- Take frequent breaks from continual standing or sitting and elevate the feet as much as possible while sitting. A stool under the desk works well.

MASSAGE

Light touch massage. Use this concentrated massage oil for local areas, such as the feet or hands, when swelling is a problem due to poor circulation. For chronic problems you can use this preparation daily to help prevent symptoms. Lemongrass is included in this remedy because it tones skin that has stretched from frequent swelling of the tissues.

❧ Hand-and-Foot Massage Oil ❧

12 drops lavender essential oil
5 drops cypress essential oil
4 drops lemongrass essential oil
4 drops grapefruit essential oil
1 tablespoon arnica infusion oil
1 tablespoon vegetable oil or unscented lotion

In a 1-ounce amber glass bottle, add the essential oils. Then pour in the arnica and vegetable oils. Note: If using a 1-ounce bottle, simply fill the bottle with the oil; there is no need to measure it. Label contents.

This oil can be used daily by massaging it into the affected area (feet, ankles, or hands). Always apply with hand strokes and circular massage in the direction toward the heart. This encourages bloodflow return and decreases swelling. Use an unscented base lotion (without mineral oil) if you plan on wearing this daily under hosiery. Lotion is water soluble and more readily absorbed by the skin.

Use fancy footwork. An ankle filter treatment can be self-administered by following the easy instructions detailed in the section on Circulation Problems. This massage technique, called Creative Healing, assists in draining this major circulation filter area of the foot and helps to prevent swelling and poor circulation.

Yoga and Movement

Make like a butterfly. This yoga pose will help prevent and reduce swelling of the lower extremities. This pose can be adapted for pregnancy states, so do not be afraid to attempt it. It relieves lower back pressure, aids the return of blood back to the heart, and assists lymphatic drainage.

The Wall Butterfly Pose

In this pose, you will be lying on the floor with your legs raised vertically above you, resting on a wall. Wear comfortable clothing and remove your shoes.

To begin, lie on your back on the floor, perpendicular to a wall, raising your legs vertically so that they are flush with the wall. Your buttocks should also be pressing against the wall so that you are in an inverted sitting pose. Bend your knees to either side and press the soles of your feet together. Try to keep your knees against the wall. Rest your arms out to your sides on the floor, palms open and facing the ceiling. Breathe deeply and slowly through your nose. If needed, you can use your hands to press your knees apart and down, allowing you to stretch completely. Close your eyes, concentrate on your breath, and relax. Rest in this pose for several minutes or as long as it is comfortable for you.

An adaptation of this pose is to simply leave your legs in the vertical position against the wall or drop them apart into a V formation. Or you can put your legs up on a chair seat, bending at the knees, if this is more comfortable for you.

Real–Life Cure

AMAZED, ELATED, AND DEFLATED

Sophia, a delightful, kind, and caring sixty-seven-year-young woman, had experienced ankle and foot swelling for years when she came to me for a solution.

She had a history of arthritis in her hands and occasional constipation. She was under routine care by a physician and was on prescription medication for high blood pressure, which included a diuretic. However, she was still bothered by moderate to severe swelling of her feet and ankles, especially during hot, humid weather.

Sophia continued to follow the advice of her physician, which was to avoid sodium in her diet and to remain on her drugs. The only thing she did differently was add essential oils to her life. She put them in footbaths and lotions. To her amazement, the swelling went down as quickly as it started.

See also Circulation Problems.

Forgetfulness

MEMORY MAKERS

Your brain is your primary health-maintenance organ.

Scientists are still puzzled about the multitude of functions and capabilities the human brain possesses, and the mind/body connection is one that's just beginning to be accepted by Western cultures.

Considering that only a very small percentage of the brain is actually utilized, there is much left to discover through research. What is known about the brain is that every detail of our lives is recorded in this astonishing "computer." Just like your computer system at work, every message or thought you process gets encrypted somewhere in the system.

Even when you delete (or, in your brain's case, forget), it remains somewhere "out there." The possibility of retrieval is very real.

Just like the clues hackers use to retrieve protected or deleted information, your mind responds to cues to help retrieve a memory. These cues are often sensory. In fact, it's believed that there is an intimate relationship between the limbic system of the brain that is responsible for memory and the olfactory system—the sense of smell.

That's why the scent of baking bread or warm oatmeal cookies can trigger a memory of your mother working in the kitchen when you came home from school as a child. Or an old boyfriend may be suddenly remembered when you smell the cologne he used to wear. Studies show that a memory link to scent is recalled more easily than any of the other senses. This is due

This Lemon Works!

A Japanese study involving keypunch operators found that, when lemon scent was piped into the ventilation system, errors were decreased by 53 percent. Lemon is an uplifting scent that is used for memory stimulation and mental alertness. Use lemon essence in a diffuser and spray it periodically in your work or study space.

The Estrogen/Memory Connection

We know forgetfulness is a common side effect of the aging process, but are women in menopause the most likely to forget? Some studies suggest they are. Memory loss has been linked to low estrogen levels.

I, however, believe there is an antidote to this problem: essential oils that mimic estrogen. These include aniseed, basil, chamomile, clary sage, cypress, fennel, geranium, nutmeg, and star anise. Interestingly, three of these oils are also ones shown to help enhance memory: basil, clary sage, and cypress. Use them to your mind's content!

to the fact that the limbic, or "old," brain is so closely associated with the sense of smell, and to some degree conditioning has taken place.

Memory can also be triggered visually—say, by a familiar landscape or a person's facial expression. Music and sounds can also trigger memories and specific times in a person's life, such as a special song or a first school dance.

AROMATHERAPY

Remember this. Essential oils that promote wakefulness, readiness, and concentration are basil, cypress, eucalyptus, ginger, juniper, lemon, lemongrass, peppermint, pine, and rosemary. These aromas can be diffused in the air by an electric unit or a room spray, or inhaled from a tissue.

Clear the mind of clutter. The reason so many people are forgetful is simply because they have too much on their minds. Stress and a hectic lifestyle—not to mention remembering things like home, work, and cell phone numbers and a variety of passwords—put your mind on overload. Studies have found that a meditative state is a great way to clear the mind of clutter and to get your thought and recall processes in order.

The focal point of meditation is breathing, deep relaxation, and centering. But I've found that essential oils can enhance the meditative state, especially when high stress levels and jangled nerves are interfering with your ability to think.

The essences used in this recipe induce a meditative state and are used by many followers during prayer, meditation, and yoga. They were often used for ceremonial rituals in ancient times. They are cedarwood, clary sage, eucalyptus, frankincense, lavender, myrrh, neroli, patchouli, pine, rose, sandalwood, and ylang-ylang.

ॐ Meditation Memory Oil ॐ

Clearing the mind with meditation oil will refresh your memory.
Carry it with you in a vial and breathe it in whenever you feel brain weary.

18 drops frankincense essential oil
10 drops lavender essential oil

10 drops sandalwood essential oil
5 drops cedarwood essential oil
5 drops ylang-ylang essential oil

In a small amber glass bottle, add the essential oils one by one using an eyedropper. Cap securely and shake to mix well. Label. Add a few drops to a potpourri burner or aromatic lamp. Lie down in a comfortable place, close your eyes, and clear your mind of all thoughts. Repeat a word (practiced meditators call it a "mantra") or pray for 15 minutes or longer. Practice daily.

It Takes Scents to Ace an Exam

I wish I had had this synergy blend around when I had to take state boards and certification tests!

Basil, lemon, and rosemary essential oils are great for memory recall, and feedback tells me that they really work at exam time. Here's what to do: Combine five parts lemon, three parts basil, and two parts rosemary essential oils in an amber glass bottle. Put them in an aroma lamp, potpourri burner, or diffuser while studying.

At test time, put a few drops on a handkerchief or tissue and sniff it periodically during the exam or when your memory needs a jolt. By utilizing the same scent while studying and then again during the exam, a conditioned response of scent and memory is produced, thus making it easier to recall information.

Keep in mind this isn't a miracle oil. You still have to study. Good luck!

Diet

Be the designated driver. Alcohol kills brain cells. It also impairs memory, concentration, and reaction time. If you must drink, limit it to three to four drinks a week.

Cut the fat. A high-fat diet makes your mind and body foggy. Opt for a diet based on fresh fruits, vegetables (especially sea vegetables), and whole grains.

Adrenal–Stimulating Aromas

The hormone pregnenolone, normally produced in the brain and adrenal glands, may help brain cells communicate better, thereby increasing memory and learning ability. It is also being investigated for its possible usefulness in treating Alzheimer's disease.

If this theory proves accurate, adrenal gland–stimulating essential oils may be helpful, namely cedarwood, citronella, clary sage, and geranium. More research is needed for this to be conclusive, but it won't hurt to use them now.

Get your Bs. Vitamins B_6 and B_{12} fight stress, enhance oxygen flow, and help brain function. Foods rich in vitamin B_6 include bananas, avocados, organic eggs, brown rice, and walnuts. Vitamin B_{12} is found in many animal sources, including salmon, tuna, herring, clams, crab, and ham.

Got nuts. Eating raw nuts and seeds and taking flax oil and wheat germ have been shown to enhance mind power by helping brain cells communicate better.

HERBS

Remember to take your ginkgo. Ginkgo biloba and ginseng are the best-known memory-enhancing herbs on the market. Get a bottle of each, and don't forget to take it every day!

A recent analysis done by Jorg Grunwald, Ph.D., in Berlin, shows that ginkgo biloba and ginseng are the two leading European plants produced for phytomedicines (which include herbal and essential oil preparations). They are primarily used by the aging population as circulatory and brain functioning aids.

And in second place . . . Other herbs used as memory enhancers are basil, blessed thistle, ginger, hawthorn, lemon balm, rosemary, and sweet marjoram. These herbs can be made into herbal infusions (tea) or taken in tincture or capsule form. Also, basil, ginger, lemon balm, marjoram, rosemary, and sage are commonly used in cooking. Use them generously.

SOUND AND MUSIC THERAPY

Now hear this. Sound therapy for clear thinking can be extremely helpful, especially if you prefer background music for concentration. The following should prove positive:

J. S. Bach—*Brandenburg Concertos*
Weber—*Oberon Overture*
Brahms—*Violin Concerto*
Scarlatti—*Harpsichord Sonatas*
Handel—*Water Music*
Soundtrack—*Born Free*
Tibetan Bells I and II
Harmonix Ensemble—*Ginkgo Biloba*

Growing Pains

⚕

NIGHTTIME ACTION

Growing up can be painful in more ways than one.

What our grandmothers used to call "growing pains" is very real. Growth, like healing, takes place while we're in a state of sleep. This is why young children are apt to wake up at night complaining of cramp-type pain, usually in the leg.

Here's what you can do to calm them down, ease their troubles, and get them back to sleep.

AROMATHERAPY

Rub it in. Keep a small bottle of muscle-relaxing aromatic oil handy for you (but not for them) near the child's bed. When they wake up, rub some on the "hurt" and massage them back to sleep. For younger children, applying the oil before bedtime or after a warm bath will help. Here's the recipe I used on my kids.

✺ Growing-Pain-Go-Away Oil ✺

6 drops lavender essential oil

4 drops basil essential oil

4 drops sweet marjoram essential oil

2 drops eucalyptus essential oil

2 drops chamomile (Roman) essential oil

2 tablespoons St. John's wort infusion oil or vegetable oil

In an amber glass bottle, add the lavender, basil, sweet marjoram, eucalyptus, and chamomile oils one by one using an eyedropper. Cap securely and shake to mix. Add the infusion oil, cap, and shake again to mix. Label.

To use, warm the bottle of oil in a warm water bath or simply put a few drops in your hands and rub them together to warm. Apply a small amount to the affected muscles and joints and massage lightly.

Note: This oil is meant for application to small areas and should not be used for a whole body massage.

Mix your own. If you want to make your own preparation, the oils noted for their muscle-soothing quality are basil, bergamot, chamomile, clary sage, cypress, eucalyptus, fennel, geranium, grapefruit, hyssop, juniper, lavender, marjoram, neroli, peppermint, rosemary, and sandalwood.

These oils can also be used in baths and compresses as well as massage oils and lotions.

HYDROTHERAPY

Take this bottle to bed. The good old-fashioned hot-water bottle is an effective treatment for muscle spasms and is especially soothing following a gentle massage and aromatic oil rub to the affected area.

See also Muscle Cramps.

Hair Loss
✍

HERE TODAY, HERE TOMORROW

Hair loss ranks right up there with wrinkles when it comes to giving aging a bad name. Those who experience it may say it's even worse!

Nobody wants to change the thick colorful locks of youth for thinning pates. Many men experience premature thinning or balding because of their genes—the ones inherited from their mother. If your mother's father is bald, bet on it that you will be, too.

But hair thinning and loss aren't only an inherited malady. Imbalances in the body can cause it, too, such as vitamin deficiencies, thyroid or pituitary disorders, and certain illnesses such as scarlet fever. Stress, overshampooing, and frequent swimming in chlorinated pools can also affect the hair. Then there's the hair thinning and loss that can result from chemotherapy and radiation treatments.

There are no home treatments that will make a bald head sprout new follicles, but there are things you can do to bring back luster to a thinning mane.

AROMATHERAPY

Treat the scalp. Essential oils remedy hair thinning because they nourish deep into the dermal layers of the skin and in tiny blood vessels where the hair follicles are located. This aromatic scalp treatment oil is effective when used over two to three months. This period of time will allow several hair growth cycles to take place, and an improvement in hair growth will be visible.

Use this oil several times weekly, after hair care, leaving it in to be absorbed into the scalp. It is called a scalp treatment because the hair itself is not the focus, but rather the scalp—more specifically, the hair follicle and microcirculatory system. Using warmed oil will increase the absorption of the oils considerably.

Scalp-Conditioning Oil

1 tablespoon jojoba oil

1 tablespoon calendula infusion oil or sesame oil

½ teaspoon carrot seed oil

10 drops lavender essential oil

6 drops clary sage essential oil

4 drops cedarwood essential oil

4 drops rosemary essential oil

In a small amber glass bottle, add the jojoba, calendula, and carrot seed oils. Add the essential oils and shake to mix. Label. Warm the oil before application by placing it in a warm water bath. To use, massage a few drops into the scalp area before retiring to bed so it can absorb overnight. Shampoo it out in the morning. Apply several times weekly.

Try your own. Essential oils known to be useful in counteracting hair loss are cedarwood, chamomile, clary sage, cypress, grapefruit, juniper, lavender, lemon, lemongrass, patchouli, rose, rosemary, and ylang-ylang. Carrier oils or infusion oils to use as part of your aromatic blend include borage, calendula, carrot seed, castor oil, evening primrose, jojoba, St. John's wort, and sesame. Try your own blend following the ratios given above.

Traditional Indian technique. A simple yet famous hair tonic from India calls for sesame oil and rosemary and lemongrass essential oil. Try your own homemade version by mixing 10 drops of each essential oil in 2 tablespoons of sesame oil.

Diet

Add oil internally. Taking natural flax oil daily, in addition to eating more raw nuts and seeds, will help lubricate your hair and scalp from the inside.

Hang Your Head in Hope

A simple way to maximize blood flow to the scalp, which is essential to spur hair growth, is to lie horizontally on your bed and hang your head over the side for about 10 minutes once or twice per day. Slant boards and headstand stools are also part of some treatment regimes. Also, sleeping with your window open will keep the air and your head cooler, which may speed hair growth.

Eat sushi. If an iodine deficiency related to a thyroid condition is causing your hair loss, eat sea vegetables such as kelp and dulse, which are high in naturally occurring iodine. Sea vegetables, as well as chlorophyll-rich sources of spirulina and chlorella, are excellent mineral and protein building blocks for hair growth. You can find them in natural food stores and Asian markets in condiment form and in soup and sushi ingredients.

Get your Bs. B-complex vitamin–rich foods are used for treatment of hair loss and include brewer's yeast, lecithin, raw wheat germ, and sunflower seeds. Taking 1 to 2 tablespoons of these B-complex foods should be adequate.

Get extra E. Vitamin E may prove useful due to its hair-growth promoting factors: 300 to 600 international units is typically recommended for this problem.

Don't go crazy dieting. Avoid restrictive or crash diets that can cause long-term deficiencies and rob your body (and hair) of vital nutrients.

Herbs

Get back in circulation. Good circulation is essential to hair growth, so reach for botanicals known for improving circulation. These are cayenne (capsicum), chamomile, ginger root, Ginkgo biloba, rosemary, sage, and turmeric. Additionally, herbs rich in minerals and vitamins are also worth a try: alfalfa, borage seed, dandelion root, horsetail herb, lemongrass, nettles, parsley herb, and yellow dock root. Use them in teas and tinctures or add them to your own hair treatment products.

LIFESTYLE

Best time to brush. A thorough nightly brushing with a good natural bristle brush is essential to bring health back to your hair. Bend over, hanging your head lower than your heart, brush your hair for several minutes, and then massage your scalp with your fingers.

Go nontoxic. Avoid hair chemical treatments, swimming in chlorinated pools (or wear a cap), and overshampooing, especially with harsh detergents and synthetic fragrances.
  See also Dull Hair.

Hay Fever

〜

NO MORE SYMPTOMS

Ahhhh—chooo! It's the calling cry that spring is in the air.

If seasonal changes leave you with the sneezing, itchy eyes, and runny nose of hay fever, here's what to do.

HYDROTHERAPY

The French connection: treat the feet. A surprisingly effective remedy for allergy-related symptoms is the footbath. It comes from Maurice Messegue, a French herbalist, who believes the feet are the best way to absorb natural medicines such as herbs and essential oils. For additional benefit, you can also use reflexology of the foot to aid in lung and sinus complaints.

This footbath can be done three times a day during allergy attacks or occasionally when early symptoms begin to surface. Try it daily for prevention when you expect seasonal changes to trigger symptoms, and see if you can observe a more diminished allergic response than usual.

Hay Fever Foot Formula

3 drops lavender essential oil
1 drop rose essential oil
1 drop geranium essential oil
2 tablespoons Celtic Sea salt or bath salt

Fill a foot basin or tub half full with tepid water. Add the essential oils to the salt and mix before adding to the water basin. Soak your feet while sitting, for at least 15 to 20 minutes. Pat feet dry and put on warm cotton or wool socks.

MASSAGE

Following, or in lieu of, the foot soak, try this massage oil, which is applied to the feet, head, and chest. This is the same recipe given in the Allergies entry, but the amount is larger and the blend more diluted because it covers more skin surface.

Clear–Head Blend II

1 drop Bulgarian rose essential oil
1 drop peppermint essential oil
3 drops lavender essential oil
2 tablespoons olive oil or arnica infusion oil

In a small amber glass bottle, add the essential oils. Add the olive oil and shake gently. Label the contents. To use, simply apply a small amount of this blend to your fingertips and massage into the scalp, temples, and cervical neck area as well as the upper chest. Inhale the essences from your hands following the application. Also apply to the soles of your feet, especially following the aromatic footbath treatment. Put on warm cotton or wool socks. Take a few minutes of quiet time to relax and close your eyes. This comforting treatment can be done twice daily, preferably in the morning and nighttime.

See also Allergies *and* Nasal Congestion.

Headache

ᕼᕲ

MASSAGE AWAY TENSION

Headaches come in many varieties, but the one that's most likely to strike is the tension headache.

Tension headaches are more common than the common cold. They are typically slow to develop and can leave their tightening arrival sign on the forehead, temples, and back of the head or neck. The throbbing and sometimes squeezing sensation ranges in intensity from mild to severe. If ignored, these headaches can be quite debilitating.

Overstimulation, such as loud noise or eye straining, can cause a tension headache. So can long hours of unrelieved work and emotional stress. In fact, anything that causes stress in your life can leave you with a tension headache. Fortunately, there are ways to send it packing.

AROMATHERAPY

Essential oils useful for headaches are numerous and include many of the antistress essential oils, including basil, bergamot, chamomile, clary sage, geranium, juniper, lavender, lemongrass, marjoram, sandalwood, and ylang-ylang. Analgesic and antispasmodic essences are also useful to remedy headaches. They include chamomile, eucalyptus, juniper, lavender, marjoram, peppermint, and rosemary. These oils can be used as massage oil blends, compresses, and in inhalation therapies.

HERBS

Get to the root of the problem. There are many herbs that offer headache relief, especially if the headache is caused by nervous tension. Garden-variety headache herbs are black cohosh, catnip, chamomile, feverfew, Ginkgo biloba, rosemary, skullcap, and valerian root. Herbs that aid in relieving headache pain are the analgesic herbs kava kava, St. John's wort, white willow bark, and wintergreen. Calming botanicals are catnip, hops, oatstraw, passionflower, skullcap, and valerian root. Muscle-relaxing and antispasmodic herbs are also beneficial and include hops, kava kava, lobelia, rosemary, valerian root, wild lettuce, and wood betony. Use in tincture or capsule form according to the labeled product directions.

Eye up lavender. If you get a headache as a result of eyestrain, relax your eyes with the Eye Pillow recipe containing lavender on page 250. It offers relief for mild symptoms and can be kept by the bedside or in an office drawer.

Hydrotherapy

Foot to head relief. An excellent remedy for headaches is the cold footbath with essential oils. I know it sounds strange, but by soaking your feet in cold water you draw blood from the head, which brings immediate relief for some headaches. If you are familiar with reflexology, manipulate the key points in the hands and feet to enchance the treatment.

⟲ Headache Relief Footbath ⟳

The key is to get comfortable and relax during this treatment.

2 tablespoons Celtic Sea salt
4 drops lavender essential oil
2 drops peppermint essential oil

Fill a tub or basin large enough to hold both feet comfortably half full with cold water (55 to 70 degrees). In a small bowl, mix the salt and oils. Add to the water and stir with your hands. Soak both feet in the cold aromatic water for 15 to 20 minutes. Sit comfortably while doing the footbath. Concentrate on breathing slowly and deeply. Relax.

Cool the forehead, warm the neck. Cool or warm aromatic compresses can be used for effective headache relief as well. If you have forehead pain, add a few drops of lavender to a basin of cool water. Put a washcloth in the water, wring it out, and lie down with the cloth on your forehead. Replace with a fresh one once it warms.

For a headache at the base of the neck and back of the head, a warm compress will aid blood flow and give relief. Follow the directions above.

MASSAGE

Go to the temple of pain relief. This recipe is for a stress-induced headache. It is an oil concentrate that is massaged on the temples and hairline. Although either lavender or peppermint essential oil works well singly, I choose to use them together in this blend. Lavender is known for its soothing properties on the nervous system, while peppermint is a mild analgesic and anti-inflammatory agent. They work synergistically to remedy a headache.

Headache Oil

10 drops lavender essential oil
5 drops peppermint essential oil
1 tablespoon vegetable oil
1 200-IUs vitamin E capsule (optional)

In an amber glass bottle, add the essential oils and vegetable oil. If desired, add the vitamin E. If using the gel capsule form of vitamin E, cut off one end and squeeze the contents into the oils. Shake well to mix completely. Label with directions for use.

To use, warm the bottle in a warm water bath and place a few drops on your fingertips. Apply in light, small circular motions to the temples of the head and just below the hairline. Typically this area is sore to the touch if the headache is severe. Gently massage this area with light pressure for a few minutes.

Inhale the essences from your cupped hands following the massage. Breathe deeply and slowly and concentrate on your breath.

SOUND AND MUSIC THERAPY

Anti-tension toning. In addition to tension headaches, this technique also helps migraines and headaches caused by TMJ pain. Practice making the sounds *ya, you,* and *yai.* To do, take a deep breath and exhale making the sound *ya.* You should feel a resonance in the head region. Repeat with the other two sounds. Make each sound individually three times. For best results repeat three times per day.

The same music used to induce relaxation and meditation may be helpful to ease a tension headache. Among my selected favorites:

Narada Collection Series—*Earth Songs*
Hennie Bekker—*Spa*
Harmonix Ensemble—*Kava Kava*

Real-Life Cure

SEEING IS BELIEVING

Dena always looked a little tense to me, but the day she burst into my classroom late she looked particularly frazzled and stressed. She started sputtering about the string of mishaps leading up to that moment, plopped herself into a seat, and exclaimed, "Does anyone have anything for a headache?" Her head, she said, was throbbing painfully.

Ah-ha, I thought. A real life lesson. I told her to close her eyes, relax her muscles, and concentrate on her breathing. Then I took a little headache oil from my stash, warmed a bit with the palms of my hands, and started to tenderly rub it into her temples. After a few minutes I could actually feel her tension releasing. I put my cupped hands under her nose and told her to take a deep breath. Dena's headache was gone.

If there were any doubting Thomases in class that day, they walked out totally convinced.

TEAS AND TONICS

Treat yourself gingerly. A simple tea made with fresh ginger root has proven to be very effective for most general types of headaches. The ginger improves circulation and reduces muscle tension and inflammation. Ginger is alkalizing, so if your body is too acidic (as is common), then here is another reason to give this tea a try. It is very safe and can be used long term without side effects of any kind. It is warming to the body and especially welcome during the cooler weather.

∞ Ginger Tea ∞

Make gingered iced tea as a warm weather option.

4 cups hot water
1 to 2 teaspoons freshly peeled and grated ginger root
   (preferably organic)
Stevia or Ginger Honey (page 48) to taste (optional)

Bring the water to a simmer on the stove. Add the ginger to a teapot and pour the water over it. Let it steep for 5 to 10 minutes. Strain and sweeten, if desired. This is also good cold.

YOGA AND MOVEMENT

Shrug it off. Neck and shoulder pain is a common cause of tension headaches. This tension-releasing exercise is easy to perform and can be practiced anywhere, even in the car. It eases tension, increases flexibility, and tones the neck and shoulder muscles. This is particularly effective if you have suffered whiplash from an automobile accident or find you carry a lot of your stress in your neck and shoulder regions.

Sit or stand with your back straight. Focus your attention on the back of the neck and shoulder areas. Gently draw your shoulders up as close to your ears as possible while inhaling. Hold for 15 seconds. If you experience discomfort, lower your shoulders a bit and hold the position for only 5 to 10 seconds. Drop your shoulders, letting out a loud, audible sigh as you exhale. Repeat this movement several times at your own pace.

See also Eye Strain *and* Stress.

Heartburn

ꞙ

PUTTING OUT THE FIRE

Are antacids a common staple in your diet?

Heartburn and indigestion are common health complaints that needn't be common at all. The burning may be felt in the chest, but the problem originates in the stomach, where gastric acid (hydrochloric acid), digestive enzymes, and various hormones are supposed to go to work on the food you just swallowed. Sometimes, however, either too much or too little of these secreted substances rises to the occasion.

Indigestion is linked to both physical and emotional factors. The physical factors can be overeating, overuse of antacids, eating too quickly, or consuming a meal high in fats or dairy products (milk neutralizes stomach acids). Stress or any kind of emotional upheaval in your life can also cause indigestion. Whatever the cause, heartburn means food consumed is not being adequately digested and therefore not properly assimilated into "usable" fuel or energy.

AROMATHERAPY

Sweet-scented solutions. Basil and peppermint essential oils are the most popular for treating digestive problems. Lavender soothes the nervous system in general and is antispasmodic. Bergamot and neroli help with anxiety and nervous tension. Other essential oils that can be beneficial to the digestive system include anise, black pepper, chamomile, fennel, ginger, hyssop, juniper, lemon, and lemongrass.

BREATH WORK

Get centered. Full and relaxed breathing aids many imbalances and is particularly useful for the nervous or stressed person troubled with indigestion. Breathing properly for 3 to 4 minutes prior to mealtime will calm the nerves.

The proper breathing technique is diaphragmatic breathing. It takes some practice but is easy to do. Get into a comfortable position. Place one palm at the center of your chest and the other at the lower edge of your rib cage where the abdomen begins. As you inhale, the lower edge of the rib cage should expand and your abdomen should rise. As you exhale, the opposite will happen.

DIET

Get to the source. Bloating, belching, a feeling of fullness after eating, flatulence, and digestive pain are common side effects if your problem is caused by a food allergy, high-fat diet, or acidic foods. If the problem continues and cannot be corrected with natural remedies or elimination of certain foods, you should see a specialist to get to the root of the problem. Dietary changes are essential to a cure.

Cumin: Secret Stomach Spice

Beans are among the most notorious of stomach abusers. Even if they don't cause you indigestion, they probably bring other woes like flatulence and bloating. The people of Mexico and India, however, have the answer to this problem: cumin.

Cumin is added to legume dishes because it counteracts stomach upsets. You can also get the same result by adding a whole onion studded with a few whole cloves or a piece of Kombu seaweed to the pot while beans cook.

Combine, feel fine. Natural Hygiene is a philosophy and lifestyle based both on principles of proper food combinations to aid the digestive process and following the body's natural cycles of elimination, appropriation, and assimilation.

Help your stomach out. Eating more naturally fermented foods, such as raw cultured vegetables, sauerkraut, and kim chi, will promote optimal digestion.

HERBS

Take a lesson from history. The medicinal power of herbs was first discovered when man took a bite of a medicinal plant and his stomach pain disappeared. I'm not sure what plant brought on the cure, but many other herbal cures for indigestion as well as other illnesses quickly followed.

International Flavor Aids

Many cultures have their own custom of easing digestive upsets.

In Italy, where meals can be a multiple-course social event, anise is the cure-all. It's an ingredient in many after-dinner liqueurs and is popular in desserts for this reason.

In India and some Asian countries, where dishes are famous for their strong, spicy flavor, fennel is the digestive herb of choice. Caraway is also used for the same reason.

If you have digestion problems, experiment in the kitchen using these spices.

Tip: Candlelight and Comfort

In our home we dine by candlelight almost every night. This has a quieting and calming effect and definitely encourages a relaxed atmosphere. It also demonstrates energy conservation and honors our special family time together. Try it tonight at your dinner table and notice the difference a little thing like this can make.

Among the traditional herbs and spices used for indigestion are basil, caraway, chamomile, cinnamon, clove, coriander, fennel, garlic, ginger, licorice, onion, peppermint, rhubarb root, sage, savory, and slippery elm.

Herbs known for their calming effect on the nervous system are also used for indigestion: hops, lavender, valerian and the aforementioned chamomile, rosemary, and tarragon.

Water and spice makes tummy feel nice. For a quick first-aid remedy for indigestion, gas, and upset stomach, try a cup of warm water with a pinch of the following spices: cinnamon, cloves, ginger, and nutmeg.

MASSAGE

Balance the solar plexus. The solar plexus is a major chakra or energy central governing digestion. It is located directly below the sternum (breast bone). This chakra is known as the energy distribution system, which involves collecting energy and sending it to where it is needed. When your chakra is functioning properly, you will experience good digestion, assimilation of nutrients, emotional flexibility, and overall mind/body harmony.

To perform chakra balancing of this area, gently massage in a circular motion with your palm. Start with small circles, gradually enlarging and returning back to the center point. This can be done over your clothing or with an aromatic massage oil or lotion on your skin. Concentrate on relaxing your breath and balancing this area.

> ## Tip: Head-to-Toe Relief
>
> An old naturopathic remedy for indigestion is to rest the soles of your feet on a hot-water bottle. This aids the digestive process, creates warmth, and increases energy flow. Try it while at the dinner table or immediately following your meal.

The following massage lotion can be used for the chakra massage and is most effective half an hour before meals. Apply over the solar plexus as well as the stomach area and backs of the hands. Use sparingly, as this is a concentrated blend. Inhale as needed from the backs of the hands.

ᎧᎧ Digest-Ease Massage Lotion ᎧᎧ

4 drops lavender essential oil

3 drops bergamot essential oil

2 drops peppermint essential oil

2 drops basil essential oil

1 drop neroli essential oil or chamomile essential oil

1 tablespoon vegetable oil or natural lotion

Combine the essential oils in a small amber glass bottle. Add the vegetable oil to use as the carrier or use a nonscented base lotion. This is a massage concentrate and is designed to use for specific and localized areas, not the entire body.

SOUND AND MUSIC THERAPY

Sounds the stomach loves. Research shows that soft melodies have a calming effect on the body, which in turn can relax the clench that stress has on your stomach. The music selections recommended here are specific to aiding digestion and improving the overall dining experience.

Vivaldi—*Lute Concertos; Oboe Concertos*

Handel—*Harp Concerto; Flute Sonatas*

Mendelssohn—*Songs Without Words*

Grieg—*The Last Spring; Heart Wounds; Holberg Suite*

Koto Flute

Mozart—*Concerto for Flute and Harp*

Chopin—*Piano Concerto No. 1*

Telemann—*Table Music*

Tone this tune. According to Deepak Chopra, a leading authority and researcher on Ayurvedic medicine, certain toning sounds can bring relief to stomach problems. The sound "huh" is prescribed for indigestion, heartburn, and abnormal appetite. Simply take a deep breath and on the exhalation make the sound "huh." Repeat this three times daily following meals.

TEAS AND TONICS

Be a tea sipper. Green tea has many healing benefits, and aiding indigestion and pain associated with chronic stomach problems is at the top of the list. To multiply its healing benefit, I added peppermint, lemon balm, anise seed, and Ginger Honey to this recipe because of their direct beneficial effects on the digestive system. Herbs for nervous tension, such as tarragon, rosemary, chamomile, and are included for their calming effect and antispasmodic properties. Rosemary also is helpful as an antioxidant and for digesting fats and lowering cholesterol levels.

This is an excellent remedy you will want to keep stocked in your pantry. Make this herbal tea mixture ahead and store in a clean glass jar.

❧ Digest-Ease Tea ❧

2 parts peppermint herb
1 part tarragon herb
1 part lemon balm herb
½ part rosemary herb
1 part chamomile flowers
1 part anise seeds or fennel seeds
1 part loose green tea leaves
Stevia, Ginger Honey (page 48), or plain honey to taste (optional)

Mix the herbs, chamomile flowers, anise seeds, and green tea leaves together in a bowl. Store in glass jar and label with directions for use. To make 1 cup of tea, add boiling water to 1 to 2 teaspoons of the herbal tea mixture. Let it steep for 5 minutes. Sweeten if desired. Strain and sip slowly and inhale from the cup. Best taken immediately following meals to aid in digestion.

Chew seeds after meals. The Sweet-Breath Seed Mix given on page 114 helps to prevent indigestion and relieves its symptoms. Simply chew the special mix of digestion-aiding seeds following a meal.

When to Call the Doctor

If you experience heartburn several times a week for no apparent reason, it's time to see a doctor. This could be a sign of acid reflux or an ulcer.

Heartburn has also been known to mimic signs of a heart attack. If you're not sure, make a safe call: go to the emergency room.

Real-Life Cure

This story is a prime example of how emotions affect the digestive system.

Vanessa, a stay-at-home mother of two young schoolage children, began experiencing an increased number of stomach complaints, including indigestion, bloating, and a feeling of fullness immediately following meals, especially dinner.

Upon questioning, she revealed that she was very stressed preparing dinner because of her children's "negative behavior" about eating. As a result of the tension at the dinner table, she ate quickly and overate. Her nervous tension continued through most evenings, which interfered with her ability to relax before retiring.

While she got many recommendations for dealing with the children at this "witching hour," she found the most relief when she addressed herself. To relieve her stress and nervous tension, she practiced stress-relief techniques such as deep breathing. She also put a diffuser containing the Slow-Down-and-Relax Blend (page 351) in the kitchen and dining area while she prepared and served meals. She found this helped calm her kids, too. During the day, she sipped on Digest-Ease Tea and even used the Digest-Ease Massage Lotion. Both, she reported, "worked like magic."

Feeling more relaxed, Vanessa found she had more patience with the children, and her husband noted she was in better spirits when he got home. She started enjoying the evening meal more, so she ate more slowly and ate less. Within days, the indigestion complaints disappeared, and over the following two weeks she noticed she had even lost a few pounds!

See also Stress.

Hemorrhoids

SOOTHE AND HEAL

No thanks, I'd rather stand.

If you have hemorrhoids, there's no such thing as taking a load off your feet. Mere contact with a chair, even a comfy down cushion, can make you squirm and wince in pain. But there's no reason to fear your wallflower status. There are millions of others who feel your pain.

Also called piles, hemorrhoids are one of the most common ailments known to mankind (yes, they are more common in men). Hemorrhoids are varicose veins that swell and blister on the interior anal wall. They itch, hurt, and sometimes bleed. Sometimes they can "pop out," creating even more discomfort to an ailing bottom.

Hemorrhoids are created by extraneous stress on the colon and rectum. Constipation, heavy lifting, sitting for long periods of time, lack of exercise, obesity and a low-fiber diet are common causes. They're also common in the last trimester of pregnancy when there is additional weight and pressure on the bowels and pelvis.

Hemorrhoids are relatively easy to take care of and prevent. But to completely treat the problem you must address the habits that are contributing to this ailment.

AROMATHERAPY

Alleviating oils. Essential oils that help tone blood vessels and decrease inflammation are used in remedying hemorrhoids. The most common oils include bergamot, cypress, frankincense, juniper, and myrrh.

Witch it gone. To eliminate the swelling and soothe the itching and pain, generously douse a cotton pad with witch hazel and dab it on the sore spots. Repeat several times a day. Instead of witch hazel you can use aloe vera gel.

Keep on truckin'. This cure is even more effective. In fact, many elderly clients have used this recipe with great success. It also has been used effectively by truck drivers who commonly have hemorrhoids due to their continual long runs.

🕮 Hemorrhoid–Relief Pads 🕮

Keep moistioned cotton pads in a Ziploc plastic bag for convenience when traveling. For home use, they are especially soothing when stored in the refrigerator.

8-ounce bottle distilled witch hazel
5 drops cypress essential oil
5 drops lavender essential oil
1 to 2 tablespoons aloe vera gel (optional)

Pour out about 1 ounce (a shot glassful) of the witch hazel from the bottle. Add the essential oils and, if desired, the aloe vera to the witch hazel bottle. Cap securely and shake. Label. Shake the contents well before each use.

To use, dampen a cotton pad with the lotion and gently pat the affected area. I recommend you use a pad following each bowel movement and a few times during the day if you are experiencing any of the annoying symptoms (burning, itching) that accompany this ailment.

Tip: Go All Natural

Buy the round, 100 percent cotton, cosmetic-type swipes or pads that are sold in pharmacies. All cotton is the least irritating to delicate, swollen tissue. Many so-called cotton balls are not made of cotton but of synthetic fibers, which may be irritating and are not as absorbent.

DIET

Get with the flow. Roughage (high-fiber foods) and plenty of water are needed to keep elimination in motion through the intestinal tract. Increase dietary fiber by eating more fresh fruits, vegetables, and whole grains. Supplement your diet with bran, psyllium seed powder, and flaxseed. Increase fluids, at least 8 glasses of pure water, herbal tea, fresh fruit, and vegetable juices per day. Avoid caffeine and alcohol, which act as diuretics. The Guaranteed-to-Work Bran Muffins on page 191 will help a lot toward preventing constipation in addition to the Restorative Flax Seed tea on page 186.

HERBS

Pile up on these. Seek out herbs that aid in rebuilding a strong, healthy bowel and colon structure. These include alfalfa, aloe vera, bee pollen, chlorella, kelp and sea vegetables, Siberian ginseng, and slippery elm. Other herbs that are traditionally used for hemorrhoids are dandelion root, goldenseal, pilewort (*Ranunculus ficaria* or *lesser celandine*), and yarrow. Garlic and onion have also been proven useful. Use the above by including in your diet and/or take as an herbal supplement.

HYDROTHERAPY

Sitz it out. A sitz bath is the ultimate healer as it is very soothing, alleviates itching, and works surprisingly fast.

You can use any of the suggested essential oils given above in the Aromatherapy section in place of those recommended here. They will work just as effectively.

Use only warm water (92 to 100 degrees) in this bath. Hot water on hemorrhoids encourages the dilation of blood vessels.

✑ Aromatic Sitz Bath for Hemorrhoids ✑

2 tablespoons baking soda
2 drops frankincense essential oil
2 drops cypress essential oil
1 to 2 cups strong herbal tea of calendula,
   chamomile (optional), or comfrey

Fill the tub with several inches of warm water, just enough to cover your bottom. Place the baking soda in a small bowl. Mix the essential oils into the baking soda and add to the warm water. Pour in the herbal tea if you have made it.

Sit and relax, doing some deep breathing exercises for 15 minutes or longer. Following the sitz bath treatment, apply a soothing swipe to the area. Do this bath treatment twice daily during flare-ups.

Lifestyle

Don't sit still. During the healing process, you need to keep from sitting for long periods of time. If you have a desk job, take breaks as much as possible.

Use soothing soap. Avoid harsh toilet soaps until the hemorrhoids have healed. Most soaps are very drying and cause further itching and irritation because they contain chemical deodorants and fragrances.

See also Constipation.

Hiccups

✍

Sniff and Stop

People display many peculiar behaviors when trying to get rid of hiccups, especially in barrooms, where unusual behavior is not necessarily out of the norm. All kinds of contortions are attempted, potions are swigged, and fright gestures are tried. But the hiccers just keep on hiccing.

When people in my family get the hiccups, however, they don't last very long. That's because I know the best way to relieve hiccups, and I'm ready to share it with you. Don't snicker. At least I can explain scientifically why my remedy works. So, you can either pull on your right ear while hopping on your left foot or try this.

Aromatherapy

Hiccups are intermittent spasms of the diaphragm that cause the audible "hic" when it contracts. So, it only makes sense that hitting that diaphragm with something that's antispasmodic should do the trick. Essential oils that fit this category include anise, basil, chamomile, fennel, lavender, mandarin, and sandalwood.

❧ Hiccup Potion ❧

Keep in a handy vial, ready to use at any time.

1 teaspoon vegetable oil
1 drop basil essential oil* or 1 drop chamomile essential oil

Mix the essential oil into the vegetable oil. Rub on your palms and hold your hands over your mouth and nose. Inhale very slowly and deeply a few times. Then rub the oil over the upper chest area just below the throat, as well as over the solar plexus area (just below the sternum). This main area is directly over several nerves that run through this region. Preferably use your left hand and rub in a counter-clockwise direction.

Note: For small children, I do not recommend using basil essential oil; instead, use chamomile or mandarin essential oil.

It's in the bag. Breathing into a paper bag is still an old standby remedy, but it can be more effective if a drop of one of the above essential oils is placed inside. Concentrate on slow, deep breathing to relax your diaphragm.

High Blood Pressure
❧

GAUGING YOUR OPTIONS

Silent, mysterious, insidious. These are the adjectives most often ascribed to high blood pressure. "Silent" refers to its common description as the silent killer. It's mysterious because no one knows for sure why we get it and why it's so hard to keep under control. And it's insidious because of the fear it instills in those who have it. Just the mention of high blood pressure is enough to make the sphygmomanometer rise for some people.

Blood pressure can vary greatly depending on the time of day, the activities we do, and our emotional state. Textbook perfect blood pressure is considered 120/80. A blood pressure reading over 150/90 is considered by many health-care practitioners to be high blood pressure—the danger zone.

Elevated blood pressure is most common in the elderly and overweight. Over 60 million Americans—that's two-thirds of those over the age of sixty-five—have high blood pressure. And its dangers are very real. It's a leading cause of heart attacks and strokes. Numerous studies show that it's a disease found primarily in developed countries, so diet and lifestyle clearly are a link. Blood pressure medications are among the most prescribed drugs in this country, and most have serious side effects. Changing your diet and lifestyle are the two most important changes you can make in taking the pressure off.

What the Numbers Say

When you hear the term *normal* blood pressure, normal is considered a range, not a specific number. The number to be most concerned about is the bottom number. It's the one that indicates wear and tear on your heart.

Normal reading = 120/80 to 140/85 or less
Borderline reading = 140/85 to 150/90
High reading = 150/90 or higher

AROMATHERAPY

Hypotensive oils. The essential oils used to help decrease blood pressure are known for their relaxing and sedating properties. It makes sense that if high blood pressure is a result of too much stress and stimulation of the nervous and circulatory systems, then calming these systems would be appropriate and beneficial. Essential oils that fall into this category include chamomile, clary sage, lavender, lemon, mandarin, marjoram, neroli, nutmeg, rose, and ylang-ylang.

BREATH WORK

Regulate more than your breath. Full, deep breathing exercises and stretches are highly recommended, since performing these simple exercises encourages relaxation and regulation of blood pressure. Read the section on breathing to get a better understanding of the importance of proper breathing and how to do it effectively.

DIET

Shun major suspects. Avoid table (refined) salt, fats, and stimulants such as caffeine, nicotine, and alcohol. Caffeine has been shown to contribute to hypertension, and alcohol temporarily raises blood pressure. Sugar and salt have also been found to be culprits in raising blood pressure.

Eat more vegetables. Vegetarians have shown considerably lower risk for hypertension; therefore, a diet based on high-fiber, low-animal fats, and low refined sugar is advantageous to lowering blood pressure.

This lean green is great. Asparagus is especially helpful for high blood pressure as it aids the removal of fluids and impurities from the body.

Do your heart good. The following food guidelines are a good guide for preventing heart disease and, by extension, are helpful in high blood pressure as well:

- Avoid hydrogenated oils: margarine, vegetable shortening, and lard.
- Eat more potassium-rich foods: dark green leafy vegetables, bananas, and sea vegetables.
- Increase omega-3 fatty acids: coldwater fish, raw nuts, and flaxseed.
- Maximize magnesium-rich foods: wheat germ, broccoli, and dark leafy greens.
- Use Celtic Sea salt instead of refined table salt (see "Much More Than a Grain of Salt" on page 262).
- Favor calcium-rich edibles: collard and mustard greens, kale, and broccoli.
- Drink plenty of pure water and herbal tea: Mineral water high in magnesium is best.
- Eat alum family foods: onions and garlic.

HERBS

Find a good herbalist. There is a plethora of evidence that herbs are effective in fighting the causes of heart disease, including high blood pressure. They include arjuna bark, basil, black cumin seeds, black pepper, cayenne, dandelion, European mistletoe, fennel, garlic, ginger root, Ginkgo biloba, hawthorn leaf and berry, Indian snake root, kudzu, motherwort, olive leaf, onions, oregano, saffron, Siberian ginseng, skullcap, tarragon, valerian root, and yarrow.

If you have high blood pressure and want to try herbs, I recommend you consult a qualified herbalist concerning dosages and the proper use of the herbs.

HYDROTHERAPY

Soak stress away. If you like to take baths, you already know the relaxation and calm they can bring. Imagine adding essential oils that are known to decrease blood pressure, promote relaxation, and enhance your feeling of well-being. It's a powerful combination!

Sip a cup of herbal tea made from one of the herbs listed above, light a candle, and play some soft background music. You will feel the stresses of the day melting away. But don't just take my word for it. Try it yourself.

Be sure to draw the correct water temperature. If the water is too hot (above 101 degrees), it has the effect of increasing blood pressure and circulation.

ℒℴ No-Tension Hypertension Bath ℴ⅃

> 4 tablespoons Celtic Sea or Dead Sea salt
> 3 drops lavender essential oil
> 2 drops marjoram essential oil
> 2 drops mandarin essential oil
> 1 drop geranium essential oil

Add the salt to a small dish. Mix in the essential oils and stir. Add the aromatic salt to a warm bath. For a simple carrier, use cream or honey. Recipes for different carrier options are given in Appendix B on page 500. Use warm water (92 to

100 degrees) to promote relaxation. Soak and relax for 20 to 30 minutes three times a week.

Go for variety. Other aromatic baths that have calming and sedative benefits are the Serenity Blend (page 147), Stress-Relief Retreat (page 460), Milk and Honey Lover's Bath (page 428), and Child's Play (page 350). Also, the alkalizing aromatic bath on page 350 is beneficial to those with an acidic body system, commonly linked to hypertension.

INHALATION

Breathe and relax. Since stress release is so important to relieving high blood pressure, I recommend filling the room air with calming essential oils. Inhalation is so advantageous because it directly goes to the nervous, circulatory, and respiratory systems.

An electric diffuser is the most effective way to introduce healing benefits of essential oils via inhalation. The following recipe can be used in a diffuser by preparing a greater quantity of blended essential oils. For inhaling from a tissue or putting a few drops in an aroma lamp, make this recipe in smaller amounts.

〰 Pressure's–Off Oil 〰

4 parts lavender essential oil
2 parts ylang-ylang essential oil
1 part clary sage essential oil
1 part nutmeg essential oil

Mix the essential oils in an amber glass bottle. Use drops if a small amount is needed, and teaspoons if a large amount is needed for diffuser use. Use in moderation by diffusing three to four times per day in 10-minute durations. For even more benefit, practice breathing exercises while the diffuser is on.

LIFESTYLE

Make the effort; it's worth it. Many studies have proven that lifestyle changes in and of themselves can lower blood pressure naturally. Blood pressure medication doesn't have to be an automatic sentence. Below are recommendations based on scientific studies:

- *Exercise.* Just walking briskly for twenty minutes a day can bring pressure down.
- *Check your emotional triggers.* As many as one-third of people with hypertension may have repressed emotions. Fear, anger, chronic anxiety, and psychological and social stress can contribute to hypertension, in addition to intimate relationship and job-related stress.
- *Stop smoking.* Nicotine constricts the smaller blood vessels and tends to raise blood pressure, in addition to increasing your risk of heart attack.

TEAS AND TONICS

Drink to your health. This herbal tea blend was developed especially for people with high blood pressure. It is a safe combination of diuretic, antioxidant, vasodilating, adrenal-stimulating, cardio-tonic, and stress-relieving herbs. The added vitamin C, in the form of rose hips, has been proven effective in scientific studies in lowering blood pressure on its own. This is a dynamic yet simple herbal tonic you can make at home and sip throughout the day.

_◌_ Pressure–Ease Formula ◌_

1 part hawthorn leaf and berry

1 part Siberian ginseng

1 part licorice root

1 part valerian root

1 part dandelion leaf and root

1 part butcher's broom

3 parts ginger root

3 parts rose hips

Stevia as sweetener (optional)

Mix the dried herbs in a plastic bag or glass jar. Label. Place 1 to 2 teaspoons per cup of water in a pot. Simmer over low heat for 5 minutes. Strain and sweeten with stevia if you wish. I suggest that you make at least 3 to 4 cups at a time and keep it in the refrigerator. Drink 2 to 3 cups daily.

Yoga and Movement

Go flat out. This yoga pose effectively removes stress, lowers blood pressure, and slows the respiration and pulse rate. It is called the "corpse pose" and is one of the classic and most popular yogic poses. Studies have shown that performing this pose helps to relieve high blood pressure and assists in regulating heart conditions due to its profound relaxing effect on the entire body. Complete directions on how to fully relax into this easy lying posture are given on page 84.

When to Call the Doctor

Do not take an elevated blood pressure lightly. Consult regularly with your health care practitioner.

If you are currently taking medication, you should not discontinue it or substitute any natural treatments without the knowledge and consent of your physician.

Hyperactivity

Keeping Kids Calm

Throwing a tantrum, wailing, cranky, excitable, overtired, testy. Describe it as you will; every mother will know what you're talking about.

Hyperactive behavior in a child is quite common (granted, more common in some than others). But an overactive child isn't necessarily "hyperactive" or overly active all the time. Sometimes children are overactive only at certain times of the day, or after eating certain foods, or in response to the current environment. "Overactive" doesn't mean abnormal or that something is wrong. In most cases, it's family business as usual. That doesn't mean you have to grin and bear it. When all-out bedlam breaks loose and your patience won't allow you to wait it out, here are some tactics to bring peace and calm.

AROMATHERAPY

The road to tranquillity. A child in a state of overstimulation and excitement can benefit from relaxation and sedative essential oils. These oils can also help ease tantrums, anxiety attacks, and overtiredness. Aromatherapy works on a subtle level and is very unlike medicinal drugs that tend to take over the body's normal rhythm. Relaxation oils are natural plant derivatives that aid the body in relaxing, slowing the respiratory and heart rate, and soothing an overstimulated nervous system.

Essential oils that can help the overactive child—in fact, anyone in an excitable state—are cedarwood, chamomile, clary sage, cypress, hyssop, juniper, lavender, mandarin, marjoram, neroli, orange, sandalwood, tangerine, and ylang-ylang. These oils can be used in baths, massage oils, or for inhalation. Most of these essences should only be used on children between six and twelve years of age. You can use the chamomile, lavender, orange, and tangerine on slightly younger children (between three and six years).

DIET

Compare intake to outburst. Is there any correlation between the foods your child eats and his hyperactive behavior? If so, your child could have a food allergy. Likely suspects include foods and drinks containing sugar, synthetic sugar substitutes, caffeine-containing foods like colas and chocolate, milk, wheat, oranges, yeast, and food additives.

If you suspect a certain food is contributing to cranky behavior, eliminate the food from your child's diet and observe the results. If you suspect an allergy, it's best to discuss it with your pediatrician.

HYDROTHERAPY

Calm with water. Aromatic baths can be very relaxing and calming for the overactive child. One of the single essential oils listed in this section can be used, or one of the other relaxing recipes given in this book, specifically the Serenity Blend (page 147), and Child's Play (page 350). Be sure to use half the adult dose for children, as many of these are given in amounts for adults.

INHALATION

It's in the air. A good and safe way to calm a child with essential oils is to get to the brain via the olfactory system with a simple mist. With every breath, essences are having a direct effect on the nervous system.

Use this aromatic water to mist a room, furniture, pillowcase, or telephone.

❧ Mellow Mist ❧

1 cup distilled water
20 drops mandarin essential oil
10 drops lavender essential oil
5 drops marjoram essential oil
5 drops sandalwood essential oil

Fill a spray bottle with the distilled water. Add the essential oils. Shake well before each use, as the essential oils float to the top of the water and are not soluble in water on their own.

Diffuse trouble before it starts. This blend is good for a diffuser or an aroma lamp. Turn the diffuser on 15 minutes before your child arrives home from school.

❧ Slow-Motion Oil ❧

4 parts lavender essential oil
1 part clary sage essential oil
1 part cedarwood essential oil
1 part sandalwood essential oil

Mix the essential oils in an amber glass bottle. Shake gently and cap securely. Label contents. Diffuse 10 to 15 minutes prior to your child coming home from school or use as needed for overactivity. Diffuse for 15 minutes at a time. The essences will last several hours in the room air. May be diffused up to three times per day.

Moderation is key. When using therapeutic essential oils for relaxation, or for any other psycho-emotional problem, you must make sure that the essences are used within normal dosages and not overused. If too much essential oil is used or if it is abused, the opposite effect of overwhelming the nervous system (and other systems involved) will result.

Real-Life Cure

MOM WINS THE TEST OF TESTINESS

A friend of mine was troubled by her teenage daughter who was coming home from middle school every afternoon acting "very hyper." She described her as "loud, obnoxious, and testy." It began to bother her so much that she asked me if aromatherapy would help.

I gave my friend a recipe for a room mist and an aromatherapy blend for use in her diffuser. I suggested a massage with calming oils, but this clearly was not an option for this girl, who could barely sit still.

Unbeknownst to her daughter, my friend diffused the essential oils in the kitchen and family room right before she came home from school. The room mist was used in her daughter's bedroom and even sprayed on the phone! Before long, her daughter was coming home from school, cool, calm, and smiling.

When the secret came out, the daughter took it well. She even admitted she noticed a difference in her ability to concentrate. She looked forward to the relaxation of being home after a hectic day at school. She called the room spray Mellow Mist, as this was the effect it had on her. Months later, my friend used the same recipes for her husband, who was experiencing a lot of stress at work. It helped him, too!

Insomnia

❧

Sweet Smell of Sleep Ease

It's 2:00 A.M. You're lying in bed, eyes wide open, and your mind is racing with thoughts about how to get a good night's sleep. It's insomnia—again. And you are not alone.

Approximately 40 million Americans have a chronic sleep disorder; another 20 to 30 million experience occasional bouts of sleep disturbance. If you have insomnia, it's important to realize that it is a symptom, not an ailment, associated with poor-quality or disturbed sleep. It doesn't equate to the number of hours you sleep, but rather to how you feel when you wake up the next day.

We have a vital need for sleep. Without good-quality sleep, energy is not restored and rejuvenation is impossible. Trouble falling asleep or getting back to sleep once awakened during the night interferes with quality sleep. It means starting a new day feeling fatigued and possibly irritable. If insomnia lasts for long stretches of time, it can affect health in general and compromise the immune and nervous systems. Recent studies have found that natural killer cell activity (immune defenses) is lowered in people deprived of sleep. It's common for bad sleepers to get more colds than good sleepers.

There is no single answer to insomnia, but there are plenty of things you can try that should affect your sleep in a positive way. First, you need to find the reason why you are not sleeping.

Nervous tension, mental exhaustion, environmental stress, worry, anxiety, depression, and relationship problems are all stress-related conditions capable of causing you to lose a full night's sleep.

Another factor is a high body temperature. Normally, body temperature becomes cooler as metabolism and digestion slow down. A cooler body temperature is associated with deep sleep. Some water beds that do not have the ability to naturally adjust (lower) can affect sleep and possibly inhibit a deep state of sleep. Exercising in the evening can cause the same problem; it can take hours for body temperature to decrease.

Eating a heavy meal or drinking large amounts of liquid right before bedtime is almost always a guarantee of sleep disturbance because of the need to get up and urinate during the night. Drinking coffee or smoking cigarettes can interfere with sleep, as they are stimulants.

AROMATHERAPY

Slumber enhancers. Essential oils are commonly used for insomnia because they have relaxing and sedative characteristics. They are basil, cedarwood, chamomile, clary sage, cypress, frankincense, helichrysm, hyssop, laurel, lavender, lemongrass, marjoram, neroli, petitgrain, rose, sandalwood, spikenard, and ylang-ylang. Many of these oils work by stimulating the production of serotonin, a naturally occurring brain chemical that helps induce sleep. Lavender and chamomile are by far the most popular essential oils for encouraging relaxation and sleep.

The English Hospital Cure

Patients in hospitals in the United Kingdom have a wonderful way of falling asleep. Rather than dispense sleeping pills, nurses routinely sprinkle a few drops of lavender essential oil on bedsheets or offer aromatic baths or massage. Because it also has an analgesic effect, lavender is especially helpful to those who can't sleep due to pain.

Cool your calves. A surprisingly easy remedy for promoting sleep and alleviating restlessness is to spray your legs with cold water and lavender essential oil. This is especially welcoming during hot, humid summer evenings but can be just as effective during the drier winter months.

⁄⊘ Sleep-Ease Leg Spray ⊘⁄

Store this spray in the refrigerator to stay cold and bring it to your bedside at night.

1 cup cold water
12 to 16 drops lavender essential oil

Add the water and essential oil to a plastic spray bottle with a fine mist. Shake well. Label. Spray on your lower legs. I suggest that you sit at the bedside and spray your legs over the floor rather than above the sheets to prevent the bedding from getting damp.

HERBS

Take a natural sleeping pill. Traditional herbs that have sedative qualities are catnip, chamomile, hops, kava kava, lavender, lemon balm, passionflower, skullcap, and valerian. These herbs can be taken in the form of herbal infusion, herbal capsules, or tincture form according to the manufacturer's directions.

Try nutmeg and milk. A warm glass of milk is an old folk remedy to help induce sleep, and it works for many people. Unless you are lactose intolerant, milk is calming. Ground nutmeg contains minute amounts of myristicin and elemicin, which can encourage sleep and dreaming. I suggest you sprinkle a little nutmeg (a pinch is all it takes) in the cup and then add the warm milk. It is very comforting and will help ease muscle tension as well.

INHALATION

Timed dispersion. Inhaling of essential oils prior to going to bed and diffusing the oils again while you sleep can be extremely effective in preventing you from waking during the night. Bedrooms are a convenient place in which to use diffusers because they are usually small and you spend a lot of time there.

This inhalation blend is designed for general use—that is, it aids in promoting relaxation and sleep by calming the nervous system. An aromatic diffuser is the most effective method to use with essential oils for inhalation; it runs by electricity and can be connected to automatic timers to go on while you are asleep.

⟡ Peaceful Sleep Spray ⟡

Spray a few drops on your pillow and sheets.

7 parts lavender essential oil
2 parts marjoram essential oil*
1 part clary sage essential oil

Mix the essential oils in an amber glass bottle. Put in a diffuser and time it according to your sleep pattern. For example, if you consistently wake up at 2:30 A.M., set the timer to turn on at 2:00 A.M. Alternatively, add 20 drops (or double this recipe) to 4 ounces of water to make a room mister. Shake before each use.

Note: Marjoram oil may have the ability to lower blood pressure, so this blend is not recommended for regular use by anyone with this condition.

The Perfect Rest Cushion

Could your bed pillow be contributing to your troubled sleep? Your place of rest should be as inviting and comfortable as possible. Try one of these bedfellows:

- Body pillows—feather and goose down huggers
- Buckwheat pillows—firm; molds to your head and neck
- Eye pillows—lavender and flaxseed to relieve tension
- Goose down pillows—the plushest, in very soft or firm
- Herbal sleep pillows—lavender scented (recipe on page 310)
- Hypoallergenic pillows—100 percent synthetic for allergy sufferers
- Pregnancy pillows—shaped in a wedge design to support the abdomen
- Swedish foam pillows—conforms to your head; heat sensitive

Bedtime Tips for Children

THE 4 BS B 4 BEDTIME

For a child who can't sleep, encourage a positive bedtime routine by practicing these gentle approaches to promote sleep for your little ones. The structure makes them feel safe and cared for. Taking the time to prepare your child for bed, by following a routine, can save hours of restless and sleepless nights for both of you! This custom has worked for our family (and many others).

1. A warm aromatic **B**ath: Children relax and get clean while playing with bath toys.
2. Read a **B**ook: When they get older, they can read to you.
3. Go to the **B**athroom: They don't wake to void during the night.
4. A **B**ear hug and **B**utterfly kiss: A big hug and a delicate butterfly kiss (brushing your eyelashes by blinking against the child's cheek).

MASSAGE

Comfort kids with touch. Children are great fans of foot or hand massages. Favorite scents include lavender and mandarin essences. When they get into bed, massage their feet or hands with a little aromatic massage oil to promote relaxation and deep sleep. When the feet are warmed by local massage it seems to be especially comforting.

This recipe is very basic and simple to prepare. It is also useful during the day or early evening when children tend to be overactive or overtired.

✒ Sleep Oil for Children ✒

3 to 6 drops lavender or mandarin essential oil (or combination)
2 tablespoons warm vegetable oil

Mix the child's favorite essential oil (or combination of the two essences) in the warm vegetable oil. This can be made ahead and kept in an amber glass bottle or prepared in a shallow dish in half the amounts given. Massage the feet, working toward the heart. Use gentle but firm pressure.

Sleep Pillow Recipe

Keep this small pillow sachet inside your pillowcase to encourage sleep and peaceful dreams. To refresh them simply put a few drops of lavender and chamomile on the pillow. Fluff in the dryer for a few minutes along with a damp washcloth.

✧ Sweet Dreams Pillow ✧

This makes a great gift.

4 parts sweet woodruff (smells like fresh-mown hay)
2 parts lemon balm
2 parts lavender
1 part each of the following herbs and spices:
    chamomile, cinnamon, hops, marjoram, mugwort, rosebuds,
    rosemary (grind the leaves so they don't poke through
    the pillow), sage, southernwood, and thyme
1 part orris root (powdered or finely grated)
Chamomile, lavender, and marjoram essential oils

Mix the above combination of sleep-inducing herbs, flowers, and spices in a large bowl. If you are making one pillow, the portions can be 1 tablespoon = 1 part. If you are making enough for gifts, use 1 cup = 1 part. However, when it comes time to add the essential oils, add about 3 to 5 drops per pillow. To do this, simply

continued . . .

count out the drops onto the orris root and mix well with a spoon or mortar and pestle. Then add this to the premixed herbs in the bowl. Put about 1 to 1½ cups of herbs into each pillow, depending on the size. Sew up the opening. Now tuck your sleep pillow inside your bed pillow.

Sweet dreams.

SOUND AND MUSIC THERAPY

A sound sleep. Restful vibrations that encourage sound sleep are ever so soothing and lullabylike. They'll also help you fall asleep quickly. The following selections are recommended:

Roth—*You Are the Ocean*
Night Music
Massenet—*Meditation*
Brahms—*Lullaby*
Schumann—*Traumerei (Dreams)*
Debussy—*Prelude to the Afternoon of a Faun; Clair de Lune*
Barber—*Adagio for Strings*
Environments—*Psychologically Ultimate Seashore; Optimum Aviary*

Jet Lag

GLAD TO BE BACK

With more and more people frequently traveling and making worldwide destinations within a day's time, jet lag and travel stress have become common ailments. It takes a good balancing act to avoid them.

Jet lag leaves you feeling in a fog. You're physically exhausted and mentally dull, and your appetite is in a total state of confusion. It can leave you with a headache, insomnia, and a weakened immune system. It's why so many travelers end up with a cold or other infection.

AROMATHERAPY

Balance the body. Essential oils that are recommended for jet lag help regulate and balance the mind and body. They are bergamot, frankincense, geranium, lavender, and rose. Many of the citrus oils can be used to refresh the mind and body, and the stimulating essential oils used to combat fatigue and lethargy are also helpful. These include basil, bergamot, clary sage, lavender, lemon, lemongrass, orange, peppermint, rosemary, spruce, and ylang-ylang.

Air treatment. This facial spray will help prevent dry skin as well as perk you up. Keep in mind that all essential oils are antibacterial in nature and will also help purify the air you breathe. Mist your face with it freely before boarding and while on the airplane. Spray your hotel room and rental car with it as well.

The Plane Facts About Jet Lag

There is a good reason why travel stress is called jet lag. And it is only partially due to traveling through time zones at 500 miles an hour.

The biggest cause is airplane environment. Many airplanes recycle and recirculate up to 50 percent of the cabin air. This air is dry and has a higher content of carbon dioxide and airborne bacteria levels. There is also a higher concentration of positive ions (as opposed to negative ions, which are health promoting) on airplanes.

Jet lag is so common that many airlines try to ease the problem with fresh food, wider seat spaces, and sleep aids such as blindfolds. But this is usually in business or first class. One British airline offers aromatherapy oils to all its travelers.

❧ On-the-Go Oil ❧

6 drops lavender essential oil
1 drop bergamot essential oil
1 drop lemongrass essential oil
½ cup distilled water or mineral water

Mix all the ingredients in a plastic spray bottle for travel. Shake well before each use, as the essential oils do not get dispersed in the water without a carrier. Spray over facial area with eyes closed. Inhale deeply with each application.

DIET

Plan ahead. Eating the right foods before and during a flight goes a long way toward preventing jet lag. Here are some commonsense rules:

- Eat light on the day prior to and the day you are traveling. This means avoiding high-fat foods, sweets, and alcohol.
- Eat a full, low-fat meal with plenty of fresh vegetables before boarding. This will help you avoid airplane fare.
- Avoid plane fare if you can. If not, order a special meal—either the diabetic or vegetarian meal.
- Avoid drinking alcohol and caffeine, as they are dehydrating in an already dehydrating environment. Plus, the altitude can make you feel the effects of alcohol faster.
- Drink plenty of pure water and juices to counteract the dry air and physiologic stress that come with traveling.
- Eat foods rich in antioxidants, especially vitamin C, and bring these supplements with you.

HYDROTHERAPY

Make time. Aromatic baths are excellent ways to recover from jet lag and travel stress. When my husband was traveling frequently on the job, he tried many blends, but this was one of his favorites. I believe he liked it not only because the familiar fragrance was comforting but also because it became a conditioned response.

⟨𝒪 On-the-Go Bath Blend 𝒪⟩

7 drops lavender essential oil
2 drops geranium essential oil
1 drop bergamot essential oil
4 tablespoons Celtic Sea salt
or Dead Sea salt

Draw a warm (92 to 100 degrees) bath. Mix the essential oils with the salt and pour into the bath. Dim the lights for a soothing, quiet, peaceful time alone. Place a cool washcloth on your forehead. Sip some fresh lemon water or chamomile tea. Get to bed a little early tonight.

INHALATION

Keep the right company. This aromatherapy blend can be your best traveling companion on long trips. Saturate a few cotton balls and keep them in a plastic bag or bring a small vial of oil to inhale while traveling. Rosemary essential oil eases disorientation, stimulates the brain, and has antioxidant properties. Lavender and bergamot essential oils help regulate the body and reduce stress. The citrus oil is uplifting and purifying, which are additional benefits to this blend.

⟨𝒪 Time in a Bottle 𝒪⟩

An inhalation blend for travelers.

4 parts lavender essential oil
2 parts lemon essential oil
1 part rosemary essential oil
1 part bergamot essential oil

Mix the essential oils in a small amber glass bottle. Use a few drops on a tissue to inhale while traveling.

MASSAGE

Reset your body. You will find it very helpful to reset your electromagnetic body, which is often out of balance after flying. To do this exercise and keep the energy (*chi*) flowing, simply massage the breast bone area located about an inch below your clavicle, near the hollow of your neck. This is the main switch for energy flow in your body. With two fingers, press firmly on both sides in a circular motion for 20 to 30 seconds to stimulate these areas.

For other remedies that can help this condition, see Stress *and* Lethargy.

Laryngitis

CURES THAT SPEAK TO THE PROBLEM

Open wide and say—nothing!

Hoarseness or a lost voice is caused by overextending your vocal cords, a common occurrence, for example, after a night of cheering at a ballgame or talking over loud music at a local club or party.

The larynx, or voice box, houses the vocal cords, hence the term *laryngitis.* So, laryngitis is an inflammation of the larynx. The symptom is a change in the normal voice; typically, a hoarse, rough, or low voice is experienced. Laryngitis can occur with no other symptoms or with a sore throat.

AROMATHERAPY

Speak easy. Essential oils known to help with this ailment are chamomile, cypress, frankincense, geranium, ginger, lemon, pine, sandalwood, and thyme. These soothing essences decrease inflammation and tone throat tissues. The best essential oil applications for laryngitis are gargles, lozenges, and compresses. Additionally, throat drops can be made to soothe swelling in the throat region. Sugar cubes are used as the carrier. The lozenge is a good way to get medicine to the throat slowly. The following recipe should not be used more than three times per day and in conjunction with the other remedies.

✏ Laryngitis Lozenge ✑

1 drop geranium essential oil
1 sugar cube or zinc lozenge

Put 1 drop of geranium essential oil on the sugar cube or zinc lozenge. Gradually melt the lozenge in your mouth, allowing the medicine to slowly soothe the throat. Avoid eating or drinking immediately following. Do not exceed three per day.

Irrigate your throat. A gargle of geranium essential oil in water is another extremely effective and simple treatment for hoarseness. It's especially helpful for people who must use their voice a lot, like teachers. Mix 1 drop of geranium essential oil in ½ teaspoon of honey and stir into a cup of cool water. Gargle well for as long as possible.

Hydrotherapy

Pack it on. A cold compress is very helpful in alleviating the swelling that is sometimes part of laryngitis. The essential oils chosen are ones that are anti-inflammatory and work especially well on the throat and larynx.

✏ Adam's Apple Compress ✑

1 to 2 cups cold water
4 drops lavender essential oil
2 drops geranium essential oil
2 drops frankincense essential oil

Pour the cold water into a bowl. The temperature should be 60 to 70 degrees. Add the essential oils and swish the water to disperse them as much as possible. Soak the cloth in the aromatic water. Remove the cloth and wring most of the moisture from it. Apply to the Adam's apple area. Re-apply after it becomes warm/body temperature. Leave on a total of 15 to 20 minutes for the full benefit. Lie down during the compress application. Repeat three times per day.

LIFESTYLE

Nurse your voice. For the speediest recovery, do the following:

- Rest your voice. The less you talk, the faster you will heal.
- Avoid dairy products; they increase mucus formation.
- Increase fluid intake by sipping cold liquids. Avoid hot temperatures, which can be irritating.
- Get more rest.
- Make a big pot of Old-Fashioned Garlic and Onion Soup (page 137) and sip it freely. Be careful that it isn't too hot when you eat it.

MASSAGE

Balance your throat chakra. For laryngitis (and virtually all respiratory ailments), the throat chakra can be stimulated or balanced through massage. Located in front of the throat, this area can easily be massaged with an unscented lotion mixed with an appropriate essential oil of your choice. Sandalwood is one of my favorites. Massage gently in a circular, clockwise direction for a minute or longer. Concentrate on your breath and the intention of healing your voice.

Real-Life Cure

AN OPERA SINGER'S SCARE

Adolfo, a friendly sixty-two-year-old opera singer, heard about aromatherapy through a friend who had taken a class of mine. He did not have laryngitis when he consulted with me, but he wanted information and guidance as to what to do the next time he experienced voice loss or hoarseness. As you might imagine, this was his greatest fear.

He took excellent care of his health and was very oriented toward preventive health. He had experienced laryngitis, which he described as "disastrous," several times in his opera career.

A good year or more passed without hearing another word from him. Then he called while on an engagement in San Francisco. It was a good-news call.

Adolfo told me that he carried the essential oils I recommended with him every time he went out of town so he was always prepared for the worst. When he arrived in San Francisco, he developed early signs of laryngitis. He gargled with geranium oil and water and used the Adam's Apple Compress. His symptoms decreased in a little less than a day, and he was able to sing the following evening, with his best voice. He was elated!

For other remedies, see Colds *and* Sore Throat.

Lethargy

⟋◌

INVIGORATING PICK-ME-UPS

Do you struggle to get started in the morning? Sneak a catnap in the afternoon or reach for a caffeine rush to stay tuned? Do you fall asleep in the evening while watching television before you find out "who done it?"

We all get fatigued from time to time, but lethargy that feels everlasting, especially when we wake in the morning, is a real handicap to living life as we are meant to.

Lethargy is a broad term covering a universe of ailments. Virtually any type of health condition sooner or later flashes fatigue as a warning sign. But stress and a hectic lifestyle can also leave us drained when we need to be awake. Resolving disease-caused lethargy requires getting to the root of the problem. But, for run-of-the mill fatigue, there are some pleasant and effective ways to perk yourself up.

No Fatigue in the Forest

Walk in a forest on a cold crisp day and I bet you'll start feeling a surge of energy within minutes.

It's no surprise that many of the energy-producing oils come from oxygenating forest scents. Cedarwood, cypress, eucalyptus, fir, juniper, pine, and spruce all possess stimulating, mentally invigorating properties. Every Christmas when we sit around the decorated evergreen tree, I am reminded of how excited and happy I feel when in the presence of these scents.

AROMATHERAPY

Better than coffee. Eucalyptus heads the list of essential oils that give a quick energy hit. In one study, long-distance truck drivers were asked to inhale the eucalyptus oil whenever they felt tired. It was found to be more effective than caffeine and other stimulants—without the side effects!

Real-Life Cure

SLEEPY IN SEATTLE

I was part of a small study investigating the stimulating properties of black spruce essential oil. Following a long hot day of note taking, lectures, and discussion, many of us were lethargic, to say the least. Some people were even napping!

A naturopathic physician went around the room applying the essential oil of black spruce to each sleepy student. Within what seemed like seconds, many of us felt a surge of energy. We were wide-eyed, invigorated, and mentally alert, myself included.

My husband and I always use essential oils to help keep us awake and invigorated on long car trips. In addition to increasing alertness, aromatherapy offers a pleasant and aromatic environment within the confines of an automobile.

Other oils that have stimulating qualities are basil, bergamot, cedarwood, cypress, eucalyptus, fir, ginger, grapefruit, juniper, lemon, lemongrass, lime, peppermint, pine, rosemary, and spruce. Essential oils that produce a feeling of euphoria are also helpful for their invigorating effect. These include clary sage, grapefruit, jasmine, rose, and ylang-ylang.

BREATH WORK

Breath as art. The act of respiration is not just an automatic function of life as many assume. It is actually a nonphysical phenomenon and bio-energetic function. To me, breathing is an art form. Your breath is intimately connected to your body and mental realms. Breath energy flows through your body in waves, energizing and supporting metabolic processes and restructuring your energy (*pranic*) body. This is very important in counteracting lethargic states. To fully understand the value of breathing and for instructions on proper breathing techniques, read the section starting on page 18.

DIET

Nourish your body. A poor diet is a chief contributor to fatigue. Too much fat, too much sugar, and too much food in general only make you ache for a good nap. Treat your body kindly. Eat well-balanced, healthy, regular meals based on plenty of green leafy vegetables and sea vegetables, citrus fruits, and berries. Eat only low-fat, high-fiber foods that are fresh and organic.

Alcohol, caffeine, black tea, and sugar may give you an initial rush of energy but will result in a backlash of greater fatigue.

HYDROTHERAPY

Foot soak that gets you dancing. Stimulating scents come in handy when, at the end of the day, you find yourself tired and run-down when you're supposed to be getting ready for a night out. My savior of the night is this stimulating footbath. It'll get you out of your loafers and into your dancing shoes in no time.

Dancing Feet Treat

2 drops pine essential oil
2 drops rosemary essential oil
1 drop clary sage essential oil
1 drop peppermint essential oil
2 tablespoons Celtic Sea salt or
    Detoxifying Bath Salts (page 128)

Mix the essential oils in the sea salt. Add the aromatic salt to the basin of cold water and stir with your hands. Sit comfortably in a chair, allowing your feet to soak in the footbath for 20 minutes. Sit quietly while doing some deep breathing exercises. To make this aromatherapy treatment even more exhilarating, place a bag of marbles or small pebbles at the bottom of the basin while you soak, for an instant acupressure/reflexology treatment.

Splash in the tropics. This full-body bath treatment is my sister's favorite pick-me-up. It is a blend of citrus fruit and the leaf from the orange tree, so it naturally has a tropical, breezy scent.

Revival Bath Blend

5 drops bergamot essential oil
5 drops petitgrain essential oil
4 tablespoons Celtic Sea salt
    (or other carrier of choice)

Draw a tepid to warm (80 to 100 degrees) bath. Perform dry skin brushing for an added benefit. Add the essential oils to the salt and pour into the bathwater. Relax and soak for 15 minutes or longer. Dry briskly.

INHALATION

Breathe in the energy. Whenever you need to stay awake, alert, and mentally stimulated, you will want this diffuser synergy in the air. It is very useful for people who work indoors and must read, study, or work numbers all day, to aid in preventing mental and physical exhaustion. Put on a nature video and diffuse this blend for the next best thing to being outdoors in the fresh air.

❧ Invigoration Oil ❧

2 parts eucalyptus essential oil
2 parts juniper essential oil
2 parts grapefruit essential oil
1 part clary sage essential oil
1 part ginger essential oil

Combine the essential oils in an amber glass bottle. Use in a variety of ways for inhalation, such as a diffuser, humidifier, room spray, aroma lamp, or tissue.

MASSAGE

Reset your zones. If you're low on energy all the time, you may need to reset your *chi*—your energy flow. You can do this by locating the acupuncture points below the hollow area at the base of your throat and an inch to each side. Use firm rotary pressure to stimulate this area for 20 to 30 seconds. The areas may be sore to touch—an indication that they are out of balance. These points are the energy centers for the kidney meridian and keep the chi energy flowing through the electromagnetic body.

SOUND AND MUSIC THERAPY

Vivacious vibrations. Marches were originally written in an upbeat arrangement to stimulate action in the soldiers. These selections definitely have a pronounced, stimulating effect. *Caution:* This music, in combination with aromatherapy, may cause you to start dancing around the room!

Respighi—*Ancient Dances and Airs; Pines of Rome*
Suppe—*Poet and Peasant Overture; Light Cavalry Overture*
Lyre Bird—(Concorde, Hastings)
Sousa—*Stars and Stripes Forever*
Schubert—*March Militaire*
Beethoven—*Turkish March*
Clarke—*Trumpet Voluntary*
Erica Azim—*Mbira* (Zimbabwe music)

TEAS AND TONICS

Tune-up tonic. This simple blend of stimulating herbs is packed with potency. It makes a nice cool beverage on a hot summer day. Garnish with fresh lemon peel and mint leaves for a festive drink. Try to find organic sources for the green tea and herbs.

℘ Vitalitea ℘

To health and vitality!

1 cup loose green tea
⅓ cup peppermint herb
¼ cup lemon balm herb or lemon verbena
2 teaspoons rosemary herb
2 cups boiling water
4 ⅛-inch slices fresh ginger root
    or 2 teaspoons powdered ginger
Fresh lemon peel and mint leaves (optional)
Stevia or Ginger Honey to sweeten (page 48)

When to Call the Doctor

One in seven visits to the doctor involves chronic fatigue and lethargy that won't go away. Some forms of fatigue can indicate an underlying disorder, such as a dysfunctional thyroid, weakened immune system, diabetes, or iron deficiency. So it is a good idea to get checked by your physician if your fatigue doesn't improve after making the recommended lifestyle changes.

Mix the green tea, peppermint, lemon balm, and rosemary in a jar and label. To prepare, bring 2 cups of water to a boil. Add 2 to 3 teaspoons of the herbal tea mix, grated ginger, and fresh lemon peel and mint leaves (if desired) and simmer gently for 3 minutes. Remove from the heat and strain. Add the stevia or Ginger Honey to taste. Drink hot or cold.

Loss of Appetite

🌀

STIMULATE THOSE TASTE BUDS

This is a condition dieters would kill to get—until they got it. It wouldn't take very long to find out how unpleasant this condition can be.

Loss of appetite deprives us of one of the joys of life—eating. But for those truly afflicted, it can leave them open to immune problems, fatigue, and anemia. Loss of appetite, in fact, can be a sign that something serious is happening in the body. Emotional upheavals can leave us without an appetite as well. Certain drugs, or combinations of drugs, can kill our appetite. But it's also a temporary side effect of common conditions that affect the respiratory and digestive systems, like a cold or flu, sinusitis, and gastritis.

Loss of appetite linked to physical or emotional problems needs to be addressed professionally. Otherwise, these remedies will help get those appetite juices flowing.

HERBS

Herbs that work on digestion and appetite are called carminative herbs, meaning they are digestive stimulants and increase appetite. Among the most common are burdock, ginger, goldenseal, hops, Oregon grape, and quassia. Other herbs known to do the same and also help improve nutrient absorption are alfalfa, barley grass, dandelion root, fennel seed, ginger root, licorice root, nettles, and parsley leaf. These herbal remedies can be taken in the form of teas, tinctures, or capsules.

Cooking with clove, fennel, garlic, ginger, lemon, nutmeg, and orange will help spur a sluggish digestive system.

LIFESTYLE

Put appeal on the menu. People who must cook for themselves or eat alone are often poor eaters. This is because much of the pleasure of a meal is absent. They often eat prepared food and consume it in front of the television.

Make an effort to prepare a fresh cooked meal. Set the table, invite a friend, put flowers on the table, or go out for a meal at least three times a week.

MASSAGE

Stimulate your sternum and your appetite. The solar plexus is a major chakra that governs digestion. It is located directly below the sternum (breast bone). This chakra is known as the energy distribution system, which involves collecting energy and sending it to where it is needed.

When this energy center is functioning properly you will experience mind/body harmony, emotional flexibility, and a good appetite. To perform chakra balancing of this area, gently massage in a circular motion with your hand. Start with small circles, gradually enlarging and returning back to the center point. This can be done over your clothing or with an aromatic massage oil or lotion on your skin. Concentrate on relaxing your breath while doing this.

This chakra massage is most effective half an hour before meals. Apply over the solar plexus as well as the stomach area and backs of the hands. Use sparingly, as this is a concentrated blend. Inhale as needed from the backs of the hands.

⚭ Before-Meal Massage ⚭

1 drop bergamot essential oil
1 drop ginger essential oil
1 drop of chamomile, clary sage, or rose essential oil
1 tablespoon warm vegetable oil

Mix a total of 3 drops of essential oil in warm vegetable oil. Rub on your palms, hold over your mouth and nose and inhale for a few seconds, then rub the oil over the solar plexus (just below the sternum), backs of hands, and back of neck. When working over the solar plexus area, go in a counterclockwise direction to promote relaxation. Do this 30 minutes or more prior to your largest meal of the day.

Is It Anorexia?

Anorexia nervosa is a serious eating disorder characterized by self-starvation brought on by a skewed self-perception. It is most frequently seen in teenage girls; however, recent information shows a rise in adolescent males as well.

Anorexia nervosa occurs in people who are thin or normal weight but see themselves in the mirror as fat. It's a life-threatening condition. Signs of a problem include significant weight loss, amenorrhea (absence of a normal menses), obsession with body weight and size, excessive dieting and exercise, dry skin, abnormal hair growth, cold hands and feet, and sleep disturbances.

TEAS AND TONICS

All of the herbs and spices included in this recipe are known to stimulate appetite.

Taste Tea

Guaranteed to stimulate your appetite.

¼ teaspoon caraway seed
¼ teaspoon cardamom
1¼-inch slice fresh ginger root or ¼ teaspoon dried ginger
¼ teaspoon dried Gentian root
1 cup water
Ginger Honey (page 48) or plain honey to taste (optional)

Gently boil the herbs and spices, covered, for 5 minutes in 1 cup of water. Strain and sweeten if desired. Sip at least 30 minutes before meals.

For other remedies, see Anosmia.

Low Blood Pressure

THE PERFECT TUNE-UP

Given a choice—which, unfortunately, you don't have—you're better off having low rather than high blood pressure. High blood pressure, known as the "silent killer," can lead to heart disease or stroke due to the constant pounding on the arteries. It's called "silent" because it doesn't show any symptoms.

Low blood pressure, however, usually isn't life threatening, though it does make its presence known. It can leave you light-headed, dizzy, or faint. Low blood pressure is diagnosed after a concurrent reading of 90/60.

AROMATHERAPY

Put the pressure on. Essential oils increase blood pressure by stimulating and toning the function and activity of the circulatory system. Known as cardio-tonic oils, they are hyssop, lemon, and rosemary. These essences can be inhaled from a tissue or diffused in the room several times per day. Black pepper, cypress, ginger, and peppermint are essential oils that help constrict the blood vessels and can be used in combination with hyssop and rosemary.

HERBS

Go with tradition. Most herbs have a regulatory effect on blood pressure, but only a handful are well known for affecting low blood pressure. They are cinnamon, clove, ginseng, oats, rosemary, sage, and thyme. Cook with these herbs and spices regularly.

HYDROTHERAPY

Turn off the hot water. If a hot shower or bath makes you dizzy, it could be a sign of low blood pressure. Hot water relaxes you and slows your pressure. This bath, using tepid water and aromatics, will gently stimulate circulation. Optimal temperature for stimulating circulation is a tepid bath temperature of approximately 80 to 101 degrees.

✍ Pressure-Boosting Bath Salts ✍

4 drops rosemary essential oil
2 drops geranium essential oil
1 drop hyssop essential oil
1 drop eucalyptus essential oil
4 to 8 tablespoons Celtic Sea
   or Dead Sea salt, bath salt, or honey

Simply add the essential oils to the carrier of your choice and mix well before adding to the bathwater. For low blood pressure I recommend a tepid water temperature (80 to 92 degrees) as this is stimulating in general. Soak for 20 minutes or longer.

Shower it on. In lieu of the bath, you can opt for an aromatic shower. Mix 6 to 10 drops of any of the essential oils listed here with 2 tablespoons of Castile Soap or an unscented shower gel, and apply in the shower. End your aromatic shower with cool water to further stimulate your whole body.

Stimulate the skin. Prior to a bath or shower, get your circulation moving with dry skin brushing. This vitalizing treatment boosts circulation, tones organs, and refreshes the entire body. It makes you feel very alive! Be sure to use only a natural bristled brush. See Dry Skin Brushing on page 40.

If you do not have a skin brush, you can substitute a dry washcloth. A new one is best, as it is a bit coarser for skin stimulation.

Tip: Cold-Feet Cure

If you have perpetual cold feet, try warming them in a small basin of tepid water (80 to 92 degrees) spiked with Pressure-Boosting Bath Salts. Simply decrease the amount in the recipe by half. For a footbath, you can even make the temperature cooler than recommended for a full bath. It will actually warm your feet by stimulating circulation.

INHALATION

I love this blend because it's a delightful herbal garden scent. It's best used in a diffuser. If using an electric diffuser, I recommend leaving it on for 10 minutes each time. The essential oils will last several hours in the room air, so no need to turn it on again for several hours.

Increase the benefits of the inhalation by performing deep breathing exercises throughout the day to boost circulation and increase oxygen to the cells.

✒ Garden–Scented Room Spray ✒

A perfect blend to increase circulation.

2 parts rosemary essential oil
2 parts hyssop essential oil
1 part cypress essential oil
1 part peppermint essential oil

Mix the essential oils in drops for inhaling from a tissue or make it in larger amounts for diffuser use by measuring in teaspoon amounts.

Note: Moderation in all things. Do not overdo it with natural cures. Too much of a good thing can be harmful or can even have the opposite effect! Moderation and balance are keys to success with aromatherapy and other forms of botanical medicine, especially when it comes to the circulatory system.

MASSAGE

Balance the heart chakra. This massage involves a heightened mental focus that can be extremely effective for balancing the heart and nerve plexus and the heart chakra. The heart chakra is the body center closely linked to the bloodstream and the immune system.

The area to massage is directly over the heart. Use a gentle clockwise motion with your mental focus on balance and regulation. Unscented lotion can be combined with the essential oils listed in this section. Pick scents you like the best. You will notice many of the oils for regulating low blood pressure are derived from stimulating spices and herbs.

SOUND AND MUSIC THERAPY

The sound of pressure rising. There is a wonderful assortment of fine music, as well as fun and lively selections that are useful for raising blood pressure and energizing the body. A list of selected marching tunes can be found on page 323. Or try some of your old favorites that will get the blood pumping, such as ragtime, boogie-woogie, rock 'n' roll, bebop, or swing. Native American and African music with drumming also can be invigorating.

For other remedies, see Lethargy.

Memory Loss

❧

SEIZE THE SENIOR MOMENTS

Seldom do people talk about all the benefits of aging, like a larger vocabulary, greater understanding of the written word, an elevated ability to reason, spiritual growth, and the accumulated wisdom based on life experience. These are significant cognitive achievements that can only be acquired through living a long, meaningful, full life. These achievements, unfortunately, are overshadowed by fear—the fear of senility and Alzheimer's disease.

Dementia is defined as the gradual lessening of reasoning ability, concentration, and memory. Some memory loss is normal as we age; however, the ravaging effects of senility and mental decline are not inevitable. That's why the old adage—"Use it or lose it"—has been linked to our minds.

Our brains slow down as we age because nerve cells weaken and die. There are a hundred billion neurons, with a trillion connections within each cubic centimeter of brain tissue, firing ten million billion times each second. The interaction of these neurochemical connections (synapses) forms the crucial basis of what we know as stored memory. It boggles the mind just thinking about it!

Scientific evidence shows that the best way to protect our brain cells is to keep them active. An active brain is a healthy brain.

BREATH WORK

Brain fuel. Oxygen is brain fuel and is absolutely essential to keeping brain cells alive. Proper deep breathing increases life force energy, stimulates hormones in the brain, increases alertness and clarity, and decreases fear and insecurity.

Older people tend be shallow breathers and thus need to be sure to practice deep breathing in order to exercise their lungs and brains. Follow the instructions for The Healing Breath on page 216 to stimulate and invigorate memory.

DIET

Feed the brain. You have the opportunity to design a dynamite program for yourself when you combine positive lifestyle habits with proper nutrition. Moderation in your eating, by decreasing fatty, non-organic meat consumption and eating more organic vegetables, including sea vegetables, is a good idea.

Feed your brain the needed nutrients for optimal functioning: antioxidants (such as pycnogenol), B complex vitamins, coenzyme Q10, omega-3 fatty acids, selenium, vitamins C and E, and zinc.

HERBS

Ayurvedic advice. According to the ancient science of Ayurveda, there are two primary herbs that are essential in the treatment of memory loss: ashwaganda and brahmi. The aromatic root of ashwaganda, more commonly known as Indian ginseng (*Withania somnifera*), is often prescribed as a general tonic that nurtures and clears the mind. It is known to calm and strengthen the nervous system, promote sound sleep, and rejuvenate tissues throughout the body.

The other plant is brahmi (*Bacopa monniera*). Known as a smart nutrient or brain food, brahmi is said to improve intellectual thought processes. It is categorized as an adaptogen, meaning it has the ability to balance all the body systems (including the immune system) and help the body cope with stress. These Ayurvedic herbs can be purchased in capsule form in health food stores.

Cerebral energizers. Because the brain is sensitive to nutritional deficiency, it stands to reason that we should take advantage of the nourishing energy that herbs provide. They strengthen and sharpen the mind and encourage emotional balance without side effects.

The antioxidant herbs are intelligent choices and include capsicum, Ginkgo biloba, gotu kola, rosemary, and sage. Brain tonic stimulants are damiana, ginger, Ginkgo biloba, gotu kola, lemon grass, licorice, peppermint, rosemary, Siberian ginseng, and spearmint. Herbs and sea vegetables high in nutrition and minerals are also a good idea: alfalfa, bilberry, dulse, kelp, nori, and other sea vegetables.

Other herbs useful in preventing memory loss and general effects of aging are elderberry, green tea,and hawthorn berry as well as the traditional Chinese herbs—androvian (Chinese orchid), astragalus, Chinese ginseng, lycee root, and shizandra.

HYDROTHERAPY

Soak in O$_2$. The skin, the largest organ of the body, acts as a secondary respiratory system and readily absorbs this vital nutrient. Your body and brain need oxygen to function properly. To revitalize your mind with oxygen, try the Oxygen Spa Soak on page 95.

INHALATION

Clear mental cobwebs. I use this spray in my office for mental and memory stimulation. It clears out mental cobwebs, makes me feel alert, and helps me focus. It can be used in a diffuser or aroma lamp, as a room spray, or simply sprinkled on a tissue and inhaled.

∞ Mint Conditioner for Mind and Memory ∞

> 5 parts lemon essential oil
> 2 parts spearmint essential oil
> 2 parts peppermint essential oil
> 2 parts black pepper essential oil
> 2 parts rosemary essential oil

Mix the essential oils into an amber glass bottle and label. Fill your electric diffuser with the blend according to the manufacturer's directions. Alternatively, you can make a room mist by placing 10 to 20 drops and 4 ounces of distilled water in a spray bottle. Shake well before using.

LIFESTYLE

Get in the game of life. Avoid depression and stay mentally active by learning new skills and challenging yourself. The expression "use it or lose it" applies here. Engage in mental activities such as reading, thinking, and creating. Take an acting or computer class, dance lessons, involve yourself in group activities, and take excursions to new places.

Top-Ten Memory Makers

Following is a collection of recommendations from health specialists, psychotherapists, and fitness experts.

- Relax and cope with stress effectively (see the section on Stress).
- Stand in the Forward Bend posture.
- Practice slow, deep breathing (see The Healing Breath on page 216).
- Pay attention and focus.
- Minimize distractions and noise.
- Write things down.
- Take your time and be organized.
- Repeat new information (like new names, addresses, etc.).
- Believe in yourself.
- Avoid harmful substances (chemicals, pollution, toxins).

Get enough sleep. Studies show that, if you get deep sleep after learning something new, it may help you remember the new information better and lock in the memory.

Stay clear of aluminum. Aluminum has been linked to Alzheimer's disease. Autopsies have shown high aluminum levels in the brains of victims. Avoid cooking in aluminum and read labels carefully (cosmetics, foods, drugs).

TEAS AND TONICS

The best brain food. The following recipe is for a stimulating herbal tea that you can prepare at home. The herbs were chosen for their antioxidant and brain-fortifying properties.

✒ Memory Tonic ~

2 parts spearmint herb or peppermint herb
2 parts lemon balm herb
2 parts gotu kola nut
1 part rosemary herb
1 part Ginkgo biloba
1 part ground Siberian ginseng root
1 part licorice root ground
2 cups water
Ginger Honey (page 48) to taste (optional)

Mix the herbs and ground root into a jar and label. To prepare, bring 2 cups of water to a boil and add 2 to 3 teaspoons of the herbal tonic mix. Reduce heat and simmer, covered, gently for 5 minutes. Remove from the heat and allow to steep for another 5 minutes. Strain and sweeten if desired. Drink 2 to 3 cups per day.

See also Stress.

Menopause
~

GREAT WAYS TO WELCOME CHANGE

Menopause is the transition from the stage of childbearing to a state of greater maturity. You may have heard menopause referred to as "the change of life" or "the change"—meaning a decline in the hormone levels responsible for producing eggs in the ovaries. The possibility of pregnancy has come to an end.

While many women have different personal feelings about this reality, the changes that come with menopause present women with a series of new challenges. Menopause can trigger a host of symptoms and changes in your body, emotions, and outlook on life.

Periods of Menopause

The changes a woman goes through actually start many years before she reaches an "official" state of menopause, and they continue for years afterward. Here is what is considered the average onset of the different stages.

- *Premenopause:* Still experiencing regular periods. Average age forty-five to forty-eight.
- *Perimenopause:* Experiencing irregular periods for previous twelve months. Average age forty-nine.
- *Menopause:* Twelve consecutive months without a period. Average age forty-nine to fifty.
- *Postmenopause:* No period for one to five years. Average age fifty-three to sixty-one.
- *Surgical menopause:* Have had both ovaries removed. Not age dependent.

The average age at which a woman enters menopause is between forty-nine and fifty years, though it can start as early as forty or as late as the late fifties. Perimenopause, which is the time between normal cycles and the cessation of menstruation, can last several months to several years. Some women experience their most intense and frequent symptoms during perimenopause rather than menopause.

The list of symptoms a woman can experience is exhausting, and each woman experiences them differently. Some of the most common physical symptoms are headaches, hot flashes, night sweats, weakness, fatigue, water retention, weight gain, abdominal cramping, vaginal dryness, decreased libido, irregular menstrual spotting, nausea, palpitations, and restless sleep. As if these weren't enough, the psychological symptoms include irritability, weepiness, concentration problems, forgetfulness, sensation of heat, altered perceptions, mood swings, anxiety, and depression.

Here I offer solutions for as many of these symptoms as possible.

AROMATHERAPY

Customized symptom relief. There are many essential oils that can help prevent or ease the symptoms of menopause. Those that contain hormone-like chemicals can be used to support the body, while other essences can be used to relieve water retention, flushing and sweats, and emotional changes.

Essential oils that have a hormone-like effect on the body are aniseed, basil, chamomile (Roman), clary sage, cypress, fennel, geranium, nutmeg, star anise, and vitex/chasteberry.

Here's what to look for when dealing with other symptoms:

Insomnia: To ease restlessness and encourage a peaceful sleep, try basil, bergamot, chamomile, lavender, mandarin, marjoram, neroli, petitgrain, rose, sandalwood, and ylang-ylang.

Night sweats: To prevent and ease night sweats, try cypress, grapefruit, lemongrass, lime, and petitgrain.

Water retention: Bloating and headaches are symptoms caused by water retention. Try cypress, fennel, geranium, grapefruit, juniper, lavender, lemon, mandarin, orange, and rosemary.

Depression: To treat mood swings and the blues, try basil, bergamot, clary sage, grapefruit, jasmine, lavender, neroli, rose, sandalwood, and ylang-ylang.

Disinterest in sex: Try the oils that act as aphrodisiacs. They are black pepper, carrot seed, clary sage, fennel, frankincense, geranium, ginger, hyssop, jasmine, juniper, myrrh, neroli, patchouli, pine, rose, rosemary, sandalwood, and ylang-ylang.

Keep a journal. You will want to give aromatherapy and other natural remedies time to take effect. It may take one to several months to notice a difference. I suggest you keep a journal to record all of your symptoms and complaints so you will be better able to evaluate your progress. Make notes of which remedies you enjoy and which are most effective. As all women are different, so, too, will be their reactions to the different remedies.

DIET

Think phytochemicals. Eating a low-fat, mostly vegetarian diet, including more soy products such as tofu, soy milk, and soy cheese, in addition to yams, may decrease menopausal symptoms due to their phytochemical content, which is similar to our own naturally occurring hormones lowered during menopause.

Eat less salt. Lowering your refined salt intake will diminish water retention and weight gain.

Watch what you drink. Avoid alcohol and caffeine, as these stimulants put additional stress on the body. Some evidence suggest that alcohol may contribute to bone loss.

Care for your bones. The biggest physical drawback of decreased estrogen levels is the gradual thinning of your skeletal structure. Estrogen protects the bones. Without it, women must depend on the mineral calcium to keep their bones strong.

Take calcium supplements to ensure you are getting adequate levels, but you should also get calcium naturally through your diet. My recommended food choices include:

- Vegetable greens: broccoli, bok choy, collard greens, beet greens, kale, okra, watercress, and dandelion greens
- Black-eyed peas and turnips
- Sea vegetables: nori, kelp, dulse, and wakame
- Seeds and nuts: sesame seeds and raw almonds
- Soy milk or rice milk
- Blackstrap molasses
- Figs and dried apricots
- Whole grains, especially amaranth and quinoa

HERBS

A host of helpers. Menopause is certainly not lacking in botanical supporters. There are just about as many, if not more, herbal remedies to counteract symptoms as there are es-

The Dairy Dilemma

Many doctors and researchers (and the dairy industry) would like you to believe that the answer to protecting bones against the onset of osteoporosis is to eat plenty of dairy products. I, for one, do not agree.

Dairy products are not a source of healthy calcium because cow's milk is loaded with artificial estrogen, which is given to female cows to fatten them up and produce more milk. Artificial estrogen has been linked to rising rates of breast cancer.

I say play it safe. Stay away from cow's milk and get your calcium sources from plant foods and soy products that are easily digested, organic, and readily absorbed by your body.

sential oils. In fact, books have been written on herbal support for menopause: It might be wise to get one.

Some of the principal herbs for menopause relief and general support are hormone precursors or balancers, nervous system relaxants, mineral rich and alkalizing herbs, and/or gland toners. Leading the list are anise seed, black cohosh, blue cohosh, burdock root, celandine, chamomile, chasteberry, chickweed, cleavers, dandelion root, dong quai, evening primrose, fenugreek, Ginkgo biloba, hops, kava kava, licorice root, maca, milk thistle, motherwort, nettles, Oregon grape root, passionflower, red clover, red raspberry leaf, sage, St. John's wort, shepherd's purse, Siberian and American ginseng, uva ursi, valerian root, and wild yam.

HYDROTHERAPY

Soak away night sweats. The following bath treatments were created for evening use. They will help ease night sweats and promote restful sleep.

⌒ Peaceful–Sleep Bath ⌒

The lemon makes this bath especially refreshing. Select cream as your
carrier if your skin is dry. Honey is soothing and antibacterial.

2 to 4 tablespoons Celtic Sea salt,
heavy cream, or honey
4 drops lavender essential oil
3 drops marjoram essential oil
3 drops lemon essential oil

Put the salt, cream, or honey in a dish. Add the essential oils and mix thoroughly. Fill the bath and add the aromatic mixture. Stir with your hands. Soak for 20 to 30 minutes.

Hot flash! Temperature topples. This bath is designed to regulate hot flashes. While you are taking the bath, read poetry or an empowering book or listen to some relaxing music or nature sounds. Sip some soothing herbal tea. You'll get a complete spa experience.

⌒ Menopause Bath ⌒

3 drops geranium essential oil
2 drops clary sage essential oil
2 drops lemon essential oil
1 drop bergamot essential oil
4 tablespoons Celtic Sea or Dead Sea
salt (or carrier of choice)

Add the essential oils to the salt. Pour into a bath of warm water (92 to 100 degrees). Soak and relax for 20 to 30 minutes.

Take a pelvic splash. In addition to the baths given above, it is helpful to always end a hydrotherapy session with a cold water application to the pelvic region. This can be done in the bath by splashing cold water onto the pelvic region in, or in the shower by targeting the cold water application to this area. Cold hydrotherapy in short durations promotes circulation and directly stimulates and tones the female organs.

INHALATION

Get a night of undisturbed sleep. Fall asleep at night while inhaling the fragrances of menopause-relieving oils and it's very likely you will not be interrupted by night sweats or other disturbances. I recommend using an electric diffuser, which can be connected to an automatic timer. Ideally, the diffuser should go on every 3 to 4 hours for 10-minute durations. The essential oils will last several hours in the room air, and you will be inhaling them while you sleep.

Take care to not exceed the recommended amounts and time limits. Too much can have the opposite effect by waking you up. The goal is to have a subtle background scent, not one that is overbearing.

Alternatively, you can use an aroma lamp or potpourri burner, although these methods require a lit candle. For a simpler method of inhalation, place a few drops on your pillowcase. However, the diffuser is the most therapeutic for night sweats and sleep disturbances.

❧ Perfect-Sleep Blend ❧

3 parts lavender essential oil
2 parts marjoram essential oil
2 parts lime essential oil
1 part mandarin essential oil

For the diffuser: Measure each part with an eyedropper or teaspoon to make a large amount. For an aroma lamp or room mist: Measure each part by drops.

LIFESTYLE

Check your mental outlook. Women who are in denial regarding their age and youthfulness seem to be more susceptible to the side effects of aging, which include the onset of menopause. Another group that may have a difficult time emotionally are those who have

Power Surges

It's not uncommon for a woman to get hot flashes so badly that you can literally see her temperature rise as she turns redder and redder. Not only is this uncomfortable, it can be embarrassing if it happens in public.

It's hard to control when and where a heat surge will develop, but there is something you can do to stop the temperature from rising: Sniff peppermint. Carry a vial of the essential oil in your purse or put a drop or two of the oil on a small folding fan or a handkerchief.

If peppermint is not to your liking, try clary sage, cypress, or fennel.

dedicated their entire lives to rearing children. Their personal identity became focused on child rearing and childbearing, and it may be difficult for them to rediscover their focussed center.

Choose to be positive. A positive outlook is helpful in dealing with this challenging phase of a woman's life. Many women enjoy this new phase, focusing on studies or projects they were unable to tackle when their children were small. I am reminded of the question posed of perception: "Is the cup half full or half empty?"

How do you perceive your reality? Do you view menopause as a sort of death sentence or as a new beginning? Research and poll studies say that your outlook and belief system make a difference.

Vanquish stress. There is a strong correlation between stress levels and the degree of severity of menopausal symptoms. Exercise helps in several ways: It increases metabolism, aids in stress relief, helps to lift depression, and relieves sleep disturbances. Daily exercising for at least 30 to 45 minutes and maintaining sexual activity will increase circulation to the pelvis and stimulate vaginal secretion.

Seek support. Seeking support for yourself while experiencing this transitional phase of your life is important. Communicate with your spouse. Talk with your friends. There are even newsletters, menopause support groups, and Internet connections (groups, newsletters, informative sites to visit) you can be part of.

Also paramount in your self-care plan is finding practitioners who are knowledgeable in natural alternatives. Nutrition (including vitamin and mineral therapy), herbal medicine, homeopathy, and aromatherapy are examples of integrative therapies that can be utilized for wellness support at this time.

SALVES

Come to the aid of your pelvis. A natural vaginal salve or cream, which you can purchase or make, should be used on a regular basis to help replenish the vaginal wall lining, which starts to thin during menopause. Daily application will minimize inflammation and discomfort caused by intercourse. Exercise, including sexual activity, encourages circulation to the pelvis and helps women who are experiencing changes in this area.

Make your own. This make-it-yourself vaginal cream is effective and relatively easy to make. It has all-natural ingredients, and it is unlikely that you will be able to find a better vaginal preparation.

❧ Sexual-Salvation Salve ❧

2 ounces natural vaginal cream
    (comfrey salve) or 2 ounces Heavy-
    Duty Ointment (page 240)
5 drops frankincense essential oil
5 drops sandalwood essential oil
5 drops myrrh essential oil
800 international units vitamin E

Place the cream in a clean amber glass jar and mix with the essential oils and vitamin E. Please note that only 15 drops (total) of essential oils are needed for this preparation. That is about a 1.5 percent dilution ratio, which is adequate for vaginal application. Apply a small amount daily.

Teas and Tonics

This herbal tea contains many traditional herbs helpful in relieving the common symptoms of menopause. Some are relaxing, diuretic, and fortifying. This tea can help ease hot flashes and night sweats if taken regularly.

🖎 Menopause-Support Tea 🖎

2 parts chamomile flowers
1 part ground ginseng root
1 part ground dandelion root and leaf
1 part ground licorice root
1 part ground valerian root
1 part garden sage
Honey to taste (optional)
Fresh lemon juice (optional)

Mix the dry herbs in a jar with a tight fitting lid. To make 1 cup of herbal tea, place 1 teaspoon of the herbal mixture in 1½ cups of boiling water and simmer (covered) gently for 10 minutes. Strain and sweeten if desired. Drink 1 cup per day. If bloating is a complaint, add fresh lemon juice, as it is a mild diuretic.

Menstrual Cramps

🖎

Relief in an Instant

Menstrual cramps can range from mild to downright debilitating. If you're looking here for help, I'm assuming your discomfort is somewhere in between. Here's what I can do to help.

AROMATHERAPY

Easing aromas. Essential oils useful in easing menstrual cramps are basil, carrot seed, chamomile, clary sage, cypress, frankincense, jasmine, juniper, lavender, marjoram, nutmeg, peppermint, and rosemary. These antispasmodic and pain-relieving essential oils are best utilized in compresses, massage preparations, and baths.

HERBS

Traditional Western herbal medicine used for menstrual cramping are black cohosh, chasteberry, chaste tree (vitex), cramp bark, dong quai, juniper, kava kava, squaw, valerian root, wild yam, and yarrow. Valerian and kava are especially calming to the nervous system.

HYDROTHERAPY

Pamper in the tub. This bath is so helpful for relieving menstrual cramps! Several of my clients use it on a regular basis as a "goddess" bath ritual to honor their femininity. Both Epsom salt and sea salt are useful in preventing muscle cramping.

⌒ Femininity Bath ⌒

*I like this bath so much I take it just for pleasure. I substitute
my own bath salts in place of the Epsom or sea salt.*

5 drops lavender essential oil
2 drops cypress essential oil
2 drops nutmeg essential oil
2 drops peppermint essential oil
Celtic Sea salt, Epsom salt,
   or Detoxifying Bath Salts (page 128)

Add the essential oils to the salt. Combine well and add to a full, hot (100 to 104 degrees) bath. Soak for 20 to 30 minutes. Do not stay in longer than 30 minutes, as it can have a draining effect on you. Wrap yourself in a warm terry bathrobe or towel and rest for approximately 20 minutes by lying on a bed and elevating your legs and feet above heart level with pillows. This is very relaxing, takes the burden off the lower back, and encourages good blood flow.

MASSAGE

The touch of comfort. This massage oil can ease most cramps and aches caused by menstruation. It is made with the analgesic, antispasmodic, and anti-inflammatory essential oils. Borage and arnica oils are used as a base for their benefit in prostaglandin production.

Massage yourself with this oil twice per day to relieve discomfort in the pelvic region and lower back. Follow with a hot-water bottle over the abdomen for additional relief and to increase the absorption of the aromatic oils.

Caring-for-Me Massage Oil

26 drops lavender essential oil
6 drops rosemary essential oil
6 drops marjoram essential oil
6 drops basil essential oil
4 drops chamomile essential oil
2 tablespoons arnica or St. John's wort infusion oil
2 teaspoons evening primrose or borage oil
2 tablespoons vegetable oil
400 international units vitamin E (optional)

Put the essential oils in an amber glass bottle. Then add the infusion and vegetable oils. Add the vitamin E if desired. Shake gently to mix well. Label contents with directions for use. To apply, massage a small amount of the oil into the lower abdominal region and lower back area. Apply the aromatic oil with gentle hand pressure, working toward the heart to encourage blood return and increase lymphatic drainage. Inhale essences from your hands after application. Apply daily during episodes of menstrual cramping.

TEAS AND TONICS

Fruit of the vine. I call this infusion Indian Maiden's Tea because of all the berries and woodland herbs it contains. Also, it is very popular among young women. This is an excellent substitute for caffeine and sugar-laden drinks that make cramping and other menstrual symptoms worse. It seems to take the edge off premenstrual symptoms as well.

When to Call the Doctor

Painful periods, called dysmenorrhea, can be caused by an underlying condition such as endometriosis, pelvic inflammatory disease, or fibroids. Extremely painful periods are not normal and should be checked by a health practitioner.

❧ Indian Maiden's Tea ❧

Enjoy it hot or cold, depending on the weather and your preference.

> 1 part juniper berries
> 1 part chasteberry
> 1 part ground cramp bark
> 1 part blue cohosh
> 1 part squaw vine
> 1 part ground valerian root
> 1 part yarrow
> Stevia or honey to taste

Mix all the ingredients except the stevia or honey into a clean glass jar. Label with directions for use. Use 1 to 2 teaspoons per cup of water and simmer for 5 minutes. Strain and add sweetener to taste.

Mental Exhaustion

Oh, My Aching Brain!

First, the bad news: Most people today appear to be under a great deal of stress most of the time. They drive themselves to get as much done in as short a time as possible, depleting their energy reserves and exhausting their minds.

Now, the good news: There is an antidote to all this lunacy. It's called relaxation, and it's a skill that can be learned. Its positive effects last throughout the day. When relaxation is experienced on a regular basis, pain is decreased, illness is less likely, and stress is lowered.

What causes mental exhaustion? At the top of the long list, we have job pressures, work deadlines, financial obligations, unemployment, marital strife, family dysfunctional issues, lack of proper rest, and physical fatigue, all of which take their eventual toll on the nervous and immune systems as well as the entire body chemistry.

Aromatherapy

Mental clearinghouse. Useful oils for mental fatigue are basil, bergamot, ginger, grapefruit, lemon, peppermint, rosemary, and sweet thyme. The same oils that are recommended to counteract stress can also be used. They are basil, bergamot, chamomile, clary sage, geranium, juniper, lavender, lemongrass, marjoram, neroli, rose, sandalwood, and ylang-ylang.

Diet

Counteract chemicals. Between our food and air, we unfortunately take in more toxic chemicals and pollutants than we should. Prescription medications, caffeine, alcohol, tobacco, and food preservatives are all too common and overused. To counteract some of these insults to the nervous system (and the entire body), we should eat more nerve-calming vitamin B–rich foods such as royal jelly, parsley, watercress, and sea vegetables (kelp, dulse, and wakame).

Eat alkalizing foods. Mental exhaustion is a form of stress, and stress causes the body's pH balance to get out of whack. It becomes acidic. Since an acidic condition is the primary cause of illness, an anti-acid, or alkalizing diet, is essential.

There are many books written on the subject of pH balancing, and I recommend you learn more about it. A partial food list is given here to get you started eating less acid-forming items. Ideally, your diet should consist of 20 percent acid-forming foods and 80 percent alkaline-forming foods. Alkaline-forming foods include most land vegetables, all sea vegetables, millet, quinoa and amaranth grains, Celtic Sea salt, herbs and herbal teas, seeds, lemons and limes, raw apple cider vinegar, raw cultured vegetables (natural sauerkraut), kefir, sprouted almonds, and sunflower seeds.

HERBS

Choose mineral-rich botanicals. For stress-related conditions like mental exhaustion, you'll want to take herbs that help nourish the nervous system. These include herbs rich in the minerals iron, magnesium, and zinc. They include black cohosh, burdock root, dong quai, ginseng, marshmallow root, oat straw, and parsley leaf. These calming herbs are also good to include for obvious reasons: hops, kava kava, lady's slipper, passionflower, skullcap, and valerian root.

Take alkalizing herbs. Plants that aid in balancing the body back to a healthy alkaline state are numerous and easy to find. They include alfalfa, aloe vera, burdock root, chamomile, chlorella, dandelion root, fennel seed, ginger root, lemon balm, and peppermint herb. Rose hips is the alkalizing form of vitamin C and is recommended instead of the acid-forming kind.

HYDROTHERAPY

Bubble your troubles away. Are there times when you wish you could be a kid again and live a carefree life? Then this bath may be just what you need. It is for the young at heart, or the ones who wish they were (like you).

By mixing this recipe in an unscented bath or shower gel, baby shampoo, or Castile Soap, you can make your own customized bubble bath that is perfect for what ails you. Don't forget to add the fun bath toys!

✍ Child's Play ✍

Take this bath whenever you feel mentally taxed.

6 drops lavender essential oil
6 drops mandarin essential oil
4 tablespoons unscented shower gel
(or carrier of choice)

Fill the tub with warm to hot water. Mix the essential oils with the carrier. Add to the bathwater and mix well. If using gel or a foaming soap, mix and pour while the tub is filling to get the most bubbles.

The serene scene. If you cannot relate to Child's Play, then this will take care of you. Just the opposite of the citrus scent, this bath has a deep, rich, provocative aroma that you can get lost in. For sensory overload, and to further quiet your mind, try turning off all the lights in the room and light one candle. A neutral water temperature (94 to 98 degrees) will further encourage a sedative effect. It is nonstimulating to the skin's nerve receptors. Incorporate appropriate music selections for a soothing spa escape and give yourself plenty of time to relax.

✍ Quiet Moments ✍

4 tablespoons honey
(or other carrier)
6 drops sandalwood essential oil
2 drops bergamot essential oil
2 drops ylang-ylang essential oil

Pour the honey into a small dish. Mix in the essential oils and combine well by stirring. Add to a full warm bath. Soak for as long as you desire. This is your time.

Get some oxygen therapy. The peroxide bath called the Oxygen Spa Soak featured on page 95 is an exhilarating whole-body treatment with a giant dose of this vital nutrient. This profound spa treatment will give you a general energy boost. Do not do this therapy too late at night, as the energizing effects are most noticeable a few hours after the soak.

INHALATION

Unwind and recharge. Hook up a diffuser in your work area to combat stress and purify the air. Inhalation of essential oils during the day is one of the most effective and easiest ways to enjoy the benefits of aromatherapy.

Room sprays are another simple method to encourage relaxation in the office. They can also be used in the home, psychotherapy setting for hypnosis, medical treatment exam rooms or hospitals, and other places where stressful conditions are present.

Since these recipes are made of pure essential oils without a carrier, they are to be used in a diffuser, aroma lamp, or simply inhaled from a tissue to which you have applied a few drops. For diffuser use, you will need to make a substantial amount to run through the machine. Alternatively, only a few drops are needed for the aroma lamp or handkerchief methods.

∾ Lavender Fields ∾

6 parts lavender essential oil
1 part sandalwood essential oil

∾ Slow-Down-and-Relax Blend ∾

6 parts lavender essential oil
5 parts ylang-ylang essential oil
3 parts sandalwood essential oil
3 parts marjoram essential oil

Measure the essential oils into a small amber glass bottle. Cap securely and label.

The Sanity Test

Make two lists: One list should include all the things you do that bring joy and health to your life; the other should include the things you spend your time doing, including responsibilities, work, errands, etc. Compare the lists. Which one is longer? If it's the second, you need to do something about it.

What items can you let go of and cross off the list? What items can you delegate to someone else? There is more to life than work. As the old saying goes, "Stop along the way to smell the roses."

MASSAGE

An extrasensory experience. For someone with mental exhaustion, touch is especially affirming and grounding. This massage oil is designed for a full-body massage. Take it with you to the massage therapist or use it at home. The oil should be warmed prior to using; the warmth will give the skin an extrasensory experience. The woodsy aroma will help ground your energy and enhance the sedative effect.

ᐯᐁ Earthbound Balm ᐁ

This has worked effectively for some of the most stressed-out individuals I know!

> 15 drops lavender essential oil
> 7 drops sandalwood essential oil
> 5 drops frankincense essential oil
> 1 tablespoon hazelnut oil or sesame oil
> 1 tablespoon hypericum infusion oil or hazelnut oil

In a 1-ounce amber glass bottle, add the essential oils and vegetable oils. Shake gently to mix. Label. This amount will be enough for two or three full-body massage applications. Place the bottle of blended oils in a hot water bath prior to using to warm the balm.

SOUND AND MUSIC THERAPY

Hum a happy tone. Toning is vibratory sound that is produced by making sounds with the mouth through breathing on exhalation. These healing sounds resonate through a specific body region and are known to restore and balance certain states. To positively affect the skull region, the sound is "hum." Take a deep breath and make the sound "hum" while exhaling. Repeat the sound three times and practice it daily for best results.

YOGA AND MOVEMENT

Still the mind. The yogis perform an exercise called the "Easy Pose" and claim that it not only straightens the spine but also slows metabolism and stills the mind. It is the latter benefit that will be most valuable for mental exhaustion.

To perform the Easy Pose, find a comfortable place on the floor to sit. Bend your knees to your chest and clasp your arms around them. This straightens your spine to prepare you for the pose. Release your arms and cross your legs (Indian style), letting your knees drop down toward the floor. Keep your head and body straight.

If you find that holding this pose is uncomfortable, place a folded towel or blanket under your buttocks. Practice slow, deep breathing and concentrate on slowing your mental thoughts. You can also do the toning described above while in this yoga posture.

Morning Sickness

SCENTS THAT SETTLE THE STOMACH

What a way to start the day! Morning sickness has got to be the least pleasant side effect of pregnancy (at least it was for me).

The nausea, the queasiness, and the stomach-churning smell of food are enough to make you, well, sick. What's worse is that morning sickness can happen at any time of day. The good news is that it usually goes away after the first trimester.

Pregnant women, however, have an extremely keen sense of smell all the time. Perhaps it is a safety feature nature has programmed into the female's system to protect mother and baby. Certainly, with all the physiologic changes taking place, in addition to this heightened odor awareness, nausea is not surprising.

Morning sickness can possibly be the result of vitamin B_6 deficiency or a low blood sugar level. However, during this trimester is when the placenta becomes seated within the uterus and is probably the most likely cause of the nausea.

Aromatherapy

Antinausea scents. Essential oils that help to prevent nausea and ease morning sickness are ginger, lavender, lemon, peppermint, rose, and sandalwood. There are others for general nausea, but these are considered safer and gentler for pregnancy. These are best applied in diluted massage oils (back of hands), compresses, and in inhalation methods (tissue, room mists). You can also make aromatic smelling salts (see page 357).

Diet

Avoid whatever ails you. Steer clear of any foods and odors that are unpleasant to you. These may include rich, highly spiced, and oily foods. Don't be surprised if one of your favorite foods suddenly starts to turn your stomach. Don't worry—your taste for it will eventually return. Small, frequent meals may be more appealing than larger, heavy ones. Avoid highly refined foods that contain sugar, salt, and fat.

It goes without saying that you should avoid alcohol, tobacco, coffee, and black tea.

Herbs

Herbs that ease. Traditional herbs used to treat this discomfort are catnip, chamomile, fennel, ginger, orange blossom, peppermint, raspberry leaf, and spearmint. Consult your doctor before using concentrated forms of these herbs, although they are regarded as safe to use as infusions (tea). Sipping cool peppermint or a warm cup of ginger tea is very comforting at this time.

Hydrotherapy

Treat your head when you get out of bed. If nausea greets you first thing in the morning, have your partner make this preparation and have it ready for you when you get out of bed. The compress should be made with warm water and applied to the forehead.

The lavender soothes the nervous system, while the lemon (or peppermint) is gently refreshing, an excellent combination for preventing or relieving morning sickness.

ᴏ No-More-Nausea Compress ᴏ

4 cups warm water
3 drops lavender essential oil
1 drop lemon or peppermint essential oil

Add about 4 cups of warm water (92 to 100 degrees) to a sink or bowl. Add the essential oils and stir with your hands. Soak the washcloth in the aromatic water. Gently wring the cloth until it is moist but not too wet. Apply to your forehead. Keep your eyes closed. Leave the compress on for 10 to 15 minutes or until you have obtained relief.

Inhalation

Quick relief. One of the simplest ways to relieve morning sickness is to inhale the essence of peppermint essential oil. It can bring immediate relief. It should be used in moderation during pregnancy because of its stimulating effects on the central nervous system. Therefore, do not use it in large amounts. Lavender, as well as lemon, has also been employed with success for nausea, either individually or in combination.

For inhalation, mix 4 parts lavender essential oil with 1 part lemon or peppermint essential oil. Put a few drops on a tissue, in an aroma lamp, or run through a diffuser. This will help to minimize other unpleasant odors that may be triggering the nausea.

For other remedies, see Motion Sickness *and* Nausea.

Motion Sickness

⋏ℴ

EASE THE QUEASIES

Leave it to the ancient Greeks and Romans to tell it like it is. In Greek, the root of the word *nausea* means "sailor"; in Latin, it translates to "seasickness."

In reality, it's that uneasy, queasy, stomach churning and turning, can't-move-a-muscle feeling that makes you want to beg for anything but this!

Any kind of motion—car, boat, amusement park ride—can cause this worse-than-death, sick-in-the stomach feeling. Other notable causes are food poisoning, gastritis, putrid odors, hangover, and early pregnancy.

When you've got it, all you really care about is getting rid of it. Here's what to do.

AROMATHERAPY

Get back with mint conditioning. The mints—peppermint and spearmint—are prime soothing scents for nausea. Smelling the essences from a vial or tissue works surprisingly well. Ginger is another powerful and helpful oil.

Other useful essential oils are basil, cardamom, coriander seed, fennel, lavender, lemon, mandarin, melissa, Roman chamomile, rose, and sandalwood.

MASSAGE

Head off trouble. If you know you are prone to travel sickness, do the following massage 30 minutes before traveling. You can also try this if peppermint aromatherapy does not work.

Apply the oils according to the directions and inhale the aroma from your warmed hands after the massage. It is a very soothing and relaxing treatment. For further relaxation after the massage, place a warm-water bottle over your tummy and lie down for 20 minutes.

Aromatic Smelling Salts

To make your own personalized aroma salts, simply fill a small bottle (¼-ounce size is nice) with rock salt. Count out 10 to 20 drops of one of the essential oils into the bottle (see list of oils above). Cap tightly and label contents.

When you feel stomach queasiness coming on, open the bottle and inhale deeply several times. The salt holds the scent very well. This is easy to carry and is not apt to spill in your purse or briefcase.

No-More-Nausea Massage Oil

Eliminate the oil and use the essential oil mixture as an extra-strength inhalation.

5 drops lavender essential oil

2 drops peppermint essential oil

2 drops mandarin essential oil

1 drop ginger essential oil

1 tablespoon vegetable oil or unscented body lotion

Count out the essential oils into a small amber glass bottle that holds at least ½ ounce. Then add the vegetable oil or unscented body lotion. Shake to combine well. Rub on your hands and inhale slowly and deeply a few times. Then massage this blend over the solar plexus (below your sternum) in a counterclockwise direction with your left hand (promotes relaxation as well).

Acupressure Relief

I have found this acupressure technique extremely effective for people undergoing chemotherapy treatment, but it helps with motion sickness as well.

Locate the pressure point on your wrist by placing two fingers at the base of your wrist, palm up. The exact point where you want to apply pressure is between the two tendons. With one fingertip from the opposite hand, press firmly for approximately 1 minute. It doesn't matter which wrist you use.

This technique prompted the creation of motion sickness wristbands that many people wear to ward off this condition.

TEAS AND TONICS

Sip of relief. This pleasing herbal tea mix is especially helpful for mild cases of nausea caused by indigestion, overeating, and eating fried foods. It is also wonderful for nausea related to colds and flu since the peppermint and ginger help with sinus congestion and stomach upset. Ginger is known to help with nervous tension, so if this is a factor in the cause of your nausea, it would be very beneficial to include.

✍ Tender Tummy Tea ✍

1 teaspoon raspberry leaf
1 teaspoon peppermint herb
½ teaspoon ground fennel seed
½ teaspoon ground anise seed
1 cup boiling water
Stevia or Ginger Honey to taste (page 48) (optional)

Combine the raspberry leaf, peppermint, fennel, and anise. Put it in loose form in a teapot or use a tea strainer. Pour the boiling water over the tea and allow to steep for 5 minutes. If desired, add the stevia or Ginger Honey to taste. Sip this tea very slowly and inhale the anti-nausea aroma from the cup.

Real-Life Cure

THE CURSE OF THE FAMILY DRIVING VACATION

Several years ago we had a firsthand experience with car sickness when we drove from Massachusetts to the southernmost tip of Florida on a family vacation. The long drive, medium-size rental car (for five people and luggage), boredom (and the kids' backseat squabbles), humid weather, and stress of traveling all took their toll.

When nausea hit our seven-year-old twin boys, I put a few drops of peppermint essential oil on a tissue for each of them to inhale. The effect on all of us was immediate! Fresh air helped, too. Turn off the air conditioner and open the car windows, even if only for a few minutes at a time.

When traveling by car, especially with kids, take along a vial or spray of eucalyptus, lavender, or peppermint essential oil. In the car, an essential oil can quickly change the environment and air quality, making you feel somewhere other than in a closed vehicle. Essential oils, especially eucalyptus, can also relieve driving stress and encourage alertness.

Muscle Cramps

SPASM NO MORE

A cramp is the result of your muscle and blood not keeping in step together. A cramp develops when muscle tissue has been contracted for a sustained amount of time, resulting in muscle spasm that cuts off the blood and oxygen supply to that area.

Every muscle in your body has the ability to cramp except one: the heart. Out-of-shape muscles, no surprise, are those most likely to cramp. Other causes of muscle cramping are fatigue, chilling, tension, poor circulation, pregnancy, and inadequate calcium levels. Some people experience cramping at night, and the most common location is the calf muscle of the leg. Muscle cramp pain can range from mild to very severe.

AROMATHERAPY

Aromatherapy massage oils encourage circulation and help relax muscle spasms. Essential oils used for cramps are basil, bergamot, chamomile, clary sage, cypress, eucalyptus, fennel, geranium, grapefruit, hyssop, juniper, lavender, marjoram, neroli, peppermint, rosemary, and sandalwood. Aromatherapy applications include baths, massages, and compresses.

DIET

Mineral robbers. By avoiding alcohol, sugar, and phosphate-containing sodas you can prevent most cramps because these substances rob the body of important nutrients. B-complex vitamins and vitamin E may be helpful, in addition to calcium and magnesium, so eat more foods rich in these vitamins and minerals. Also, by adding real Celtic Sea salt to your diet (and forgoing the refined demineralized table salt) you will be naturally providing your body with essential minerals from the sea (see "Much More Than a Grain of Salt" on page 262).

HYDROTHERAPY

Moist heat. Heat, in the form of aromatic baths or warm compresses, is often recommended as part of an athlete's treatment regime. The moist heat promotes circulation and prevents further muscle cramping.

✐ No–More–Cramps Compress ✎

2 cups warm water
2 drops lavender essential oil
1 drop marjoram essential oil
1 drop hyssop essential oil

Warm the water so you can comfortably touch it. Place the water in a bowl. Add the essential oils and stir with a wooden spoon. Soak a piece of flannel or a washcloth in the warm water and wring out the excess moisture. Apply to the cramped muscle. Cover with a towel. Place a hot-water bottle over the towel to keep the compress warm.

Additionally, St. John's wort oil can be applied to the skin before applying the compress. This will protect the skin as well as add anti-inflammatory benefits. Reapply the compress, when it becomes dry or cool, for 15 to 20 minutes.

MASSAGE

Concentrate on relief. This recipe is a concentrated massage oil intended for small areas only. This oil can also be applied before working out to prevent muscle cramping or before bedtime if that is when cramping is more apt to happen. It can also be used while experiencing a cramp. Warm the oil in a hot-water bath prior to the massage to increase the absorption of the oils and to enhance circulation.

❧ Massage Oil for Cramps ❧

8 drops rosemary essential oil
8 drops marjoram essential oil
6 drops lavender essential oil
4 drops eucalyptus essential oil
1 tablespoon St. John's wort infusion oil
1 tablespoon vegetable oil

In an amber glass bottle, add the essential oils and then the carrier oils. Shake gently to mix well. Label the contents with directions for use. Apply a small amount to the affected muscles and massage lightly.

Real-Life Cure

MASSAGE AWAY CRAMPS

Nineteen-year-old Courtney began experiencing such severe muscle cramping while playing soccer she feared her athletic life would be short-lived. Not only did they cause her to quit midgame, but she also started to get cramps at night. Even pregame stretching didn't help.

What did help, she discovered, was pregame stretching preceded by a nice muscle massage with essential oils 30 minutes before practices and games. She also applied aromatic compresses routinely.

The results were very positive; with regular use of the massage oils, Courtney noticed that her cramps were gradually subsiding. She began to focus on a more comprehensive stretching routine before games and at night before retiring. Cramps were soon a problem of the past.

YOGA AND MOVEMENT

Stretch your limits. Adequate stretching of muscle groups before and after exercise is good prevention for this type of problem. Consult a good exercise book or talk to a personal trainer about exercises that reduce muscle spasms.

Exercise in bed. A few minutes of stretching before bedtime can help prevent and eliminate nighttime leg cramps. I like this stretch because it's simple and you can do it in bed: Point your toes up while pushing the back of the knee down against the bed. Relax and repeat several times.

Seek higher elevation. To help prevent nighttime leg cramps, keep your feet and calves elevated at night on two pillows at the end of the bed.

Do the ultimate stretch. There is nothing better than yoga for stretching and toning.

Muscle Soreness

RELIEF IS JUST A BATH AWAY

A long day of spring cleaning in the yard and garden can take its toll on muscles that spend most of their winter lounging indoors with less activity.

You won't feel it at first, but hours later you can't help but feel what you've done to your poor underused muscles. They'll be so sore, stiff, tired, and swollen, just moving them will make you grimace with pain. Your muscles will remind you of what you've done to them for days unless you take immediate action.

AROMATHERAPY

The essence of pain. The therapeutic essential oils that will be most useful for overworked muscles are the anti-inflammatory, antispasmodic, and analgesic-containing type. These include basil, black pepper, cajeput, chamomile, cypress, eucalyptus, ginger, juniper, lavender, marjoram, nutmeg, peppermint, and rosemary.

If you feel achy all over your body, an aromatherapy bath is your best solution. For soreness of a specific muscle, you can treat it directly with local hand baths or footbaths and compresses.

HERBS

Herbs that help muscles recuperate are the ones that are antispasmodic and muscle and nerve relaxants. These include chamomile, cramp bark, ginger root, hops, kava kava, passionflower, rosemary, skullcap, valerian, and wild lettuce. Herbs that help with decongesting circulation are also beneficial. They include capsicum, cinnamon, garlic, ginger root, Ginkgo biloba, and hawthorn leaf and berry. Strong infusions can be made to add to the spa bath, soaks, and compresses as well as taken in supplemental form (capsules, tincture, herbal tea).

HYDROTHERAPY

Take the two-day treatment. Typically, when muscles have been improperly used and abused, the peak of soreness occurs up to two days later; therefore I recommend this bath be taken for two to three consecutive days for best results.

Following the bath, you should feel very relaxed. You can apply aromatic massage oil to any special muscles that need extra attention and then wrap up in a robe and rest. Taking time out to rest is one of the most important steps toward reversing the damage and healing your muscles. Getting out of the bath and going straight to work will undo some of the relaxing benefits of the treatment.

Epsom salt (magnesium sulfate) is recommended in this spa soak as it assists the detoxification and drainage of the accumulated lactic acid in the major muscles, which is the cause of achiness.

ᓚ The Ultimate Muscle Soak ᓂ

This bath is totally relaxing for the mind and for the muscular system.

> 4 drops lavender essential oil
> 2 drops juniper essential oil
> 2 drops rosemary essential oil
> 2 drops peppermint essential oil
> 1 cup Epsom salt

Add the essential oils to the Epsom salt and mix well. Sprinkle the aromatic bath salts into a full bath of warm to hot water (92 to 104 degrees) and stir with your hands to disperse. Soak for 20 to 30 minutes. Drink some of the Gardener's Tea (recipe on page 366) while in the tub to relax from the inside out, too! Pat dry and wrap in a bathrobe or blanket. Lie down to rest with your legs elevated (and your arms, if they have been overworked also).

The runner's special. Running a race, no matter how well conditioned you are, takes a toll on the leg muscles. This bath includes juniper and eucalyptus essential oils, which aid circulation and swelling. To speed recovery, drink plenty of liquids to rid the body of accumulated waste such as muscle toxins and lactic acid.

❧ Marathon–Man Muscle Relief ❧

4 drops lavender essential oil
2 drops rosemary essential oil
2 drops eucalyptus essential oil
2 drops juniper essential oil
1 cup Epsom salt or Celtic Sea salt

Draw a warm bath. Mix the essential oils in the salt and add to the bathwater. Soak for at least 30 minutes.

MASSAGE

Move pain out. Gently work out lactic acid accumulation in sore muscles using a light to medium touch. Long strokes are better than kneading the area. This excellent concentrated massage oil was created for use on specific muscle areas, not for a whole-body massage.

❧ Muscle–Relief Massage Oil ❧

12 drops lavender essential oil
6 drops rosemary essential oil
4 drops juniper essential oil
3 drops peppermint essential oil
1 tablespoon arnica infusion oil
1 tablespoon vegetable oil

In an amber glass bottle, add the essential oils and then the carrier oils. Shake gently to combine well. Label with directions for use. Apply a small amount to the affected muscle and massage into the skin. Apply as needed, up to three to four times per day, for soreness and stiffness.

TEAS AND TONICS

Gardener's reward. Getting plenty of fluids should include consumption of this excellent healing tea. Chamomile is key because of its anti-inflammatory and relaxing action. Drink it freely after muscle exertion.

Perhaps some of these plants are in your garden, so pick them while you're outside working so that you can make this tea as soon as your work is complete. Sip this tea while soaking in your bath or while you're sitting back and admiring your day's work.

✺ Gardener's Tea ✺

1 part kava kava
2 parts chamomile flowers
1 part rosemary herb
1 part cramp bark, ground
Pinch of cinnamon and
    ginger root powder to taste
Stevia or Ginger Honey (page 48)
    as sweetener (optional)

Blend all the herbs together. Bring water to a boil. Pour hot water over 1 to 2 teaspoons of herbal tea mix and spices and let it steep for 5 minutes. Strain and add sweetener if you wish.

Nail Infections

BACK TO PRETTY HANDS AND FEET

What price vanity? How about the cost of a visit to the doctor's office with unsightly sore nails.

Nails are not meant to be sculpted, tipped, lacquered, and layered with sparkles and fake overlays. Even polish can be harmful. Nails need to breathe. Covering them up in ornamentation traps moisture underneath, the perfect breeding ground for a fungal infection. The result? Nails can turn yellow, separate from the nail bed, lift up, and become thickened. Once a fungal infection involves a nail, it can spread, disfigure, and cause so much pain you'll want to ward off manicures forever.

AROMATHERAPY

The castor oil cure. A nail-penetrating treatment can be made with castor oil and essential oils. Castor oil has been used traditionally for its aid in healing wounds and infections.

Even if you have healthy nails, I recommend you do this treatment following any routine grooming procedure such as clipping, cleaning, and filing.

⌇ Spa Soak for Nails ⌇

An essential treatment
for both abused and healthy nails.

4 tablespoons warm castor oil or vegetable oil
15 drops lavender (preferably *L. spica*) essential oil
5 drops geranium essential oil
5 drops tea tree essential oil

Prepare this treatment by mixing the warm castor oil in a shallow dish or saucer, then adding the anti-fungal essential oils. Soak fingernails for at least 5 to 10 minutes. Discard after use.

Other antifungal oils. Essential oils used to treat fungal-type infections are angelica root, black spruce, cedarwood, fennel, German and Roman chamomile, lavenders (especially spike), lemongrass, myrrh, patchouli, peppermint, rose geranium, rosemary, sandalwood, spikenard, tagetes, and tea tree.

Nails: The Mirror to Health

According to the ancient art of Ayurvedic medicine, the nails are a prime site for diagnosing disease. The color and shape of the nail can point to particular disorders such as nervousness, malnutrition, malabsorption, chronic illness, and calcium or zinc deficiency.

For example, consistent in this tradition, if a nail is pale, it indicates an anemic state; a yellow nail is a sign of a delicate liver; while a blue nail is symptomatic of a fragile heart or lungs. Other telltale signs are ridges, a sign of poor nutrition; white spots, an indication of calcium or zinc deficiency; and clubbed nails, which often correlate to a delicate heart or lung constitution.

HERBS

Herbal helpers. Various botanicals can be used externally as salves, hand baths, compresses, and lotions, as well as taken internally in the form of herbal teas, tinctures, and capsules. Antifungal herbs are barberry bark, black walnut hulls, chaparral, comfrey root, goldenseal root, pau de arco, and roobios (Red bush).

Since fungal infections compromise the immune system, immune-supporting herbs are helpful. Astragalus, capsicum, echinacea root, fennel seed, ginger root, peppermint, rosemary, Siberian ginseng, and turmeric are included in these areas of defense.

Fill up on garlic. Get a double dose of cure with garlic, which is both antifungal and immune supporting. Eat it to your heart's content. I recommend sipping on Old-Fashioned

Garlic and Onion Soup, which can be found on page 137. Make use of pickled garlic and garlic syrup, which can be made or purchased at specialty shops.

LIFESTYLE

Prevention first and always. A fungal infection can set your plans for pretty nails back big time. Here are some secrets to healthy nails.

- Use an antifungal soap containing tea tree oil.
- Dry nails completely.
- Keep nails trimmed short.
- Change manicuring instruments once infection is gone and start new on healthy nails.
- Avoid artificial nails and nail polish.
- Wear open-toed shoes and sandals as much as possible.
- Avoid closed shoes while infection is healing.
- Wear all-cotton or -wool socks.
- Wear cotton-lined gloves while doing dishes or garden work.
- Avoid going barefoot in locker rooms, gyms, and public showers.
- Eat healthy to keep your immune system strong.
- Use aromatherapy at the first sign of a fungal problem.

SALVES

The most powerful healer. Typically, nail fungal infections involve the nail bed, making it sometimes difficult to remedy. This area of the fingers or toes is where nail growth originates. Concentrated massage oils or ointments are applied here to treat as much new growth as possible.

This ointment is designed to be applied over the nail and surrounding area, particularly above the nail bed. The recipe is for a 1-ounce salve with an 8-percent concentration of oils; therefore, it is one of the most concentrated treatments in this book. Because the balm is applied to only a very small area and necessitates powerful treatment, it is a higher than normal blend of essential oils.

⟋⟋ Beautiful–Nail Balm ⟋⟋

2 tablespoons Heavy-Duty Ointment (page 240) or comfrey salve

25 drops lavender essential oil (*L. spica,* spike lavender, is best)

10 drops geranium essential oil

10 drops tea tree essential oil

3 drops spikenard or sandalwood essential oil

2 drops chamomile (German or Roman) essential oil

If making your own heavy-duty ointment, I recommend using the calendula infusion oil as the base, to promote healing and regeneration of new healthy cells. Add the essential oils when the ointment begins to cool. Pour into a clean, widemouth glass jar. Alternatively, you may add the essential oils to already prepared comfrey salve.

Apply twice daily by massaging into the entire nail and cuticle area. Focus attention above the nailbed area.

Nasal Congestion
⟋⟋

FUEL FOR THE FLOW

Tip: Color Signs

If mucus from a runny nose runs clear, you have nothing more than common congestion. If drainage is colored yellowish-green, then it's a sign of an infection such as sinusitis.

Stuffed up and don't know the reason why?

When the nasal passages suddenly stop service of air flow, it means excess mucous has accumulated in your nose and throat. I refer to it with the old-fashioned term *catarrh*.

Any number of things can bring

it on—an allergy, something in the environment you just entered, the weather. Often it is the first sign of an oncoming cold or other virus.

The quick onset of nasal congestion, called acute rhinitis, affects some people more than others and can range from mild to severe. If a stuffed-up nose commonly gets between you and easy breathing, here's what to do.

AROMATHERAPY

Aromatherapy is such an easy solution to a stuffed-up nose because essential oils respond well to problems of the respiratory system. They are natural expectorants.

Take eucalyptus and breathe easier. The oil of the eucalyptus plant is the best natural expectorant. Many other essential oils such as cedarwood have this property as well— either used singly or in combination with eucalyptus oil. Put a few drops on a handkerchief and carry it with you to sniff throughout the day. Also, a plastic baggie holding a few cotton balls with several drops of essential oil on them makes an easy inhalation method for travel.

Other essential oils that can be used for nasal catarrh are basil, bergamot, cypress, fennel, frankincense, hyssop, lavender, lemon, marjoram, myrrh, pine, rosemary, and sandalwood. There are many choices, so if you have particular scent favorites, try them. Remember that basil, fennel, peppermint, and rosemary are possible skin irritants, so use them in small quantities.

DIET

Pass on the milk. To hasten your recovery, avoid dairy products, which are known to increase mucous production.

Lemon your best aid. Drink fresh lemon juice in hot or cold water during the day to loosen mucus, flush your system, and balance pH levels. The vitamin C in lemons will also help fight off colds.

Go for garlic and onions. Cook with lots of garlic and onions, which are natural germ fighters; these also help with catarrh situations. Make the Old-Fashioned Garlic and Onion Soup on page 137 to ward off a cold, clear the sinuses, and boost your immune system.

Do As the Yogis Do

For serious cases of congestion, the age-old practice of nasal washing can do wonders. It is used frequently by yogis who find it most helpful in keeping their nostrils clear during meditation, when it is important to breathe freely.

To do this you need a neti pot, a ceramic vessel that looks like a small Aladdin's lamp. Make up a solution of ¼ teaspoon Celtic Sea salt and enough lukewarm water to fill the neti pot. Stand over a sink and bring the spout to your nose, bending forward slightly over the sink. Tilt your head to the right and forward slightly. Pour the water into your left nostril. The water will flow from one nostril to the lower nostril and out into the sink. Adjust your head to allow the proper flow of salt water. After the pot is emptied, blow into the sink through your nose to clear any excess water from the nostrils.

INHALATION

Have a steam heat treat. To loosen and expectorate excessive mucus, the ideal treatment is steam inhalation. Steaming or vaporization offers a direct hit of heat, vapor (steam), and essential oils. This age-old treatment is still considered the best way to get the flow going again.

⟨⟩ Steam Team ⟨⟩

This method is particularly effective for upper respiratory infections.

4 cups hot water
2 drops eucalyptus essential oil
1 drop cedarwood essential oil

Bring the water to a simmer and transfer to a ceramic bowl. Add the essential oils to the water. Hold your head about 8 inches over the water, close your eyes, and cover your head with a towel to form a tent. Slowly and deeply inhale through the nose and mouth. Allow loosened mucus to drain freely into the water bowl. For maximum benefits, steam for 5 to 10 minutes. Pat dry your face and neck area with a towel. Cover your neck and chest to maintain warmth after the inhalation. Follow with the Nasal-Break Chest Rub recipe below.

Note: Keep your eyes closed during this treatment, as the volatile oils can irritate the eyes and cause tearing.

Massage

Rub here and breathe. This rub is made with powerful respiratory clearing essential oils. It has a delightfully pure and herbal scent, unlike the cloying medicinals mixed with Vaseline our mothers and grandmothers used.

✍ Nasal–Break Chest Rub ✺

> 20 drops eucalyptus essential oil
> 5 drops basil essential oil
> 5 drops peppermint essential oil
> 5 drops cedarwood essential oil
> 2 ounces vegetable oil

In an amber glass bottle, add the essential oils one by one with an eyedropper. Add the vegetable oil. Cap securely and shake well to mix. Label. Apply a small amount of the oil to the upper chest area, lower neck, and back area between the shoulder blades and the base of neck and massage in circular and downward strokes. Be sure to get under the jaw, down from the ears, where many lymph nodes are located. Afterward, inhale the essential oils from your hands. Use two to three times per day, preferably in early morning and at bedtime.

Real-Life Cure

NO MORE SCHOOL DAZE

Angela's chronic nasal congestion left the twelve-year-old girl feeling tired and "out of it" during school. She found it hard to concentrate. Fearing her grades would fall and not wanting to put her on drugs that could leave her feeling worse, her mother came to me for help.

I suggested that Angela should try a steam inhalation before she left for school in the morning. After the very first treatment, she felt her nasal passages opening up, which she described as "crackling sounds in my nose." She opted not to use the Nasal-Break Chest Rub during the day because of its odor, but she applied it after school and at night. She carried eucalyptus oil with her throughout the schoolday to inhale as needed when her stuffy nose interfered with her concentration.

After only two days, Angela was breathing better. When attacks occur, she goes right for the inhalation therapy. And she always carries her oil with her "just in case."

See also Sinusitis.

Nausea and Vomiting

❧

CURES YOU CAN STOMACH

Think of vomiting not as a sickness but as a cure. It is a cure for the nausea that got a grip on health as you knew it just a few short hours ago. Ultimately, it's a cure for what caused your nausea, mostly likely something you ate.

Vomiting may be a miserable experience, but there is no avoiding it. In fact, voiding the offensive substance in your stomach is exactly what you want to do.

Sometimes, however, nausea and vomiting are miserable side effects of a virus such as the flu; it's a feeling that can seem never-ending. But it will end—in due time. The immediate concern when it comes to vomiting is staying hydrated.

AROMATHERAPY

Stomach easing aromas. Essential oils often used for nausea, vomiting, and general abdominal upset include angelica root, basil, black pepper, cajeput, cardamom, coriander seed, fennel, ginger, lavender, lemon, mandarin, melissa, neroli, peppermint, Roman chamomile, rosewood, and spearmint. These essences aid in calming the nervous system and naturally refresh and uplift the mind and body during an uncomfortable situation.

DIET

Replace fluids. When you are vomiting, the ultimate goal is to stay hydrated. A lot of liquid is lost through vomiting. Drink clear liquids—water, juice, and weak herbal tea. Sip in small amounts throughout the day.

Reintroduce foods gradually. After a bout with nausea and vomiting, you do not want to shock your digestive system with heavy meals. Clear soups, such as my Old-Fashioned Garlic and Onion Soup on page 137, are perfect to start you back to good health.

INHALATION

Inhale a lemon drop. Specific for regurgitation or the feeling that you are ready to throw up are anise, fennel, and lemon. Simply put a drop or two of any of these oils on a tissue and inhale. Or put the drops in an electric diffuser or aroma lamp.

MASSAGE

Hold everything. This massage lotion is relaxing, slightly cooling, and antispasmodic in action. Use it when nausea is overwhelming and after the fact to provide calming relief to the nervous system. It has a refreshing scent, which will help erase the aftereffects of vomiting.

✍ Back-to-Health Lotion ✍

1 drop basil essential oil
1 drop peppermint essential oil
1 drop lavender essential oil
2 teaspoons vegetable oil

Mix the essential oils with the vegetable oil. Rub in your hands to warm. Inhale deeply over the nose and mouth area (three slow, relaxed inhalations). Then massage gently over your abdomen (solar plexus) in a circular clockwise motion.

When to Call the Doctor

If vomiting is projectile in nature, contains blood, or becomes a symptom following a head injury, seek medical attention at once. It could be an indication of something more serious than food poisoning.

Also, if vomiting doesn't ease after 24 hours, you should see a doctor. This is most important in young children and the elderly, where dehydration is a risk.

There are disease states that can cause vomiting, such as glaucoma, meningitis, hepatitis, and some gastrointestinal cancers.

Oily Skin
✍

TACKLING THE T-ZONE

The T-zone is the scarlet letter of your face.

The slick and shiny "T" that forms across the forehead and follows a midline through the nose and mouth to the chin announces that you have oily skin. It means your sebaceous glands, which manufacture the lubricant sebum in the skin, are overproducing.

Oily or greasy skin is an unwanted condition because it can cause blocked pores and inhibit the skin from performing its many functions, including elimination of waste. If pores become blocked and infected, then acne results.

People with dark complexions and dark hair tend to experience oily skin most often. The good news is they do not show signs of aging as readily as others, since the skin has an abundance of moisture.

AROMATHERAPY

Regulate sebum production. Essential oils useful for oily skin conditions include basil, bergamot, carrot seed, cedarwood, clary sage, cypress, eucalyptus, geranium, grapefruit, juniper, lavender, lemon, lemongrass, mandarin, patchouli, petitgrain, rose, rosemary, sandalwood, tea tree, and ylang-ylang. Lightweight carrier oil choices are apricot kernel, canola, grapeseed, hazelnut, jojoba, kukui nut, and sunflower.

Give your face a tone-up. For oily skin, a good, all-natural facial cleanser or vegetarian soap is recommended since it dissolves and removes oil, dirt, and other impurities.

A good facial toner should be used to remove excess oil from the face and thoroughly clean the skin. Witch hazel, apple cider vinegar, and floral water combine to make a very effective facial toner. Lemon juice, astringent herbs, and infusions are very useful in toning and balancing oily skin types. This facial toner should be applied to the skin with cotton cosmetic pads that will aid in removing excess oils and in balancing the pH of the skin.

Oily Skin Facial Toner

4 ounces herbal infusion or distilled water
2 tablespoons apple cider vinegar or witch hazel
1 teaspoon honey
4 drops lavender essential oil
2 drops rosemary essential oil

In an amber glass bottle, add the herbal infusion or distilled water. Sage, yarrow, or rose petals are good choices. Add the vinegar. Combine the honey and the essential oils and mix well with the end of a spoon. Add the aromatic honey to the toner solution and shake well to mix completely. Shake well again before using. Moisten a cotton pad and wipe your face. Avoid the eyes and concentrate on the oily areas. Use three times per day to remove excess oil.

Light lotions only. Ideally you will want to use thin, easily absorbed, and light carrier oils or lotions that are water-based. You can easily add essential oils to your oil-free lotions by following the simple guide given in the General Treatment Blending Chart in Appendix B. Be sure your lotion does not contain any paraffin, mineral oil, or other petroleum by-products. These will inhibit the essential oils from getting absorbed and will promote blocked pores and greasy skin.

The recipe that follows is made with very light oils and essential oils that are specific to oily skin types. With regular use, this aromatherapy facial preparation will regulate over-active sebaceous glands and diminish oiliness.

✍ Light Moisturizing Nourishment ✍

2 teaspoons hazelnut oil
1 teaspoon jojoba oil
¼ teaspoon carrot seed oil
6 drops rosemary essential oil
2 drops geranium essential oil
2 drops basil essential oil
2 drops cypress essential oil

In a 1-ounce amber glass bottle, add the vegetable and seed oils. Add the essential oils and mix well by shaking the bottle. Label. Use twice daily after cleansing the face and use a facial mist just prior to applying. Use 4 to 6 drops and apply to the neck and face. Avoid the eye area.

Always mist first. Lotions and oils should be used sparingly and applied over a well-misted face. Facial mists can consist of floral water (hydrosols) or mineral water. They offer a thin water moisture base to glide the oils over and allow a more even distribution.

Diet

Decrease fats. We are what we eat, right? So it only makes sense that excess fat and oil in your diet can show up as excess oil in your skin. Decrease the fat in your diet, especially hydrogenated and animal products such as dairy. Eat plenty of high-fiber foods such as fruits, vegetables, and whole grains. Incorporate more herbs into your diet. Rosemary, for example, helps with fat (oil) regulation and oily skin conditions.

Grow a rosemary garden. The herb rosemary is a skin herb because it helps regulate oily skin conditions. Grow it and use it fresh in your cooking as well as in herbal infusions, facial mists, and spa baths.

Herbs

Effective herbs that aid oily skin conditions and large pores can be utilized in facial toners and moisturizing sprays. They can be used in facial masks, clay packs, and facial steams. Some astringent botanicals to choose from are blackberry leaves, hawthorn leaves, rosemary, and thyme.

❧ Pacific Island Mud Mask ❧

2 tablespoons powdered clay
2 to 3 tablespoons rosemary herbal infusion (enough to form a paste)
1 drop bergamot essential oil
1 drop cypress essential oil
2 drops ylang-ylang essential oil

Mix the clay and water to form a thick paste in a small saucer or ramekin. Add the essential oils and mix very well. Apply to your face and neck, avoiding the delicate eye area and hair line. Do not allow to dry completely. Mist the face intermittently with floral water, mineral water, or herbal tea to prevent drying. Leave on for 20 minutes. Gently remove with a cool, damp washcloth.

LIFESTYLE

Oil-free solutions. In your daily face routine, do the following:

- Use oil-free makeup and foundations or wear no makeup at all.
- Avoid using heavy oils on the skin (lanolin, mineral oil)
- Use exfoliants to keep pores clean and open, but take care not to overuse them as they can stimulate oil production when used too frequently.
- Keeps your hands away from your face to prevent clogged pores and blemishes.
- Do not use a loofah or any other harsh scrubber on the face.

Palpitations

NO MORE ANXIOUS MOMENTS

A heart that beats normally goes about its business in an unobtrusive way. You can't hear it and you usually can't feel it—unless you put an ear or hand up against your heart.

A heart that picks up speed and sound is a sign there's something stressful in your space. Anxiety and fear can fire up the heartbeat. So can apprehension of any kind such as an upcoming task or event you won't be greeting with pleasure—like giving a speech. Stimulants, such as coffee and caffeine-containing soft drinks and candy, can also give the heartbeat a rush.

Normally, this is a come-and-go event. But if you want to look and feel cool as a cucumber in the face of stress and anxiety, here's what you can do to slow down and mellow.

AROMATHERAPY

Hand-to-nose relief. Essential oils that are useful in relieving anxiety and palpitations are basil, bergamot, cedarwood, chamomile, cypress, frankincense, geranium, helichrysm, jasmine, juniper, lavender, lemon, marjoram, melissa, neroli, orange, patchouli, rose, sandalwood, spikenard, and ylang-ylang. Any of these essential oils, or a combination, can be inhaled from a tissue for immediate use when palpitations and feelings of anxiety are experienced.

BREATH WORK

Exhale slowly. Take several deep and relaxed breaths, inhaling from the nose for a count of three, and slowly exhaling from the nose for a count of six. Stand in front of an open window or go outdoors for the best oxygen-rich air you can find.

DIET

Stay away from stimulants. If an upcoming presentation or speech makes your heart race, stay away from stimulants such as alcohol, coffee, cola drinks, and chocolate the day of and the day before an event. Drink plenty of pure water and eat lightly.

HERBS

Cool and calm comrades. There are many herbs that soothe and calm. Among them are black cohosh, oat straw, passionflower, skullcap, and valerian root. Cardio-tonic herbs may be useful and include cayenne pepper, ginger root, Ginkgo biloba, gotu kola, hawthorn berry, lobelia, motherwort, peppermint, and Siberian ginseng.

Dosages vary greatly, and these herbs come in a wide variety of forms (capsules, tincture, tea), so you will want to take them according to the recommendations of your health professional and the manufacturer's labeled directions.

HYDROTHERAPY

Create your space. Aromatic baths are a very pleasant way to unwind and relax, especially for anyone with a history of anxiety and palpitations. Make sure the water temperature is just right (not too hot) to avoid increasing your heart rate. Perfect water temperature for this bath is between 92 and 100 degrees. Dim the room and light one candle. Take slow, deep, relaxing breaths as you soak. Sip herbal tea and listen to some natural sounds that encourage peaceful repose, like singing birds or waves splashing on the seashore.

Flower Power for Anxiety and Fear

Flower essence therapy is based on the belief that emotions and physical problems are interchangeable. Since emotional upheaval is the chief cause of palpitations, it only makes sense that flower essences can offer some release. Flower essences can be taken in teas or placed in the spa bath. Here's what to look for:

Anxiety: agrimony, aspen, cerato, cherry plum, chicory, crab apple, elm, heather, larch, mimulus, red chestnut, rock water, white chestnut, or the blend Rescue Remedy

Fear: aspen, cherry plum, mimulus, red chestnut, rescue remedy, and rock rose

My favorite herbal tea recipe, called Stress-Free Herbal Tea on page 465, is the perfect accompaniment to this spa experience. If you own one of those large seashells, the kind you can listen to the ocean in, then by all means find it and bring it into the tub with you!

❧ Heart-Pleasing Bath ❧

6 drops lavender essential oil

2 drops clary sage essential oil

2 drops ylang-ylang essential oil

4 to 6 tablespoons Celtic Sea or Dead Sea salt

Mix the essential oils into the salt. Pour into a fully drawn bath. Stir with your hands. Both of these naturally occurring mineral salts are high in magnesium, which promotes muscular (the heart is a muscle) relaxation and is one of the reasons it is recommended in this special recipe.

INHALATION

Automatic relaxation. When the heart starts pumping at home or in the office, spray the air around you with this mist. Keep it handy in a drawer. You'll get the most therapeutic benefit if you use an electric diffuser. You can turn it on during stressful situations and regularly throughout the day (every 4 hours), for at least 5 to 10 minutes, depending on the ventilation and square footage of the room.

When to Call the Doctor

Prolonged episodes of palpitations, rapid pulse, chest pain or tightness, shortness of breath, and dizziness are all symptoms that should be evaluated immediately by a health-care practitioner, as they are danger signals that the circulatory system is distressed.

Peaceful-Pace Mist

A very effective natural tranquilizer.

4 parts lavender essential oil
2 parts ylang-ylang essential oil
2 parts sandalwood essential oil
1 part lemon essential oil

Mix the essential oils into a small bottle, depending on the amount you choose to make. This blend can be used in a diffuser (in larger proportions) or inhaled from a tissue or small vial for immediate use when palpitations are experienced.

SOUND AND MUSIC THERAPY

Find tranquillity in music. Sound therapy can be a powerful tool to calm and balance both mind and body. Humans are sensitive to sound (energetic) vibrations. They can be used to comfort, soothe, and relax. Here are some of the most relaxing, profoundly calming harmonies I know of to recommend. They can be played softly in the background of your living or work environment to provide a soothing soundscape.

Kelly-Halpern—*Ancient Echoes*
Tibetan Bells
Young—*The Mystery of Destiny*
Nature's Symphonies—*Tropical Rainforest*
Deuter—*Wind and Mountain*
Halpern—*Gifts of the Angels*
Earth Songs—*Narada Collection*

Pollution

✐

CLEAN-AIR ACTIONS

It's an invisible, but serious, problem.

Even though public awareness is increasing, record numbers of people are getting ill from poor air quality and sick-building syndrome. Allergies related to such things as synthetic chemical exposure are mounting. With growing populations within crowded cities comes an increase in human odors, more garbage, and more human waste. This all adds up to a decline in air quality.

As incredible as it may sound, the Environmental Protection Agency (EPA) claims that the levels of indoor pollutants can be as much as one hundred times greater than outdoor levels. Also, they have documented a higher incidence of illness, as much as a 40 to 50 percent increase, if a building was found to have problems with air quality.

The World Health Organization (WHO) states that at least 30 percent of "new and sealed and remodeled" buildings have air-quality problems. Heating, ventilation, and air-conditioning systems can be breeding grounds for bacteria, viruses, and fungi. These germs prefer warm, dark, moist places to grow and live, making stagnant water, humidifiers, filters, and ducts the perfect homes for them to propagate.

Real–Life Cure

NO DRUGS PLEASE

Barbara, a strong and determined thirty-two-year-old mother of two and a full-time office manager, had recently undergone a physical exam as a result of increasing episodes of heart palpitations.

The results were great: She was found to be in excellent health with normal blood pressure, pulse, and respiratory readings. Her doctor felt the palpitations were caused by stress and recommended a mild tranquilizer, which she did not want to take. That's when she came to see me.

This was Barbara's first experience with alternative medicine. She learned new and better ways to deal with her stress levels. At first it was a challenge for her to avoid stimulants (coffee, chocolate, cola drinks) in her diet, to spend time on herself, to take aromatic baths, to receive massages, and to remember to take the essences to work with her.

Eventually (three weeks after meeting with me), she brought a diffuser to work with her. She had figured out that this was where she needed it the most! To her surprise, it was well received by her coworkers.

Today, Barbara experiences fewer episodes of a racing heart, she takes time for herself regularly, and, most important, she has never needed to take the prescription first offered to her by the doctor.

Sick-building syndrome is a transient illness with a wide variety of symptoms that disappear once the person leaves the "problem environment"—usually an airtight office building—and then reappear once the environment in question is re-entered. Symptoms include fatigue and afternoon lethargy; headaches, dizziness, and nausea; decreased creativity and productivity; concentration problems; allergies, flulike symptoms, and throat or eye irritation; dry, itchy skin; and asthma, especially if attacks are triggered by molds and fungal spores.

Environmental toxins, secondary smoke inhalation, smog, dirty air conditioners, and air vents are other health hazards. The poor air quality they create weakens and stresses our

Is Newer Better?

No. Modern homes and offices are containers of chemical hazards. Newer carpets, furniture, foam insulation, paint, fireplaces, wallpaper, solvents, machinery, adhesives, copying machines, and blueprints create poor indoor air quality.

When buildings are sealed airtight and recirculate the same air, the above pollutants can be accumulative. Some examples of invisible, harmful gases include formaldehyde, xylene, benzene, and carbon monoxide. Even some air fresheners contain formaldehyde! As little as .01 parts per million in the air can cause symptoms such as burning sensation in the eyes, nose, and throat; nausea; coughing; and skin rashes.

respiratory and immune systems. When the body is unable to detoxify and purify itself through adequate cleansing, it becomes susceptible to disease as the toxic matter accumulates in tissues.

There is a lot of work that needs to be done to correct these intrusive threats to the air we breathe. In the meantime, here's what you can do to counteract them.

AROMATHERAPY

Deodorize and kill. Scientific studies have proven that essential oils, due to their antiseptic qualities, have the potential to kill germs (germicidal), destroy bacteria (bactericidal), and eliminate offensive odors. They do not merely cover up or mask bad odors, as some might think, but actually alter the physical and chemical molecular structures. Some are very powerful.

A few of the tested microorganisms that were drastically inhibited by the diffusion of essential oils were *E. coli, Neisseria gonorrhea, Streptococcus faecalis, Staphylococcus aureus,* and *Pneumococcus.* Some essential oils work directly on neutralizing these harmful organisms. Research scientist Dr. Jean Valnet demonstrated the bactericidal properties of eucalyptus essential oil. A 2-percent dilution in spray form killed 70 percent of the airborne staphylococcal bacteria.

Scent Scaping: Pros and Cons

Environmental fragrancing is a term heard often these days, relating to the process of diffusing essential oils or synthetic fragrances into our living and working spaces. We don't even have to be consciously aware of the scent; it can be subliminal. As a matter of fact, it is best utilized when the scent scape is barely noticeable and merely in the background.

Interestingly, some private and commercial companies have studied particular scents and their effects on brain waves. Those scents that were calming demonstrated a smooth wave pattern (alpha) versus the stimulating scents that caused dramatic peaks and dips (beta patterns) in brain-wave measurement.

The actual amount of essential oils needed to induce a positive effect on us and the surrounding environment is quite small. Even if we do not consciously perceive the scent, our central nervous system continues to respond. The goal is to perceive a background scent, not one that is overwhelming.

Aromatic fragrancing, however, can be abused. Consider those individuals who may have allergies, asthma, or related sensitivities. There may be a thin line between what may be considered a positive addition to the quality of our environment and what may be viewed as a negative interference with it. Personal sensitivities, allergies, and public awareness need to be considered.

Nevertheless, I think the use of essential oils for purifying the air, naturally deodorizing and killing potentially harmful germs, and creating an uplifting aroma is a giant step toward making a positive influence on our environment and assisting humankind in staying connected to nature.

Some essential oils shown to have high antiseptic and antibacterial properties include bergamot, citronella, eucalyptus, juniper, lavender, lemon, lemongrass, orange, peppermint, petitgrain, pine, rosemary, sandalwood, and tea tree. Use these in a diffuser, room spray, inhalation, or spa bath.

Lemon fresh and natural. It is no accident that we equate lemon and pine smells with cleanliness. Just count the number of cleaning solutions and room deodorizers that include

Mood–Altering Modern Devices

Becoming increasingly popular both for commercial and personal use are the natural aromatic environmental fragrancing machines and devices. These electric-powered machines emit airborne essential oils into the atmosphere of a room, a portion of a house, or an entire office building. The chief goal is to purify and positively enhance the indoor air quality of work spaces and homes.

The fragrances can also be chosen for their beneficial effects on emotional and mental states. One extensive study, for example, found that lemon essential oil increased the acuity of typists and computer programmers when piped in through the air-conditioning system. Eucalyptus oil was found to be very effective for keeping night-shift employees awake and more alert with fewer mistakes and accidents.

In some countries, like Japan, delivery systems designed with computerized scent programs are attached to large ventilation systems. The air-conditioning system filters the air, then adds scent and recirculates it. Improving alertness and increasing productivity and relaxation can be some of the desired outcomes of this type of mass ventilation.

The scent that is emitted from these systems can be changed according to the time of day or shift. A fresh, pleasant lemon scent, for example, may be piped in during early morning to help wake up and gently stimulate workers. In early afternoon a more stimulating scent may be used; then perhaps a relaxing blend can be emitted right before the workday is over to aid in relaxation and preparation for evening.

The United States is implementing some of these ideas but on a much smaller and limited scale than in Japan, where it is more widely accepted. Large commercial systems are now being developed and implemented for the workplace. Customized "signature" scents are becoming popular and are being developed by aroma experts for large, exclusive hotels as well as commercial malls and movie theaters.

these particular scents. Unfortunately, virtually all are of synthetic origin. But don't despair! Scent your own natural Castile or castor oil–based organic cleansers with essential oils like citrus, peppermint, and pine. They will be gentler and safer alternatives to what you may be currently using and will have great deodorizing and germ-killing benefits. Use 80 to 100 drops in 8 ounces of an organic household cleaning solution.

Diet

Go green and organic. Eat fresh, raw, organic fruit and vegetables, especially sea vegetables. Green sources, such as chlorella, barley grass, spirulina, alfalfa, nettles, and dark green leafy vegetables like spinach, are excellent sources of minerals and aid in purifying the blood and vital fluids. Foods high in vitamin E are well known for their ability to boost the immune system and possess antioxidant properties. These include vegetable and nut oils, sunflower seeds, wheat germ, and whole grains.

Seek protection in the sea. Seaweed or sea vegetables are potent protective elements from the ocean that counteract the damaging effects of common radioactive and environmental contaminants. Seaweed contains more minerals than any other food and also many trace elements.

This soup is detoxifying to the body, eliminating extra fluids and contaminants. It has cleansing, rejuvenating, and energy-giving properties. It is steeped with nourishing benefits due to the high-mineral and chlorophyll-containing sea vegetables and field greens it contains. Sea vegetables, land vegetables, and the Celtic Sea salt make this an alkalizing meal. Omit the soy sauce and miso for a superior alkaline meal, as these are acidic, although they are used in very small amounts in the recipe.

⟋ Wholesome Sea Green Soup ⟍

A super detoxifying soup that you'll want to make as often as possible.

    1 cup assorted sea vegetables
        (alaria, dulse, kelp, nori, wakame) broken into pieces
    4 cups water (to soak seaweed)
    1 large onion, chopped
    2 celery stalks, chopped

6 cloves garlic, minced

¼ cup minced green onion or chives

3 tablespoons extra virgin olive oil

2 cups chopped assorted fresh greens
   (beet greens, cabbage, spinach, and swiss chard)

1½ quarts water or soup stock
   (made with 1 low-sodium vegetable bouillon cube)

Pinch of cayenne pepper

Black pepper to taste

2 tablespoons low-sodium soy sauce (optional)

5 ⅛-inch slices fresh ginger root

1 tablespoon miso (optional)

½ teaspoon Celtic Sea salt (optional)

Soak the sea vegetables in water for 10 minutes, then strain and set aside (for use in facial mist, bath, or to water plants) or discard. Sauté the onion, celery, garlic, and green onion in the olive oil until the onions are soft. Add the sea vegetables to the soup stock and simmer. Add the sautéed vegetables, along with the greens, to the soup stock. Add the herbs, spices, soy sauce (if desired), and ginger root. Simmer for 20 to 30 minutes. Combine the miso (if desired), with 1 cup of soup stock and dissolve. Return to the soup and (if desired) add the Celtic Sea salt.

For a heartier winter meal, increase soup stock to 2 quarts and add 8 ounces of whole wheat soba noodles for the last 5 minutes of cooking time.

Herbs

Herbal prevention. Traditional herbal medicine has been used for centuries for purifying the body, preventing disease, and enhancing immune system health. Antiviral, antibacterial, and antioxidant herbs provide the strongest protection.

Antiviral herbs include astragalus, myrrh gum, and St. John's wort. Antibacterial herbs include black walnut, chaparral, echinacea root, garlic, goldenseal root, and thyme. The antioxidant herbs include astragalus, chaparral, echinacea, Ginkgo biloba, hawthorn berry, pau de arco bark, and Siberian ginseng. These herbal powerhouses can be taken in capsule form, tinctures, or tea form.

HYDROTHERAPY

Wash away toxins. Specific treatment baths have been used for ages to aid the body in releasing unwanted chemicals. An aromatic alkalizing bath is recommended if you suspect you have a highly acidic body condition or if you know you need to detoxify heavy metals from your system. Baking soda is used to create the highly effective alkaline treatment that is necessary.

Try a bath with Detoxifying Bath Salts (page 128). Submerge yourself for at least 20 to 30 minutes, covering as much of your body as possible. Take a short shower following the soak, rinsing off any toxins and pollutants remaining on the surface of your skin. Be sure to drink at least 2 cups of water during and following this spa treatment.

If you have access to a sauna, you can multiply the detoxifying and cleansing effects by utilizing one. Also, by performing dry-skin brushing prior to the sauna or spa bath, you will better prepare the skin for the detoxification process.

INHALATION

Inhalation is perhaps one of the oldest ways in which aromatics were used by ancient cultures. For centuries, incense and aromatic woods have been burned in religious ceremonies and purification rites and are prime examples of inhalation methods. Today, the United States, Europe, and Japan lead the way in using modern applications of inhalation for improving air quality and enhancing workplace and home environments.

Make your own room environment. Aromatic room mists are an easy way to change the milieu of any room in a hurry without the use of electrical hookups or the danger of a burning candle. You can make your own by simply adding 10 to 20 drops of essential oil to a 4-ounce spray bottle of distilled water. Mix and match your own fragrances according to your personal preference. Make sure to shake the bottle well before each use because the oils do not mix with water naturally. Mist high over the head and about the room. The fine misters are best.

General antiseptic spray. This is an all-around general antiseptic synergy that can be mixed and placed in a diffuser or blended into a room spray with distilled water.

For the diffuser:

✍ Pure-for-Sure Synergy ✍

5 parts lavender essential oil
3 parts eucalyptus essential oil
3 parts pine essential oil

For a room mist:

✍ Pure-for-Sure Spray ✍

4 ounces distilled water or mineral water
10 drops lavender essential oil
6 drops eucalyptus essential oil
6 drops pine essential oil

Pour the distilled water into a fine-mist spray bottle. Add the essential oils. Shake well before using. Best to spray high above your head. Avoid spraying directly onto live plants.

LIFESTYLE

Protect public places. In the workplace, gyms, and schools, we often have large numbers of people and their germs contributing to health problems and infectious diseases. Prevention is the key. Proper maintenance of heat and ventilation systems must be maintained, including regular and thoroughly consistent cleaning, replacement of filters, and use of bactericidal, deodorizing, and disinfecting essences.

Fill your house with nature's number-one natural air filter. Not only do plants produce life-sustaining oxygen, they are living air filters, taking in dirty air and consuming or digesting the multitude of chemical pollutants that can cause various health problems and even cancers. They help clean the air, making it safer for us to breathe.

Currently, there are a number of biochemists and other scientists who are studying correlations between certain plant species and the toxins they are capable of digesting, making a specialized list of toxin-specific plant categories. For example, Boston ferns digest formaldehyde, while English ivy seems to be especially effective in consuming benzene. A few of the NASA plant experiments in the 1980s involved placing plants in highly polluted, enclosed rooms containing chemical toxins. Within a 24-hour period many of the toxins had been digested by the plants, and previous toxin levels were greatly reduced.

> ## Tip: Use Natural or Nothing
>
> Many fragrances used today are 90 percent synthetic in origin. These include room deodorizers, perfumes, and cleaning supplies and are a responsible cause for many respiratory allergies and stressed-out immune systems.
>
> Make natural choices in your personal-care products and cleaning solutions whenever possible to limit your exposure to these chemicals.

Some plants are especially good for filtering air pollution and cleaning the air. These are ideal for the home and office. Keep plants clean and dusted, as this increases their effectiveness. Excellent air-filtering plants include:

Areca palm	Dwarf date palm	Peace lily
Arrowhead vine	English ivy	Spider plant
Boston fern	Golden pathos	Striped dracaenea
Chrysanthemums		

Make vacuuming a pleasure. Put a few drops of grapefruit, lemon, or orange essential oil on the vacuum cleaner bag or filter for extra cleaning power and for an added uplifting scent to a not-so-uplifting chore!

Add fragrance to a room with a more potent potpourri. Potpourri, which, translated from French, literally means "rotten pot," is a medley of moist or dry ingredients derived from flower petals, herbs, woods, and spices. We are most familiar with its dry version. Many of the classic recipes include rose petals, wood shavings, spices, and herbs, and a fixative such as orris root.

Depending on its country of origin, potpourri can differ greatly. Potpourri often consists

Tip: Recycle Fragrances

In the foyer of our home I have a huge, three-foot-tall urn full of potpourri. It contains a collection of many past summers' flowers, herbs, and aromatic seeds and many past winters' preserved evergreens and cones. When I go through the pantry cupboards, instead of throwing out the old spices, herbal teas et cetera, I happily toss them in the urn and give them a stir.

of the common plants native to that region. In France, they may include roses, violets, bay, lavender, jasmine, rosemary, and various spices. From England, you might expect roses, juniper, lavender, thyme, geranium, and sweet fern. In India, sandalwood, patchouli, citrus, and spices are the dominant scents.

Potpourris comprised of mostly dried plant parts do contain a minute amount of essential oil. However, you can easily add pure essential oils to your old potpourri to refresh it, or simply add the essences to a newly made batch. Other old-fashioned ways of using aromatherapy are pomanders, sachets, herbal pillows, and homemade lavender wands for linen closets, drawers, and bedrooms.

Open doors. About 80 percent of our daily lives are spent indoors, either in our homes or at the office or workplace. Many of these indoor spaces lack fresh air. One simple way of refreshing our indoor air is to cross-ventilate the air daily by simply opening doors and windows to let in fresh air.

I make a daily habit of opening windows while I make the bed, opening doors when I sweep and vacuum, and sleeping with a window cracked.

Postpartum Depression

Zapping the Baby Blues

After nine months of pregnancy and hours of painful labor, depression is hardly a fair pay-off for the fruits of a joyful delivery. But postpartum (after childbirth) depression is common and can strike new moms anywhere from several days following delivery to one year later. Vague feelings of depression, tearfulness, feelings of being overwhelmed, resentment, anger, or deep depression can be experienced in varying degrees.

Postpartum depression is caused by a fluctuation in hormones combined with new demands of motherhood. Stress, responsibility, sleepless nights, and the change in family dynamics are all factors. Often, a mother expects perfection from herself, her spouse, and their new baby. It never works that way.

Aromatherapy

Match your scent to your emotion. The primary goal of aromatherapy support for the baby blues is to relieve stress, encourage relaxation, lift the spirits, and rebalance the body. As you might expect, there are essential oils that can do all these things. The most frequently used essential oils for this problem are bergamot, chamomile, clary sage, geranium, grapefruit, jasmine, neroli, rose, and ylang-ylang.

I find bergamot and geranium most helpful in regulating the body and emotions. Many of the florals, such as jasmine, neroli, and rose, help lift the spirits. Clary sage, grapefruit, jasmine, and rose are euphoric essential oils and can lift mild depression.

Ylang-ylang essential oil helps tame anger, which may not be a conscious feeling you are experiencing, but it is not unrealistic to feel a little resentment toward all the changes taking place around you. Indeed, experts believe some forms of depression may in fact be anger turned inward instead of outwardly expressed. If this is the case, as I have seen periodically, then ylang-ylang is the answer.

HYDROTHERAPY

Take time for yourself. I always tell new mothers and seasoned ones alike that when you fill up your own cup (take care of yourself), only then can the cup get full and overflow for the benefit of others. Therapeutic baths are a wonderful way to treat yourself. They relax and offer personal quiet time to gather your thoughts. Do make time for this special spa treat as often as you can so you can be the best mom you know how to be!

Depending on your skin's needs or what you have on hand, you can choose your bath base into which you'll mix your essential oils. For dry skin, use the cream; for oily skin or fatigue, try the sea salts. For irritated and normal skin, experiment with honey. They are all superior choices for the spa bath.

✿ New Mother's Pampering Bath ✿

4 drops lavender essential oil

2 drops ylang-ylang essential oil

2 drops clary sage essential oil

1 drop bergamot essential oil

1 drop mandarin essential oil

½ cup bath base (Celtic Sea or Dead
  Sea salt, heavy cream, or honey)

Mix the essential oils into the bath base. Blend well. Draw a warm to hot (92 to 104 degrees) bath. When filled, add the aromatic bath mix into the water and stir well with your hands. Sink into the water and enjoy your private time. Soak for as long as you desire.

INHALATION

Sniff and lift your spirits. This is a synergy blend designed for a diffuser, aroma lamp, or direct inhalation from a tissue or aromatic salts. It is a blend well liked by many; you don't have to be experiencing postpartum depression to enjoy it. It is a light, slightly fruity, heavenly scent, sure to lift your spirits and balance your emotions.

～ Baby Blues Synergy ～

4 parts lavender essential oil

2 parts ylang-ylang essential oil

2 parts clary sage essential oil

1 part bergamot essential oil

1 part mandarin essential oil

Mix the essential oils in an amber glass bottle with a screw top. For a large amount, use an eyedropper or teaspoon as the measure. If a smaller amount is needed, simply count them out as drops, using the above ratios.

LIFESTYLE

Get support. Asking for help, receiving nurturing and support (both physically and emotionally), eating healthy foods, and getting enough rest are measures new mothers must take. This type of support gives mom the chance to recuperate and bring balance to her life. When friends or neighbors offer to help, let them. Or ask for massage gift certificates or baby-sitting "coupons."

When I had my twins, I was overwhelmed and ended up hiring a teenage girl to help clean the house and play with my older child so that I could attend to the newborns more easily and be more relaxed. The fact is, when there is a new addition to the family, some of the other chores must be let go. I'm giving you permission not to do everything!

MASSAGE

A gift from me to you. The mass-produced, store-bought lotions cannot compare to a customized, perfect body silk cream. Take a few minutes to personalize your own spa product. I created this pampering lotion recipe just for you! It is lush, softly fragrant, and mood elevating.

The recipe can be easily divided in half to make 4 ounces, or ½ cup, of lotion. Just be sure to lessen the essential oil drops by half as well. The additional rose hip seed oil creates a more luxurious and moisturizing lotion. You will want to use this everyday just because it makes you feel so good!

Lavender Rose Silken Lotion

8-ounce bottle natural unscented lotion (no mineral oil)
60 drops lavender essential oil
30 drops rose geranium essential oil
12 drops rose (Bulgarian) essential oil
2 teaspoons rose hip seed oil or jojoba oil (optional)

If you have just purchased a new bottle of natural lotion, empty out or use a small amount, about 4 teaspoons, so you can add the extra ingredients to the existing bottle. This allows some extra room in the lotion bottle to add the oils and shake them to mix. Add the essential oils and, if desired, the rose hip seed oil. Shake well. Label.

Baby your hands. Make a scented hand cream by adding the above essential oils to a heavier hand cream. Keep it next to the baby's changing table or the sink and use it after motherly duties to reap the benefits of an antidepressant treatment throughout the day. Be sure to purchase an all-natural hand cream without mineral oil or petro-synthetic preservatives that can block the essences from being absorbed through your skin.

Other remedies can be found in Depression *and* Stress.

Premenstrual Syndrome

EASY SYMPTOM RELIEF

With more than 150 symptoms and still counting, it was just a matter of time before premenstrual syndrome (PMS) got subdivided.

These subdivisions, or clusters, are credited to Guy Abraham, M.D., an endocrinologist and research gynecologist from the United States, and includes two emotional and two physiological states.

Emotional PMS-A is the most common and includes anxiety, mood swings, nervous tension, and irritability. The second emotional cluster, PMS-D, is the least common of all the types. Its symptoms include depression, withdrawal, insomnia, forgetfulness, and confusion. Other psycho-emotional symptoms are anger, aggression, weepiness, sensitivity, restless sleep, and difficulty concentrating.

The first physical cluster, PMS-H, deals with the more common fluid retention such as swollen arms and legs, breast tenderness, bloating, and weight gain. The second physical category, PMS-C, includes symptoms such as craving sweets, increased appetite, palpitations, and dizziness. Other physical symptoms include nausea, constipation, cramping, headaches, diarrhea, and decreased libido.

PMS is caused by an increase in estrogen and a decrease in progesterone. It produces a wide variety of unpleasant and uncomfortable symptoms ranging from mild to severe. An estimated 30 to 40 percent of women experience some form of PMS.

Aromatherapy

Keep a journal. When incorporating aromatherapy into your lifestyle, be sure to allow two to three months before expecting dramatic results. Aromatherapy is a gentle and supportive form of natural healing. I suggest you start keeping a journal to record any symptoms you experience during the next several months, so you will be better able to evaluate your progress.

Feminine floral oils. Many of the essential oils reputed to be effective for PMS are from some of the most fragrant flowers. These include chamomile, clary sage, lavender, melissa, neroli, rose, and rose geranium. Oils with hormone-like activity similar to female hormones are also helpful. These include anise, basil, fennel, and nutmeg.

Diet

Whole foods only. Eat lots of fresh fruits and vegetables and plenty of whole grains and essential fats, especially nuts, seeds, and fish. Be sure to drink plenty of fluids such as pure water and herbal tea. Drinking a cup of hot water and fresh lemon juice in the morning helps to cleanse the entire system and decreases water weight gain, as it is a natural diuretic.

Taking a concentrated form of whole-leaf aloe vera has proven very beneficial for inflammatory conditions and constipation, two symptoms that are a problem for many women. Avoid food additives, refined carbohydrates and sugar, caffeine, alcohol, refined salt, and animal and dairy products (especially if they are not organic).

Alkalize your body. Eat more alkalizing foods and herbs, including drinking fresh lemon juice, to balance your system. They will go far in regulating your body, especially if you tend to overeat refined carbohydrates at this time. Eat plenty of mineral-rich foods such as sea vegetables (bladderwrack, kelp, nori, wakame) and the alkalizing herbs alfalfa, burdock, dandelion, nettles, and watercress. Prepare the Wholesome Sea Green Soup on page 389. Seaweed is the primary ingredient in this recipe and is high in minerals and trace elements. It is both detoxifying and alkalizing.

HERBS

Taking herbs as capsules and tinctures are effective for PMS. They include beth root, black cohosh, blue cohosh, chastetree berry, cramp bark, dong quai, false unicorn root, ginger root, maca root, raspberry leaf, squaw vine, and wild yam extract. Hormone-balancing botanicals include burdock root, damiana, fennel seed, and peony root. Mood-stabilizing herbs are also helpful and include black cohosh, black haw, lady's slipper root, licorice root, passionflower, peppermint, rosemary, skullcap, strawberry leaf, and valerian root.

HYDROTHERAPY

Broad spectrum bath. The essential oils chosen for this recipe aid in bloating and water retention and help with depression, nervous tension, and irritability. The essences are regulating and balancing for the female reproductive system and generally relaxing and euphoric. This bath treatment covers all the major symptoms of PMS. I suggest you take this bath three times per week, about two weeks prior to your period.

Natural Celtic Sea salt is the best for aiding water retention and muscular cramps and aches, but Epsom salt or honey can be used as alternatives.

✍ PMS Blues Bath ✍

5 drops lavender essential oil

2 drops geranium essential oil

2 drops grapefruit essential oil

1 drop clary sage essential oil

½ cup Celtic Sea salt, Epsom salt, or honey (as carrier of choice)

Add the essential oils to your carrier and mix well. After the bath has filled, add the mixture to the water and stir with your hands. Close the bathroom door for the full inhalation effect. Soak for 20 to 30 minutes in this warm to hot (92 to 104 degrees) aromatic bath treatment.

INHALATION

Make your own mood-improving air. Since there is such a wide variety of emotional states experienced by individuals during PMS, I have listed specific essential oils that can have a positive effect on the most common of these.

Customize your very own inhalation blend by choosing one to three essential oils from one or more groups below, depending on your specific needs. A few drops can be used in an aroma lamp or potpourri burner, or a larger amount can be placed in an electric diffuser. Mix and match as you please. Notice that some essential oils, like basil and bergamot, appear in more than one category and are considered key essences for treating PMS.

Irritability, aggression, nervous tension, anxiety	*Depression, tearfulness, decreased libido*
Basil	Basil
Bergamot	Bergamot
Chamomile	Clary sage
Clary sage	Grapefruit
Frankincense	Jasmine
Hyssop	Lavender
Jasmine	Lemon

Lavender
Mandarin
Marjoram
Rose
Sandalwood
Ylang-ylang

Mandarin
Neroli
Rose
Sandalwood
Ylang-ylang

Fatigue, lack of energy
Basil
Cypress
Eucalyptus
Frankincense
Ginger
Grapefruit
Hyssop
Juniper
Lemon
Peppermint
Pine
Rosemary

Regulating, balancing emotions
Bergamot
Clary sage
Frankincense
Geranium
Lemongrass

Tip: Go Natural

It is especially important to choose natural alternatives and products when it involves internal use, as with tampons. Nowadays, unfortunately, tampons are made with synthetic, unnatural materials such as rayon, which releases toxins linked with toxic shock syndrome. The material is usually chlorine bleached, which also produces dioxin, a known carcinogen. Also, additives to increase absorbency and to add fragrance are used and pose a health risk as well.

Use natural options, such as 100 percent cotton tampons (Natracare and Tampax Naturals) or a reusable menstrual cap (called the Keeper).

MASSAGE

Nurturing massage. A massage oil is very helpful in easing bloating, backache, and cramping. If you are not using an aromatic bath, it can be very effective for the discomforts of PMS if used daily.

Apply a hot-water bottle or hot compress for additional relief, if desired. I find the mild to moderate cases of PMS respond quite well to massage oils alone, while the more severe PMS symptoms need the additional heat application for the greatest benefit.

This recipe includes infusion oil of arnica or St. John's wort to help with muscular cramps and general inflammation. Both borage oil and evening primrose oil are known to increase prostaglandin levels, which decrease inflammation, and are of great benefit for PMS-related symptoms. This is a massage concentrate and should only be applied to local areas of the body such as the lower abdomen and back. Do not use as a whole body massage oil. Apply daily during episodes of PMS symptoms, up to two weeks prior to menses.

PMS Massage Oil

A potent premenstrual potion.

20 drops lavender essential oil
10 drops rosemary essential oil
6 drops clary sage essential oil
6 drops juniper essential oil
6 drops lemon essential oil
2 tablespoons vegetable oil
2 tablespoons arnica infusion oil
  or St. John's wort infusion oil
2 teaspoons evening primrose oil
  or borage oil

Mix the essential oils in an amber glass bottle. Then add the vegetable and infusion oils. Shake gently to mix well. Label the bottle with contents and directions for use. To apply, massage a small amount of the oil into the lower abdominal and lower back areas. Apply the aromatic oil with gentle hand pressure, working toward the heart to encourage blood return and increase lymphatic drainage. Inhale the essences from your hands after application.

SOUND AND MUSIC THERAPY

Something to harp about. Music that is soothing and promotes stress relief is most effective for PMS. Try to select feminine pieces—those that are performed by female vocalists and contain string music such as harp.

Stivell—*Renaissance of the Celtic Harp*
Lee—*Celestial Spaces for Koto*
Harpestry—*Contemporary Collection*
Halpern—*Gifts of the Angels*
Cluck, Bach & Tchaikovsky—*Flute Dreams*
Robert Gass/On Wings of Song—*From the Goddess; O Great Spirit*

TEAS AND TONICS

Productive reproductive tea. This herbal tea helps to nourish the female reproductive system during times of PMS or menopause. Because of its delightful taste and positive emotional effect on most women, I suggest you enjoy it more frequently than once per month.

✕ Goddess Tea ✕

6 parts raspberry leaves
4 parts chamomile flowers
2 parts rose petals
1 part fresh or dried ginger root
1 part ground licorice root
1 part rosemary herb
Honey to taste (try Ginger Honey, page 48) (optional)

Combine all the dry ingredients in a clean glass jar and label. If using fresh ginger root, cut a ¼-inch slice for each cup of tea. When using dried or dehydrated ginger, use ¼ teaspoon (or to taste). If using Ginger Honey, you may omit the ginger root if you wish. Pour boiling water over 2 teaspoons of herbal tea mix per cup and steep for 5 to 10 minutes. Drink hot or cold.

Real-Life Cure

NO MORE MONTHLY MOOD SWINGS

Barb would know two weeks ahead of time when her period was coming because of all the PMS symptoms she experienced, including dramatic mood swings verging on depression. She also suffered from bloating, carbohydrate cravings, and mild headaches.

Barb, who was thirty-eight at the time she came to see me, was otherwise healthy, ate a balanced mostly vegetarian diet, and exercised regularly. The problem was that her PMS symptoms usually lasted for two weeks. Half of her life was being spent in misery! Her irritability, in fact, was so bad it began to affect her relationship with her boyfriend and her coworkers.

She had tried many of the over-the-counter medicines suggested for PMS symptoms but didn't experience much improvement. She was feeling desperate and confused when she came to see me.

She began taking aromatic baths and using massage oils. She purchased and starting using a diffuser in her apartment. She used oils that directly affected her emotional symptoms. She began to feel a big difference about the sixth week, and by her second month she had very few symptoms.

By the second month, she said she had only one day of symptoms before her period came. The aromatherapy had helped balance her system, and she no longer had to spend half her life in misery. As part of her dietary change, she began taking aloe vera concentrate and herbal tea to nourish her system and help diminish water retention.

It has been a few years since her PMS problems, and she says when she starts menopause she will certainly turn to aromatherapy to help her!

Raynaud's Syndrome

WARMING TRENDS

Long, cold, wintry weather forces some people to seek refuge in warm climes. For people with Raynaud's syndrome, it's numb hands and feet.

Raynaud's syndrome is a circulatory system ailment that causes supersensitivity to cold that is felt mostly in the hands and feet. It's not just cold weather that can cause this disease to flair up but *any* contact with cold. Reaching into an ice tray or grabbing a cold glass can cause a reaction—usually cold or numb limbs that are difficult to warm up. It's caused by a decrease in the blood flow of the small vessels. Typically people with Raynaud's are less sensitive to heat and pressure and are therefore more prone to touch-related accidents, cuts, abrasions, and burns. It is not a dangerous condition but may be uncomfortable.

The Other Face of Raynaud's

There are two forms of Raynaud's disorder—primary and secondary. Often called Raynaud's syndrome, the primary form is the benign but uncomfortable disorder discussed here. It is the most common.

The secondary form, known as Raynaud's phenomenon, is caused by related health problems such as lupus, scleroderma, mixed connective tissue disease, and carpal tunnel syndrome. People whose work involves regular use of vibrating type machines or tools are also susceptible to this form. Also some medications have been linked to causing this condition, including chemotherapy agents, beta-blocker–type drugs for high blood pressure, and some narcotics and cold remedies.

AROMATHERAPY

Thawing scents. Aromatherapy can be supportive by preventing vasospasm and increasing local circulation. Essential oils are most useful when applied via compresses, bath treatments, and massage oil. Aromatherapy oils helpful in easing Raynaud's symptoms are black pepper, fennel, geranium, lavender, nutmeg, and rosemary.

DIET

Be caffeine-free. Decreasing stimulants such as alcohol and caffeine is necessary to ease symptoms of this ailment because they are vasoconstrictive and can further complicate the condition. Remember there are considerable amounts of caffeine in cola drinks and chocolate as well as in coffee.

Join the garlic-and-onion brigade. Garlic and onions are renowned for aiding in circulatory problems. If you have Raynaud's, get as much as possible in your diet.

HYDROTHERAPY

Water treatment. Excellent for increasing blood circulation and dilating the capillaries, this warming bath treatment offers short-term benefits by easing symptoms.

❧ Hand- or Foot-Warming Bath ❧

2 drops geranium essential oil
2 drops rosemary essential oil
1 drop lavender essential oil
2 tablespoons Celtic Sea or Dead Sea salt

Add the essential oils to the salt and mix well. Pour into a basin of warm (92 to 100 degrees) water and stir. Soak hands or feet for 15 to 20 minutes. Follow with treatment oil for additional relief. When the water temperature cools, replace with warmer water.

Caution! Check water temperatures. Take extreme care in checking the water temperature. People with Raynaud's cannot adequately judge the water temperature by using their affected hands. A warm-to-hot bath temperature is optimum (between 98 and 104 degrees). I recommend using a candy thermometer to measure the water temperature.

LIFESTYLE

Make the right move. Lifestyle changes can help to alleviate the intensity of symptoms often experienced by people with Raynaud's syndrome.

- Smoking causes poor circulation, and nicotine decreases skin temperature and may instigate attacks, so quit if you can and avoid secondary smoke.
- Keeping your hands and feet warm is extremely important. Layer your clothing in the cooler months, and wear gloves, mittens, heavy socks, and leggings, as appropriate.
- Regular exercise can boost total circulation, raise body temperature, and aid sleep and stress reduction. A good stretching routine can be very beneficial as well.
- If your symptoms are particularly serious and interfere with your life, you may want to try acupuncture. It has been shown to decrease discomfort in some people.

MASSAGE

Rub your hands together. This hand (and foot) oil is very effective for all types of muscular inflammations and nerve-related pain and is beneficial in reducing the symptoms of Raynaud's. It should be applied morning and night for several weeks in order to observe benefits.

This recipe can also be made with an unscented lotion rather than an oil base for quicker absorption. The wheat germ oil is high in vitamins A, D, and E and is exceptional for strengthening weakened capillaries. Vitamin E has long been used for skin rejuvenation and healing; in addition, it has antioxidant properties.

⟨ Raynaud's Hands-On Oil ⟩

Use this after a warm bath to help increase its healing power.

26 drops lavender essential oil
10 drops rosemary essential oil
7 drops geranium essential oil
7 drops nutmeg essential oil
2 tablespoons wheat germ oil
2 tablespoons St. John's wort infusion oil (hypericum)
800 international units vitamin E (capsules)

In a 2-ounce amber glass bottle, add the essential oils. Add the wheat germ oil and the St. John's wort infusion oil. Use the vitamin E capsules by cutting the end of the gel cap and squeezing the contents into the bottle. Shake gently to mix well. Label contents. Use twice daily or more often as necessary during the cold weather months and during problem attacks.

Real-Life Cure

FINE FIX FOR SPORTS FANATIC
Jeff's love of fall sports became seriously affected after he started to experience cold hands, white knuckles, and blue fingernail beds while he was playing football and soccer. The sixteen-year old was diagnosed with Raynaud's by his physician.

Willing, as he described, to "try anything," he started to use the hand oil and hand bath treatments I recommend here. After several weeks, he became less sensitive to the cold, and his symptoms began to wane.

As is typical of someone his age, Jeff doesn't spend nearly as much effort during the warmer months keeping up with his treatment, even though I recommended he do so. Nevertheless, when football and soccer season roll around, he starts up again with the oils and hand baths. To his delight, he can keep on playing!

Ringworm

✑

THE ALLOVER TREATMENT

Ringworm is not a worm. Rather, it is a superficial fungal infection of the skin. It does, however, have a peculiar "ring" formation of growth, which is how it got its name. It grows outward from the center, leaving an inactive middle portion that develops a red ring appearance on the skin. It's most common in children.

Depending on where on your body you have the fungal infection (tinea) will determine the medical name given to describe this ailment. If the ringworm is located on the scalp, it is referred to as tinea capitis. This type can be very itchy and can cause hair loss in patches. It is also contagious; infected pets, soil contamination, and person-to-person contact with someone who already has the condition are the most common sources of infection. Common use of hairbrushes, combs, and hats can easily spread this from person to person.

New Fungus Fighter

A new oil from New South Wales called Mountain or Native Pepper (*Tasmannia lanceolata*) has demonstrated potent antifungal properties in laboratory testing against several organisms, including *Candida albicans,* yeasts, as well as ringworm. Be on the lookout for it. As of this writing, it was not widely available in most health stores in the United States.

Ringworm can also appear on the body in a single ring patch or multiple patches and is called tinea corporis, or circinata. Typical locations are exposed areas of the arms, hands, and feet. It can also extend into areas of the scalp, hair, and nails.

Topical antifungal agents are necessary to treat ringworm. It can be stubborn to treat, so you must be patient and consistent with treatment and hygiene. Most ringworm conditions require 10 to 14 days of consecutive treatment. In some stubborn cases, a month may be necessary to totally get rid of the fungal growth. The important thing to remember is to apply this treatment two to three times per day, for 10 or more consecutive days. This is a challenge but must be done to be successful.

AROMATHERAPY

Aromatics that get the ring out. Essential oils that show antifungal properties are basil, cedarwood, chamomile, cypress, eucalyptus, fennel, geranium, lavender, lemon, myrrh, patchouli, rosemary, sandalwood, and tea tree. Of these, the safest for children are geranium, lavender, and tea tree. Peppermint essential oil must be highly diluted before using because it can irritate the skin. Some experts suggest you use specific essential oils "neat," or straight on the skin.

Get concentrated help. The following aromatherapy treatment oil is very concentrated and is designed for use on small areas such as ringworm. Because fungal infections can be resistant to treatment, a strong blend such as this is warranted.

I find an oil base encourages slower evaporation of the essences and is very effective. However, since this is a fungal infection, light oil is recommended rather than a heavy ointment, as fungi thrive in moist, dark, warm conditions.

Ringworm Treatment Oil

25 drops tea tree essential oil
15 drops lavender essential oil
5 drops geranium essential oil
5 drops peppermint essential oil
400 international units vitamin E (capsides)
2 tablespoons vegetable oil (sesame or soy)

In a 1-ounce amber glass bottle, add the essential oils and the vitamin E. You can use vitamin E gel caps by cutting one end and squeezing the contents into the bottle. Add the vegetable oil. Shake the bottle to mix. Use a Q-tip to apply the oil to the affected skin areas. Be sure to cover the entire patch. Apply this treatment oil three times per day for at least 10 consecutive days.

Tip: The Flax Attack

Flaxseed oil is a well-known fungus fighter. I've found that a tasty way to get it in your diet is to use it as a base for salad dressing. Add to it the antifungal-fighting herbs fennel, garlic, rosemary, savory, and thyme for a fully loaded healing recipe. To make, add 1 teaspoon of each of the spices according to personal taste to ¼ cup of flaxseed oil with ¼ cup of olive oil.

HERBS

Special skin wash. Acidophilus, aloe vera, and apple cider vinegar have been proven to be effective fungal fighters, but their benefits are multiplied when combined with one or more of the following antifungal herbs: black walnut, garlic, goldenseal, and myrrh. The easiest way to use them in concentrated form is in a tincture. I recommend combining them in a skin wash. Leave out the garlic if you are concerned about the aroma.

🖎 Fungal-Fighting Skin Wash 🖎

¼ cup apple cider vinegar
2 tablespoons aloe vera gel (whole leaf extract)
2 dropperfuls (total) of any of the following herbal tinctures:
    black walnut hulls, garlic, goldenseal, and myrrh
10 drops tea tree essential oil
¼ teaspoon Celtic Sea salt

In a 4-ounce amber glass bottle, measure out the vinegar and aloe vera gel. Add the herbal tincture. Mix the tea tree essential oil with the small amount of sea salt and then add to the bottle. Shake well to combine. Label. To use, dip a cotton swab or ball into the herbal wash and dab onto the affected area. Allow to dry.

Try the hair of the horse. Horsetail Tea is an excellent fungal fighter and can be consumed freely throughout the day. This herb is rich in minerals, including silica, which is beneficial for healthy skin and hair. You can find my recipe for making it on page 105.

LIFESTYLE

It's a family affair. Lifestyle modifications to enhance family hygiene are extremely important whenever you are dealing with a contagious ailment such as ringworm.

- Use clean towels daily, and do not share towels with other family members.
- Dry skin thoroughly after bathing to help contain the spread of the infection. Use a hairdryer on a low setting.
- Put clothes through two drying cycles in the dryer. This guarantees they will not harbor fungi. You can also place several drops of tea tree essential oil onto a washcloth and toss it into the dryer with the clothes, for additional benefit.
- Keep children's nails short to help prevent scratching and spread of ringworm.
- Use an antifungal or natural vegetable-based soap that contains antifungal essential oils.

Real-Life Cure

TYPICAL CHILD'S PLAY

Robbie, age six, had quarter-inch diameter rings on his arm and thigh when his mother discovered he had ringworm. By the time I was consulted, the rings had grown to approximately ¾-inch and multiplied to several other areas.

I presume the child got the infection from his pet dog or from playing in the woods and soil. Robbie claimed it itched only slightly and he was not bothered by it.

His mother applied Ringworm Treatment Oil (recipe on page 411) twice per day and gave him several baths weekly. The infection completely disappeared within 11 days. It has been over one year, and Robbie has not been reinfected since.

Scars

∞

A NATURAL COVER-UP

But will it leave a scar?

This is the most frequently asked question of people who show up in the emergency room with a deep wound that needs stitches or surgical repair. The honest answer is . . . it all depends.

Wounds undergo several stages of repair, including cleaning up the area and killing bacteria. Within 3 to 7 days, fibroblastic cells go to work forming the new collagen and elastin necessary for the wound to close and heal. However, in deep wounds or those that have become infected, usually fewer collagen and elastin fibers are present, giving the firmness and non-elastic characteristics to many scars.

Scars are easier to prevent than they are to erase. Once a scar is formed, the right treatment at the very least should help diminish it.

AROMATHERAPY

Wound-healing oils. Essential oils that aid healing, kill bacteria, and reduce inflammation are the ones to use to prevent scarring. They work best when used as soon as possible and before fibroblastic cells go into action. To prevent scar formation, as in thermal burns, apply two to three times daily for up to a few weeks until total healing has taken place. Once the wound has healed, begin applying the essential oils in a carrier and always include vitamin E. If a scar has already formed, aromatherapy treatments need to be applied three times daily for 3 to 6 months. It is best to use these oils in ointments that can be directly applied to the skin.

Essential oils include bergamot, chamomile, eucalyptus, frankincense, geranium, hyssop, juniper, lavender, lemongrass, mandarin, neroli, patchouli, rosemary, and sandalwood.

Carrier oil options noted for their healing properties are calendula, carrot seed, comfrey, hazelnut, olive, rose hip seed, vitamin E, and wheat germ. Mix essential oils with these carriers to make healing ointments.

Use lavender first and fast. Lavender is one particular essential oil that can be applied "neat" directly to a wound or burn without needing to be diluted in another oil or carrier. It can be applied immediately to any burn to prevent infection and scarring. Lavender can also be used in cool or warm compresses or sterile dressings.

Dress it in aloe. A wound dressing can be made by saturating a sterile gauze pad with aloe vera juice and several drops of lavender essential oil. Leave this on the wound for 8 to 10 minutes or until it has dried. Do this three times per day.

SALVES

Stick with Preparation S. After the wound has closed and healing has taken place, you can begin applying this salve to help prevent scarring and to promote healing to underlying tissues. It can be used on surgical scars, trauma wounds, and burns.

You may also use this on older scars to help soften and reduce their appearance. Remember: The older the scar, the longer the treatment will take. Allow at least 3 to 6 months of treatment to see any change in old scar tissue.

In this preparation, more than twice the normal quantity of wheat germ and vitamin E is used. It is a potent formula, so use it sparingly on scar tissue and the immediate surrounding skin. You can gently heat this oil by placing it in a warm water bath to increase absorption into the skin.

Scar–Diminishing Preparation

> 1 tablespoon calendula infusion oil
> 1 tablespoon hazelnut or olive oil
> 1 teaspoon wheat germ oil
> ¼ teaspoon carrot seed oil
> ¼ teaspoon rose hip seed oil
> 800 international units vitamin E (capsules)
> 20 drops lavender essential oil
> 5 drops frankincense essential oil

In an amber glass bottle, add the calendula, hazelnut, and wheat germ oils. Add the carrot seed and rose hip seed oils, along with the vitamin E. Vitamin E gel capsules can be used by cutting one end and emptying the contents into the bottle. Shake this mixture of oils well. Add the essential oils and shake gently to combine well. Label with instructions for use. To use, apply three times daily to closed wounds and scars.

Seasonal Affective Disorder

❦

NATURE'S ANSWER

It's SAD but true.

An estimated 35 million Americans experience some form of Seasonal Affective Disorder (SAD) in the short, gray days of winter. All because of inadequate light and sunshine.

People with SAD experience symptoms from mild to severe—from lethargy, concentration problems, irritability, and cravings for sweets and carbohydrates to tearfulness, so-

Location, Location, Location

The farther you are from the equator, the greater your chance of coming down with Seasonal Affective Disorder (SAD).

I live in the Pacific Northwest where we may only have two short days of sunshine during the month of December. No wonder Seattle is the coffee drinking capital of the United States! Daylight-deprived persons find themselves looking for external stimulation, such as caffeine, and craving carbohydrates and sweets to get through the dismal days.

It's no coincidence that the main center for SAD research is located here!

cial withdrawal, loss of libido, low self-esteem, weight gain, and depression. Difficulty getting up in the morning is common among people with SAD.

The good news is that SAD is short lived. All symptoms fade with the coming of spring and the longer days of sunshine.

AROMATHERAPY

Get some liquid sunshine. The hypothalamus is the part of the brain that is responsible for regulating moods, sex drive, sleep, and hunger. So it only makes sense that essential oils that stimulate the hypothalamus can help to counteract SAD. The big three SAD oils are bergamot, frankincense, and geranium.

Take a shine to lemon. Just looking at this shiny yellow citrus fruit conjures up thoughts of sunshine for me! Citrus oils are known for their inherent uplifting and "sunny" disposition and the positive effect they can have on us. A variety of citrus-derived oils are available including bergamot, grapefruit, lemon, lime, mandarin, and orange.

Light-Bearing Elixirs

According to the science of flower essence healing, there is a direct correlation between seasonal affective disorder and particular flower essence remedies. This may or may not be applicable to your situation, but it's worth exploring as a possibility. They can be purchased at most health-food stores and taken according to package directions.

Balsam and poplar: Synchronization of body rhythms with planet
Chiming bells: Depression due to loss of inner connection
Grass of Parnassus: Receiving nourishment from nonvisible light
Single Delight: Feeling of isolation in times of darkness
Sunflower: To receive energy from the sunlight

The oils are naturally found in the citrus fruit's outer peel, where the sun's light rays are absorbed to ripen the fruit. In a sense, these precious essences store up the sun's powerful energy. You can certainly feel a difference after inhaling one of these fresh citrus scents.

HYDROTHERAPY

Take exotic and euphoric soaks. For an allover body immersion treatment, also known as a bath, the recipes shared below are effective in toning the body and creating a euphoric mood, and are especially useful during seasonal changes.

If your skin is dry, which is all too common in the midwinter months, add 1 to 2 vitamin E capsules by cutting the end and squeezing the contents into the salts. Alternatively, half a cup of heavy cream can be substituted for the sea salt, for extra soothing and moisturizing effects.

✍ Island Retreat ✍

This is a skin toning, balancing, and regulating spa soak with a Pacific Island scent.

6 drops lavender essential oil
6 drops lemongrass essential oil
3 drops ylang-ylang essential oil
2 to 4 tablespoons Celtic Sea salt
Vitamin E capsules (optional)

✍ Floridian Sun ✍

I find the light citrus aroma slightly euphoric.

5 drops grapefruit essential oil
3 drops basil essential oil
3 drops lime or mandarin essential oil
1 drop clary sage essential oil

2 to 4 tablespoons Celtic Sea salt
Vitamin E capsule (optional)

Draw a warm to hot (92 to 104 degrees) bath. Mix the essential oils with the salt. Add to bathwater. Sink into this relaxing retreat for as long as you wish.

Create a Sultry Atmosphere

Maybe you can't make it to a tropical isle in the dead of winter, but with a little innovation you can be there in spirit. Here's how:

Gather together a collection of seashells, crystals, stones, sea sponges, seaweed, loofahs, or anything that congers up tropical thoughts in your mind. Turn on all the lights in the bathroom and play soft nature tracks in the background such as ocean sounds, dolphin music, or rainforest sounds. Slip into an aromatic spa bath. Lean back, relax, and sip on a freshly brewed glass of herbal iced tea.

INHALATION

Whiff a summer breeze. Close your eyes, set off this fragrance into your air space, and you'll feel like you're in a tropical paradise.

I recommend putting this blend in a diffuser with an automatic timer, but it can also be put in an aroma lamp, potpourri burner, or room spray.

✍ Tropical Oasis ❧

A citrus fresh reminder of summer for the midwinter doldrums.

3 parts lemon essential oil
3 parts mandarin essential oil
2 parts lemongrass essential oil

2 parts grapefruit essential oil
2 parts bergamot essential oil

Place all the essential oils in an amber glass bottle and shake well. To make a large amount for diffuser use, measure by eyedropper. If needing a smaller amount for use in an aroma lamp, count out the oils by drops.

Try this blues chaser. Chase away the blues associated with SAD by alternating this blend with Tropical Oasis, or use it on its own. Its ingredients help with mild depressive states and regulation of the mind/body continuum.

✑ Nature's Answer Oil ✑

4 parts clary sage essential oil
4 parts ylang-ylang essential oil
3 parts geranium essential oil
2 parts basil essential oil
1 part sandalwood essential oil

Mix the essential oils in an amber glass bottle. Label. To use in a diffuser, simply add to the bottle or reservoir for the apparatus. If you want to enjoy this aroma by using an aroma lamp or simmering pot, add 4 to 6 drops into the hot water chamber.

LIFESTYLE

Get outdoors. Even on cloud-covered days, you will experience more diffused sunlight out of doors than you will indoors. So plan daily walks first thing in the morning or on your lunch break. The earlier in the day you can be outside, the greater the amount of sunlight you will absorb.

Plan special activities on the weekend such as hiking, visiting botanical gardens and state parks, and bird watching. Best yet, get involved in winter sports like skiing, skating, snowboarding, and sledding. If you get to love winter activities, you just may hate to see winter end!

Avoid human hibernation. Plan activities with friends and family members, such as those listed above. Participate in group activities and social functions. Host a party in the middle of winter. I suggest a summer luau in your home in January or February, as these seem to be the dreariest months.

Stress relief is good medicine. Adopt a good stress-relief regime for yourself. Any form of exercise as well as deep breathing are important for all types of stress, including SAD.

Transform your surroundings. Invest in a light box or several full spectrum lights for your home and office space. Paint your common areas in lighter colors or change the window coverings to allow more light to filter in. Diffuse uplifting, antidepressant, and citrus scents into your environment. Play uplifting music. I find ocean sounds and nature recordings are very pleasing to many people who suffer from varying degrees of SAD.

Take a sauna. Frequent your gym more often and use the sauna. I own a sauna, which I just love, and use different aromatherapy blends in it depending on my needs. It has a very bright, full-spectrum light in it and provides lots of heat during any kind of bleak weather.

Sit by the fire under the stars. On dry winter evenings when the stars are out, our family enjoys a special time together sitting around the fire pit on our patio and staring into the bright flames of the fire. Although not as therapeutic as sunlight, candle flames and fires do provide the eyes with beneficial luminous energy.

 For other healing remedies, see Depression *and* Stress.

Sensitive Skin

✍

The Pure and Simple Solution

Delicate tissue is the issue. It doesn't matter if skin is young or mature, oily or dry. If your face suddenly appears flush, red, or irritated for no apparent reason, you have sensitive skin.

Persons who have sensitive skin are prone to allergic reactions, skin breakouts, and rashes. They may also sunburn easily. People with supersensitive skin can even develop hives or rashes when confronted with emotional stress.

It's hard to figure out what's causing your skin to blush because the attacker is often invisible, such as an ingredient in a cosmetic, soap, or skin-care product. Some people can blush from wine and certain alcohols. A skin patch test is the best way to find out what's bothering your skin.

Aromatherapy

Unadorned purity. Simplicity and pure ingredients are important in a skin-care regime for sensitive skin types. Mild cleansing, kind toners, and delicate moisturizers are the aim. Use a simple floral water, like chamomile or orange blossom, to gently tone and mist the face. Herbal infusions made from mild toning plants can be useful alone or added to floral waters and a little apple cider vinegar.

Essential oils good for sensitive skin and soothing to allergic-type reactions are chamomile, frankincense, jasmine, lavender, neroli, rose, and sandalwood.

Be kind to your skin. A good, safe, and gentle toning lotion may be difficult to find, so make your own using the recipe below. It contains simple ingredients that are effective for toning, balancing the skin's pH, and providing moisture. Chamomile and lavender are the herbs and essential oils that are most often utilized for these sensitive skin types.

✐ Gentle Toner ✑

7 ounces floral water or herbal infusion (chamomile or lavender)
1 ounce apple cider vinegar

Make an herbal infusion of chamomile or lavender flowers by pouring near-boiling water over 2 to 3 tablespoons of fresh or dried flower tops. Alternatively, you can purchase pure floral water or hydrosol of the same type to make this recipe. Simply add 2 tablespoons of cider vinegar and mix well. Pour this lotion into a spray bottle for easy application. Use daily after cleansing the skin.

Make your own moisture. Besides the toner, a good, moisture-rich aromatherapy preparation is important to complete the sensitive skin–care regime. Hypoallergenic nut and plant oils along with mild yet effective toning essential oils are used in this recipe. Carrier choices good for sensitive skin are apricot kernel, avocado, hazelnut, jojoba oil, safflower, sesame, and sweet almond.

This oil should be applied twice daily, or after cleansing and toning. The essential oils chosen make this a very emollient, gentle, and light moisturizer oil blend.

✐ Moisture–Rich Emulsion ✑

2 teaspoons hazelnut oil
1 teaspoon sesame oil
¼ teaspoon jojoba oil
400 international units vitamin E capsules (optional)
8 drops lavender essential oil
2 drops chamomile essential oil
2 drops jasmine essential oil

In an amber glass bottle, add the hazelnut, sesame, and jojoba oils. Add the vitamin E if desired. The capsules can be used by cutting the end and emptying the contents. Add the essential oils and shake to mix well. Label. To use, apply to moist skin. Put a few drops on your fingertips and smooth onto your face in an upward motion, avoiding the eyes.

LIFESTYLE

Become an alert consumer. Always inquire about and check the origin, reputation, and purity of the products you purchase for your personal use, especially when deciding on facial products.

Make sure your essential oils are genuine and authentic, 100 percent natural, and pure and have been stored properly. Avoid complex blends of aromatherapy oils and use simple ingredients. Other oils that are possible sensitizers are coconut, cocoa butter, and corn.

Avoid chemical additives such as synthetic dyes, petroleum by-products, preservatives, and artificial fragrances. Artificially fragranced bath soaps, detergents, deodorants, makeup, hair treatments, moisturizers, and shampoos should all be suspect.

Irritant-Prone Essential Oils

These essential oils can cause irritation to sensitive, inflamed, or allergic skin types.

Aniseed

Basil

Bay

Benzoin

Camphor

Citronella

Fennel

Lemongrass

Lemon verbena

Peppermint (when used
   undiluted, it will cause
   skin irritation on all
   skin types)

Rose
   (in high concentrations)

Rosemary

Ylang-ylang
   (in high concentrations)

All absolutes and concretes

Any oils produced by solvent
   (chemical) extraction

Sexual Dysfunction

✺

LOVE POTIONS

Aphrodisiacs—substances that are reputedly capable of enhancing sexual pleasure or sexual desire—go back to the beginning of time when Eve lured Adam into sin with the bite of an apple.

Folklore aside, science has found that there really is a connection between certain foods and substances that can motivate the libido. In fact, herbs have been used for centuries to stimulate circulation and cure impotence.

Experts claim that male impotence is caused by several factors, including problems within the vascular, neurological, and/or cardiovascular systems. In women, estrogen levels and insufficient foreplay may be factors in the decreased interest in sexual desire. Infections, medications, and alcohol can slow the libido in both men and women.

Opposites Do Attract

It appears true, to some extent, that opposites do attract, at least when it comes to body odor. Researchers have found that we are most sexually attracted to those whose basic body smell is least like our own.

It has also been discovered, however, that oral contraceptives reverse body-smell preferences. Additional studies show that we smell best to a person whose genetically based immunity to disease differs most from our own.

AROMATHERAPY

Essential oils are mood-enhancing substances that are capable of creating many different moods or feelings such as warmth, femininity, euphoria, romance, or spirituality. Aphrodisiacs can be used to enhance feelings of self-confidence, joy, and a general feeling of well-being. They become therapeutic when they affect the emotions and the nervous system. Aromatherapy, more than any other form of complementary system, has unlimited potential in this area.

A Kiss Is Just a Kiss?

Kissing is still one of the best ways to intimately smell others. In fact, in several languages the word *kiss* means "to smell." The face is one of the places where there are ample sweat glands, which play a key role in producing a person's characteristic smell. Regions of the body with a large number of sweat glands and hair are considered erogenous (arousing sexual feelings) body zones. It is primarily these areas, and the odors produced there, that make up the smell characteristic to each and every person.

The glandular connection. The pituitary gland, also known as the master gland of the endocrine system, is responsible for controlling hormone production of other glands. There is an association between an underactive pituitary gland and a decreased interest in sex as well. Interestingly, the essential oils that have the ability to stimulate the pituitary gland are also those that have been used in aphrodisiacs. They are clary sage, jasmine, patchouli, and ylang-ylang.

Scents that attract. Jasmine absolute (which means it was solvent extracted due to its low essential oil content) is the most sought after fragrance in the perfume industry because it has a very erogenous effect on humans. Ambrette seed (*Hibiscus abelmoschus, L.*) and angelica are two essential oils that are used in lieu of animal derivatives in perfumes and aphrodisiacs because of their musk-like scent.

Other essential oils that have aphrodisiac properties are black pepper, cardamom, carrot seed, cedarwood, coriander, elemi, fennel, frankincense, geranium, ginger, hyssop, juniper, myrrh, neroli, nutmeg, oak moss, pine, rose, rosemary, sandalwood, vetiver, and ylang-ylang.

These oils can be very effective for setting a mood, affecting the emotions, and stimulating the brain to achieve arousal. Aromatic baths, massage oils, and inhalation make the most sense as they also encourage intimacy and touch. Essential oils can also be used in the Jacuzzi, sauna, or shower. Sprinkling a few drops onto the bedsheets and using candles, diffusers, and room sprays are other ideas to experiment with.

DIET

Sexy foods choices. Eating foods rich in fatty acids, such as evening primrose oil, niacin, safflower oil, and vitamin E, has proven helpful in the area of sexual health. Nutrients that may be helpful are phosphorus and zinc. Some foods said to have aphrodisiac qualities are oysters, clams, mussels, chocolate, figs, raspberries, and elderberries.

At one time it was thought that if a particular food looked like a sex organ, it had aphrodisiac properties. But I think that only works for the highly visual person. I'll take chocolate and aromatherapy any day!

Bake cinnamon buns. Here's a little at-home experiment you can try next time you're baking in the kitchen. One study measuring penile blood flow in medical students found that the aroma of freshly baked cinnamon buns definitely had a positive effect, sexually, on men.

HERBS

Libido enhancers. There are numerous botanicals that have been used throughout history because of their purported effects on sexual health. In general, herbs that stimulate energy and increased libido in both sexes are astragalus, catuaba bark, cayenne, damiana leaf, elderberries and elder flowers, eucommia bark, ginger root, kava kava, kola nut, mandrake, muira puama, oats, raspberry seeds, red clover, sarsaparilla root, suma, Tribulus terrestris, wild carrot, and yohimbe.

Herbs that are known to regenerate and nourish the female reproductive organs and are gender specific to women are black cohosh, burdock root, damiana, evening primrose, licorice root, maca, prickly ash, and red raspberry.

Regenerative herbs for the male reproductive system are bee jelly and pollen, damiana, ginseng (American, Chinese, and Siberian varieties) and gotu kola. Pygeum bark and saw palmetto are two herbs specific to male sexual function and also aid the health of the prostate gland.

HYDROTHERAPY

Plan a lover's splash. A clean, softly scented body is very sexy. The bath can be a prelude to your special evening: Just make sure the kids are asleep and the water isn't too hot. To make your spa a special and meaningful time together, light a few candles, dim the lights, and play some romantic music. An exotic carrier-bath blend of honey and milk is used to disperse the essential oils into the water. They are luxurious additions to this special spa soak and are excellent for all skin types.

◎ Milk-and-Honey Lover's Bath ◎

6 drops ylang-ylang essential oil
3 drops clary sage essential oil
2 drops sandalwood essential oil
1 drop bergamot essential oil
¼ cup heavy cream
¼ cup honey

Pour the honey into a bowl or measuring cup. Add the essential oils into the honey, as they combine well with it. Next add the cream and mix well with a spoon. After the bath has been drawn, pour the aromatic milk-and-honey mixture into the water and disperse with your hands.

Woodstock redux. Popular among the baby boomer generation, this bath was designed with the sixties era in mind. Both patchouli and ylang-ylang essential oils are known for their powerful aphrodisiac properties.

To create a uniquely fun bathtime together, burn a small amount of high-quality patchouli incense in the next room and play some old sixties music in the background. The fragrance of patchouli has recently experienced a resurgence among teenagers. Isn't life interesting?

◎ Woodstock Whoopee Bath ◎

6 drops patchouli essential oil
6 drops ylang-ylang essential oil
2 to 4 tablespoons Celtic Sea or Dead Sea salt

Mix the essential oils with the sea salt. Pour into a fully drawn warm (92 to 100 degrees) bath. Stir with your hands to disperse.

Iɴʜᴀʟᴀᴛɪᴏɴ

Make aromatic innuendos. Care should be taken when associating scent with lovemaking, as it needs to be subtle. By incorporating essential oils into the experience, you can drift into a different state of mind. You can use aromatherapy to create a romantic retreat away from the rest of the world without ever leaving the bedroom! It is an easy way to discover new experiences. The best aphrodisiac will make use of the brain, because this is where the sexual center is located, in addition to memories and hormone regulatory functions.

You are going to thoroughly enjoy this synergy. It is an aphrodisiac and euphoric blend for special occasions. Due to the cost of the ingredients, and their viscosity, use it sparingly. Use an eyedropper to measure the oil into an aroma lamp or potpourri burner—no more than 3 to 5 drops. Because of the small amount, I don't recommend using a diffuser.

ᴗ Love in a Mist ᴗ

10 drops ylang-ylang essential oil
2 drops patchouli essential oil
2 drops black pepper essential oil
3 drops clary sage essential oil
2 drops neroli essential oil
1 drop rose (absolute or otto),
   may substitute rosewood
1 drop jasmine essential oil
   (or absolute)

Mix the essential oils in a small amber or cobalt-blue glass bottle. Keep the top tightly closed and label. This quantity is enough for four or five heightened, sensuous experiences.

LIFESTYLE

Know your body. Communicate openly your desires, preferences, and dislikes to your mate. Discuss your feelings and ask for what pleases you. You may not get it, but don't rely on hoping the other person guesses or figures it out.

Spend more time alone with your mate and focus on each other. Make a commitment to each other that your relationship is a priority in your lives. Make eye contact and listen attentively. To be a good listener doesn't mean you have to do anything but hear what the other person is saying.

Drive out stress. Stress can have a detrimental effect on your sex drive, yet it is often overlooked as a cause. Job stress, marital problems, environmental toxins, and poor sleep can all diminish the quality of your love life. I have an entire section in this book dedicated to stress as well as anxiety. Be sure to read those sections if they apply to you.

Sexual Gains

The benefits of a good sex life within an enduring love partnership go far beyond spiritual closeness and emotional riches. There are physical benefits as well. So if you're looking for reasons to get closer to your mate, read on.

Sex improves skin and muscle tone, aids sleep, increases a sense of well-being, helps burn calories, and generally improves one's self-image and self-esteem. Healthy sex can also be a factor in protecting you from heart disease, migraine headaches, pain, prostate cancer, stress, and lowered immunity.

MASSAGE

Use a slow, warm hand. The best, most effective aphrodisiacs are created with sensitivity and a delicate hand. If a massage blend is too concentrated, it will be unpleasant or repulsive rather than erotic. The aim is to create a subtle body scent, together with other pleasurable aromas that will delight and arouse. A blend of the erogenous, stimulating or calming, and euphoric essential oils makes a well-rounded aphrodisiac synergy.

This very sensual massage oil is designed for the whole body. I suggest warming the oil in a hot-water bath prior to application to increase absorption. There is enough here for two bodies, so decide who will go first.

✍ Eros Love Oil ✎

12 drops sandalwood essential oil
6 drops ylang-ylang essential oil
4 drops clary sage essential oil
2 drops rose oil (for dark hair and skin) or
2 drops neroli oil (for light hair and skin)
4 tablespoons sweet almond oil or safflower oil
½ teaspoon evening primrose oil (optional)
½ teaspoon carrot seed oil (optional)

Mix the essential oils with the warm sweet almond or safflower oil in a shallow dish. If desired, mix in the evening primrose and carrot seed oils. Apply to the body in small amounts using a comfortable pressure and working toward the heart. Avoid the face and genital area.

SOUND AND MUSIC THERAPY

Play a lover's melody. Music has been revered for millennia for its ability to woo, relax, and excite its listeners. We have all experienced firsthand how certain pieces of music can affect our emotional state as well as arouse old memories and perhaps feelings, too. Sound therapy can relax or energize, depending upon the needs of the couple. Although a highly personal choice, these selections were made because they invoke or awaken general feelings of love and devotion.

Franck—*Panis Angelicus*
Denver-Domingo—*Perhaps Love*

Herbert—*Ah, Sweet Mystery of Life*
Jessye Norman—*Sacred Songs*
Bach—*Jesu, Joy of Man's Desiring*
Mendelssohn—*Violin Concerto*
Yanni—*Reflection of Passion*
Bocelli—*Romanza*

TEAS AND TONICS

Get a tea-time high. If herbs could speak, this tea blend would be poetic. It surely is an herbal tea for romance. It smells wonderful as it is being brewed. Serve with herbal honey if you desire more sweetness in your life!

✑ Tea for Two ✑

Pick a few fresh (unsprayed) rose petals and float them in your teacups.

3 cups boiling water
2 teaspoons rose petals
1 teaspoon spearmint herb
1 teaspoon licorice root (ground)
1 teaspoon hawthorn herb
Pinch of the following: cinnamon, coriander, and nutmeg
Vanilla Honey or Ginger Honey to taste (pages 221 and 48) (optional)

Bring the water to a boil. Place the herbs in the hot water and simmer on low for 3 minutes, with cover on. Remove from the heat and allow to steep for 5 additional minutes. Strain and serve with fresh herbs or flower petals. Sweeten to taste with the honey if desired.

Make a toast to romance. This lover's tonic is a bit complicated, but it's worth the trouble. It is admirably called Love Potion No. 9 because of the nine herbs it contains and its association with the familiar song. It needs to age for 1 to 2 months—even longer is fine. The recipe can be doubled easily. Serve in a small aperitif glass. Enjoy!

❧ Love Potion No. 9 ❧

5 tablespoons angelica root

5 tablespoons astragalus root

5 tablespoons Chinese wolfberry

1 tablespoon cinnamon bark

10 tablespoons damiana leaf

10 tablespoons elderberry and/or elder flower

5 tablespoons licorice root

5 tablespoons Panax ginseng root

5 tablespoons raspberry seeds
    (or, if unavailable, use the dried fruit)

8 cups brandy, rum, or vodka

4 tablespoons Ginger Honey (page 48)
    or plain honey to taste (optional)

All roots and bark herbs should be finely chopped (but not powdered). Heat the brandy gently in a glass or enamel pot. Have a large, covered glass jar ready to hold the entire amount after it has heated. Place the herbs in the jar. Pour the heated brandy over the herbs and stir. Seal. This mixture will need to age for 1 to 2 months.

Interfering Illnesses

The following list of common health conditions are associated with sexual difficulties.

Arteriosclerosis	Endometriosis	Overweight
Cancer	Fibroids	Pelvic inflammatory disease
Cystitis	Hormonal changes	Prostatitis
Depression	Medications	Sexually transmitted diseases
Diabetes	Ovarian cysts	Stress

Shake it periodically. After the liqueur has aged, strain very well through several layers of cheese cloth or a strainer. If desired, add the honey to sweeten to taste and pour into clean bottles. Label.

Sinusitis

✑

GET ALL STEAMED UP

Our head contains four air pockets, known as sinuses, which lie behind the brow and under the cheeks. Sinusitis is an inflammation of the mucous membrane lining of these sinus cavities. Symptoms are stuffed-up nose, sinus pain, headache, mild fever, thick discharge, difficulty breathing, tooth and upper jaw pain, feeling of fullness in the face, pressure behind the eyes, and postnasal drip.

That's a lot of symptoms for such a small part of the anatomy. No wonder they make us feel all stuffed up!

Common causes include nose injury, anatomical deviations, allergies, and bacterial or viral infections. However, smoking and polluted environments, poor air quality, and sick-

Colors of the Nasal Spectrum

The color of your nasal fluid can determine whether or not you have an infection as well as reflect your general state of health.

Clear or *white:* healthy mucous
Yellow: sign of bacterial or viral infection
Green: often means chronic infection; will typically have a bad smell
Brown: sign of fungal infection or result of smoking
Gray: often thick or hardened; sign of dehydration
Red: blood in the mucous

building syndrome are also linked to sinus problems. Sinus sensitivity is so great in some people that chronic sinusitis is practically part of their lifestyles. It doesn't have to be; there are ways you can feel better fast.

AROMATHERAPY

Sinus problem stoppers. Essential oils known to benefit the respiratory system and specifically the sinuses are primarily derived from tree and herb plants. They are called pulmonary antiseptics and include cajeput, eucalyptus, hyssop, juniper, lavender, lemon, niaouli, peppermint, pine, rosemary, tea tree, thyme, and sandalwood.

Among the essential oils that aid in the thinning of mucus and aiding its discharge from the body are basil, bergamot, cedarwood, eucalyptus, fennel, hyssop, lavender, marjoram, myrrh, peppermint, pine, and sandalwood.

A few essential oils—bergamot, chamomile, eucalyptus, lavender, and lemon—are utilized to strengthen the immune system. They are often used in combination with some of the oils mentioned above for a treatment protocol. As you will see, there are many ways to use essential oils that target this condition, primarily inhalations, compresses, humidifiers, massages, and irrigations.

DIET

Soup, tea, and plenty of water. It is important to stay well hydrated while experiencing a sinusitis attack. Be sure to drink at least 8 to 10 glasses of pure water daily, as well as plenty of herbal teas. Green tea with lemon and ginger root tea are especially good for loosening mucus. Also, make the warming and delicious soup that contains a powerhouse of cold-fighting herbs and vegetables called Old-Fashioned Garlic and Onion Soup on page 137. It comes close to being a cure-all broth.

The ultimate spice mix. I created the Stay-Healthy Spice Seasoning blend after researching the numerous antibacterial spices and their effects on killing bacteria. I prepare this seasoning blend for my home cooking and use it regularly. Keep the mix in a recycled spice jar with a shaker-type lid. It is a delicious, multicultural spice combination. Use organic, nonirradiated, freshly dried herbs and spices whenever possible. Visit your local co-op or natural foods market for ingredients or order them through the mail from a reputable company. As you can see, there are quite a few ingredients in the recipe, so you may want to make a larger amount and share with family and friends. This recipe makes about ¾ cup and stores well if kept cool and dry. For a no-sodium version, omit the Celtic Sea salt.

✍ Stay–Healthy Spice Seasoning ✍

The ultimate culinary blend to keep germs at bay. Use it daily. It's delicious
as a marinade for meats, sprinkled on vegetables, and in salad dressings.

4 tablespoons finely ground Celtic Sea salt (optional)

3 tablespoons garlic powder (no salt)

2 tablespoons onion powder (no salt)

1 teaspoon allspice

1 tablespoon thyme

¼ teaspoon powdered cinnamon

1 tablespoon tarragon

¼ teaspoon cumin

Pinch of cloves

4 bay leaves finely ground

Pinch of cayenne (add more to taste if you like spicy-hot!)

1 tablespoon finely ground rosemary

1 tablespoon marjoram

Pinch of mustard powder

1 tablespoon sage

½ teaspoon finely ground fennel

¼ teaspoon coriander

1 tablespoon finely ground black pepper

2 tablespoons basil

½ teaspoon ginger root powder

¼ teaspoon finely ground anise seed

1 tablespoon finely ground red pepper flakes (optional)

Place all the ingredients in a coffee grinder, food processor, or blender to finely blend the spices (especially if you did not purchase the spices already preground). Store in clean, dry spice jars and label.

Herbs

Powerful antibacterial agents. In ancient times, before refrigeration, spices were used to prevent food from spoiling, as they killed harmful bacteria and allowed the food to be stored for longer periods of time. That's how powerful these herbs are, and fortunately they are abundant in nature. Among them are bee propolis, royal jelly, and honey, black walnut hulls, chaparral, clove, echinacea, elder (berry and flower), elecampane, garlic, ginger root, goldenseal, myrrh gum, pau de arco, and turmeric.

Dry up nasal passages. For minor sinus infections, these plant-derived decongestants will help loosen the mucus and dry the nasal passages: bayberry, eucalyptus, garlic, goldenseal, horehound, kelp, licorice root, sage, sea vegetables, and thyme.

High-Ranking Herbal Antibiotics

Here are a dozen of some of the most widely available, powerful, and effective herbs used today by herbalists and naturopaths to fight infection. Besides being used throughout history, scientific research has confirmed their potent antibiotic activity.

Acacia	Goldenseal
Aloe vera	Grapefruit seed extract
Cryptolepsis	Honey
Echinacea	Juniper
Garlic	Licorice
Ginger root	Sage

HYDROTHERAPY

Get rid of the throbbing pain. For severe cases of sinusitis or for pain relief associated with blocked sinuses, hot compresses will provide immediate relief. Care needs to be taken when applying compresses to the face. Avoid using extreme heat and keep your eyes closed. Do not allow the compresses to drain into the eye area.

With frontal headache and pain between the eyes, apply the compress to the center of the frontal sinuses, which are located on the lower forehead just above the eyes. If you are experiencing pain in the cheek, teeth, or upper jaw areas, then you will want to apply the compress to the maxillary sinuses, which are on either side of the nose and upper cheeks (below the eyes).

Sinus-Relief Hot Compress

2 cups hot water
4 drops lavender essential oil
4 drops eucalyptus essential oil

Pour hot water into a bowl. Make sure the temperature is correct (100 to 104 degrees). Add the essential oils. Swish the oils to disperse as much as possible. Soak a cloth in water. Remove the cloth from the water/essential oil bath and squeeze out most of the moisture. Lie down on a bed or couch with your head slightly elevated, at about a 30-degree angle. This position will further encourage drainage of the sinuses. With eyes closed, apply the compress over the affected sinus areas. Leave the compress on until it dries out, or for a total of 15 to 20 minutes. Cover the bowl of hot water with a lid to keep warm and remoisten the compress as necessary.

INHALATION

Get breathing again. An inhalation formula containing germ-killing essences specific to the respiratory system will break up mucous, drain your sinuses, and get you breathing easy again. Eucalyptus, pine, and tea tree essential oils are the perfect ingredients, since they are antiseptic, anti-inflammatory, and natural expectorants. The goal is to drain the sinuses and kill any germs present. This inhalation remedy will also prevent germs from taking hold in these swollen, mucous-laden cavities, where they can easily set up an infection.

Sinus Steamer

4 cups hot water
1 drop eucalyptus essential oil
1 drop tea tree essential oil
1 drop pine essential oil

Pour the hot (100 to 104 degrees) water into a bowl and add the essential oils. Form a tent over your head with a towel. Keep your eyes closed and place your head approximately 8 inches from the water level to prevent a steam burn. Set a timer for convenience and inhale slowly and deeply for 10 minutes. This steam treatment should be done at least twice a day, but three to four times a day if infection (yellow or green drainage, low-grade fever) is present.

Note: Keep your eyes closed during this treatment, as the volatile oils can irritate the eyes and cause tearing.

Diffuse daily. The use of a diffuser for therapeutic inhalation is one of the best treatment methods for indirect inhalation. For sinus conditions, I recommend the Pure-for-Sure Synergy blend on page 392 for its antiseptic and bactericidal effects. Conquer-a-Cold Combo blend on page 178 is useful as an antiseptic for the respiratory tract. Diffuse one of these blends several times during the day and night, for at least 15 minutes each time while you are in the room.

Hand-to-nose relief. Place 1 to 2 drops of any of the essential oils recommended for sinus relief on a tissue or handkerchief. Hold it up to your nose and mouth and inhale deeply several times.

Alternatively, place 3 drops of eucalyptus, pine, or tea tree essential oil on the palms of your hands. Rub your hands together briskly to create warmth and encourage the volatilization of the oils. Cup your hands, hold them over your nose and mouth, and inhale deeply. Exhale by turning your head away from your hands. Inhale again by deeply breathing the essential oil aroma into your sinuses and lungs.

Both of these methods will help the sinuses stay clear and offer protection while out in public.

LIFESTYLE

Get plenty of rest. Rest and relaxation promote a healthy immune system, which is important for beating a sinus infection. Go to bed early and take a nap during the day if you can. A hot bath at night does wonders for promoting a restful sleep.

Allergic to anything? Avoid dairy products, which can encourage mucous formation. If your sinus problem is allergy related, avoid the allergens that you have identified as triggers. Common culprits are dairy products, wheat, peanuts, corn, eggs, citrus, and sugar.

Take it one nostril at a time. The best way to blow your nose is to gently blow one nostril at a time.

Go with the flow. Keep mucous flowing and your nasal passages clear by running a cool mist humidifier containing a few drops of eucalyptus oil mixed in the water. Visit a sauna or steam room or take a steamy shower.

MASSAGE

Breathe clear at night. To keep nasal passages clear at night, try this facial massage just before going to bed. It is important that you stay clear of the areas around your eyes, since the oils in this blend are very volatile and can be irritating. This massage oil is especially useful when you do not have the time to do steam inhalation or compresses. It can be used as part of the total sinusitis-relief program or used alone for mild cases. If you are prone to sinusitis, this sinus oil can serve as a preventative.

❧ Open-Sesame Sinus Oil ❧

This can be used as a massage oil as well as nose drops for sinus relief.

> 1 tablespoon sesame oil
> 3 drops lavender essential oil
> 2 drops eucalyptus essential oil
> 1 drop peppermint essential oil

To the sesame oil, add the essential oils. Mix well. To use as massage oil, apply sparingly to the face in the areas of the affected sinuses. Avoid the eyes as much as possible. Massage into the skin until absorbed. Inhale from your fingertips before washing hands well. May be used three times per day.

To use as nose drops, tilt your head back and, using an eyedropper, place 1 drop of the sinus oil mix into each nostril. Or put a few drops on your fingertips and inhale the oil. Use up to three times per day.

SOUND AND MUSIC THERAPY

The sounds of sinus. The vibrations made by uttering specific tones are believed to help cure specific parts of the body. According to the healing art of vibrational toning or sound therapy, the sound that resonates the sinuses and nasal passages is "ma." Simply take a full, deep breath and make the sound "ma" while exhaling. Repeat this practice three times daily for best results.

Real-Life Cure

NATURAL DROPS HIS SINUS SAVIOR

Daniel spent five years on decongestants, analgesics, antibiotics, and anti-inflammatory medications to help his chronic sinusitis. Not only did they do little to relieve his headaches and stuffed-up nose, but the side effects of the drugs made him feel miserable. He was also worried about how the long-term use of the drugs would affect his health. He decided he wanted to go natural.

Daniel was somewhat addicted to nose drops, so I suggested he try my Open-Sesame Sinus Oil as his new nose drops. Undoubtedly, he was getting a "rebound" effect from the heavy-duty nose drops he was taking. He loved the scent and mild effect of my formula. He also loved the results!

Bouyed by his progress, he started on steam inhalations and hot compresses. As he started to feel better, he also started to take vitamins and improve his diet.

"I never realized how much energy this problem was taking from me," he said. "I was drained." But not anymore. Daniel still gets sinusitis but not as frequently and not as severely. Now, when he starts to get headachy and stuffy, he reaches for his natural drops.

When to Call the Doctor

If you experience a considerable amount of blood in your mucus for more than a few days or a bloody nose that will not stop, seek medical attention. Also, if your symptoms of sinusitis advance beyond facial and eye swelling, immediately visit your doctor to rule out orbital cellulitis, which can cause damage to the nerves in this area.

Sore Throat

✌

Gargle Power

Was that sandpaper you had for dinner last night?

If you wake up in the morning with that dry, scratchy, painful-to-swallow sign of a sore throat, it could just mean you're in for a few hours of punishment for some misdemeanor committed the day or night before—like talking too much or being in a smoke-filled room.

But 90 percent of the time this is not the case. A sore throat is an early warning sign that you're coming down with something, most likely the flu or another virus. Fall back to sleep for a few hours and you might wake up with a fever and swollen glands. Open wide and that throat likely will look as bad as it feels.

This doesn't mean you should just give in to what might lie ahead. The faster you take action, the quicker you'll be up and at 'em again.

Aromatherapy

Gargle first and fast. At the first sign of a sore throat, gargle with an antiseptic solution. Salt water with lemon is easy and effective. So is apple cider vinegar and water. I, however, prefer to take no chances, so I go straight for the heavy artillery. The ingredients in this recipe are well-known infection fighters and can help stop an illness before it starts.

✌ First-Sign-of-a-Sore-Throat Gargle ✌

1 cup sage herbal tea or hot water
1 tablespoon fresh lemon juice
1 tablespoon apple cider vinegar
2 drops geranium essential oil
1 drop ginger essential oil
1 teaspoon raw honey or Sage Honey (recipe on page 446)

Brew the sage herbal tea or hot water. Add the lemon juice and apple cider vine-gar. Add the essential oils to the honey and thoroughly mix before adding to the herbal tea mixture. Gargle with this recipe for 1 to 2 minutes several times per day. For optimal freshness, prepare daily or store in the refrigerator.

Add some antiviral power. For a sore throat coupled with flulike symptoms such as swollen glands, here's an even more potent remedy. It's very effective against viruses. It also uses apple cider vinegar but the oils in this recipe are antiseptic and astringent. They make a perfect team to fight viruses.

✍ Super–Strength Sore Throat Gargle ✍

1 cup sage or thyme herbal tea or water
1 tablespoon apple cider vinegar
1 drop geranium essential oil
1 drop pine essential oil
1 drop lemon essential oil
1 teaspoon Sage Honey (page 446)

Brew the herbal tea and strain. Add the apple cider vinegar. Add the essential oils to the Sage Honey and thoroughly mix before adding to the warm tea mixture. Stir well. Pour into an amber glass bottle and label with directions for use. Shake well before each use. Gargle with this several times for as long as you can. Gargle three times per day. Do not eat or drink anything immediately after gargling.

When you can't gargle, spray. This is ideal for when you're away from home and gargling is out of the question. You'll need a spray bottle in order to deliver the medicine to the back of the throat.

Note that this spray is more concentrated than my gargle recipes and uses a greater number of essential oil drops per volume. Use it as you would any medicine—with dis-cretion and according to directions.

Intensive Throat Spray

½ cup chamomile herbal tea
1 tablespoon apple cider vinegar
2 drops geranium essential oil
1 drop lemon essential oil
1 drop hyssop essential oil
1 drop tea tree essential oil
1 teaspoon Sage Honey (page 446) or plain raw honey

Brew the herbal tea and strain very well so herb pieces do not plug the spray nozzle. Add the apple cider vinegar. Mix the essential oils in with the Sage Honey, then add this to the tea mixture. Pour into a glass spray bottle and label. Shake well before each use. To use, spray directly into the back of the throat while breathing in. One to two sprays is equivalent to one single treatment application. The liquid can be swallowed. Do not eat or drink for 15 minutes after using the spray. Take three times daily.

Other sore throat soothers. Essential oils for sore throats include bergamot, black pepper, cedarwood, cinnamon, clary sage, clove, eucalyptus, frankincense, geranium, ginger, hyssop, lavender, lemon, niaouli, orange, peppermint, pine, sage, sandalwood, and tea tree.

For flu-related sore throats try benzoin, chamomile, cypress, eucalyptus, fennel, hyssop, lavender, lemon, peppermint, pine, ravensara, rosemary, sandalwood, and thyme.

DIET

Refresh your throat. Drink plenty of liquids, including herbal teas, juices, and soups. Fresh lemon juice in water, hot or cold, and ginger tea are very soothing. Suck on a Popsicle or fruit pop.

Eat gingerly. It's hard to eat when your throat is sore, but you need to get your cold- and flu-fighting nutrients such as vitamin C and zinc. Foods high in vitamin C include pineapple, cantaloupe, strawberries, oranges, kiwi, and grapefruit. Foods rich in zinc include eggs, nuts, and whole grains. Go for soft foods such as eggs, soups, and fruits and vegetables such as bananas and cooked spinach.

Avoid dairy. Milk and other dairy foods create mucous, which is tough to handle when your throat is sore.

Sweet and divine medicine. You'll find Sage Honey listed as an ingredient in many of the recipes in this book. The recipe is given here because it is so soothing on rough and raw throats. Make it as often as necessary and keep it on hand. I keep a full jar in the pantry cupboard to add to herbal teas when needed.

🖉 Sage Honey 🖎

This has such a wonderful taste, it's hard to believe it's such great medicine.

1½ cups raw honey
¼ cup fresh sage leaves (*Salvia officinalis*)

Heat the honey over low heat. Add the sage leaves and heat gently, taking care not to boil (excessive heat destroys the beneficial qualities of the honey). Heat until the sage leaves become dry. Now the herbal qualities and essential oils have been extracted from the sage herb and are contained in the honey. Strain with a slotted spoon or sieve. Pour the aromatic honey into a clean glass jar and label. You can add a fresh sage leaf or two to the final aromatic honey if you desire.

HERBS

Herbal antiviral agents. Herbal medicine in the forms of warm herbal teas, capsules, and tinctures is widely prescribed for a sore throat. Traditional used herbs are agrimony, chamomile, echinacea, fenugreek seeds, garlic, ginger root, goldenseal, raspberry leaf, sage, and slippery elm.

Herbs specifically known for their antiviral properties are especially helpful due to the high statistical probability that a sore throat is caused by a virus. Effective herbs for viral infections are astragalus, echinacea root, garlic, lomatium, myrrh gum, pau de arco, and St. John's wort.

Immune strengthening herbs include astragalus, bupleurum, chaparral, echinacea root, pau de arco, reishi mushroom, shizandra berry, and Siberian ginseng.

HYDROTHERAPY

Wrap yourself up in wet-water warmth. A warm-water bottle or heated neck wrap will be very comforting to most people experiencing a sore throat. A soothing warm pack can be applied for 15 minutes each hour as long as it is comfortable.

Get steamed. Steam heat spiked with essential oils that gets to the back of the throat is both soothing and healing. Bring a pot of water to a simmer and add 3 drops of any of the essential oils listed above. Place a towel over your head to form a tent. Keep your eyes closed and inhale the aromatic steam for 5 to 10 minutes.

Strep Warning

Strep throat is a bacterial infection that, if left untreated, can have serious consequences: It can cause pneumonia, rheumatic fever, and heart damage. Only a relatively small number of sore throats are caused by bacteria, but the only way to know for sure is through a throat culture.

Strep is often accompanied by a fever greater than 101 degrees. If you have a sore throat that doesn't respond quickly to home remedies and if symptoms worsen, go to your doctor for a throat culture.

For other remedies and information, see Colds *and* Tonsillitis.

Sprains and Strains

✍

SPEED HEALING

Is it a sprain or is it a strain? The pain is the same, so what does it matter?

Actually, it matters a lot.

When you badly twist a joint (usually an ankle or foot) in a fall or other incident, the intense pain is immediate. Rapid swelling is very close behind. It's a sprain if the ligaments surrounding a joint are injured. It's a strain if a muscle or tendon or both are damaged. The severity of the damage can range from mild to severe. If the ligament, muscle, or tendon is torn, you could require surgery.

It takes a trip to the emergency room to officially find out the site of the injury, but you can't wait that long to take action. Treatment must be immediate. R.I.C.E. is the acronym to remember when you have this type of injury: rest, ice, compression, elevation.

HYDROTHERAPY

Think cold. The faster you can get an ice pack on the injury, the better. Ice will help reduce swelling—and can even prevent it if you act fast enough. Put an ice pack on your injury for 15 minutes at a time for the first 48 hours. Make sure the limb is elevated.

Crushed ice in a plastic bag is best because it's easy to wrap around the injury. Wrap the bag in a cloth. Ice should not come in direct contact with your skin because it could cause an ice burn. If the skin is broken, the wound must be clean first.

Make a peas offering. If you happen to have a bag of frozen peas in your freezer, use it for a cold pack instead of the ice. The tiny rolling action will hug the injury well. Frozen corn can also be used.

Go cold and hot. After the first 48 hours, you can put heat therapy into action to encourage circulation and healing. A moist heating pad or a moist hot compress is best. You should alternate between heat and cold for 15 minutes every few hours for effective first-aid treatment.

First Aid for the Freezer

Rice packs are used by nurses, physical therapists, and massage therapists in hospitals, rehabilitation centers, and nursing homes. They are kept cold in the freezer for ice therapy and are microwaved for instant hot therapy.

To make a rice pack at home, fill an old but clean tube sock with rice. Tie or sew the end of the sock closed. Place the rice pack in a plastic bag and store in the freezer. It can be kept indefinitely. You now have a first-aid freezer section!

For heat therapy, put the rice pack in a microwave oven for 2 minutes (depending on the size of the pack). Be careful that it does not get too hot.

Speed the healing. You can help increase the action of a cold pack by adding special healing agents and oils. Witch hazel is an astringent and will help stop the bleeding and swelling that have likely occurred within the soft tissue. Comfrey tea is especially comforting on ligaments. Cypress will stop bleeding by constricting blood vessels. Chamomile and marjoram will help reduce inflammation.

✺ Double-Action Cold Compress ✺

½ cup cold water or comfrey herbal tea
½ cup distilled witch hazel lotion
2 drops chamomile essential oil
2 drops marjoram essential oil
2 drops cypress essential oil

In a bowl, pour the cold water or cold comfrey tea and the witch hazel. Add the essential oils and stir well to disperse. Soak a washcloth in the compress solution.

Squeeze the cloth and apply it to the affected joint. Cover with a plastic wrap. If you have an ice pack, lay that over the plastic and cover with a towel. Elevate the sprained joint during the treatment. When the compress becomes dry or warm, replace it with a fresh one. Continue the compress for 20 minutes. Do this treatment three times per day.

Second phase. The healing oils used in this moist compress are different because now the goal of treatment is to increase circulation and enhance healing, as bruising will have already taken place. Anti-inflammatory agents continue to be included in addition to analgesic essential oils.

⚬ Double-Action Warm Compress ⚬

½ cup warm water
½ cup distilled witch hazel
2 drops chamomile essential oil
2 drops rosemary essential oil
1 drop hyssop essential oil

In a bowl, pour the warm water and the witch hazel. Add the essential oils and stir well. Soak a compress cloth in the warm (92 to 100 degrees) solution. Wring out and apply to the affected joint. Layer with a plastic wrap. Place over the plastic a hot-water bottle to keep the compress warm (optional). Wrap with a towel. During compress treatment, elevate the affected limb above heart level, if possible. Replace the compress when it becomes dry or cool. Leave on for 20 minutes. Do up to three compresses per day to help dissolve bruising and relieve soreness.

MASSAGE

Concentrated salves. Gently massaging the wound after hot and cold therapy will help facilitate drainage and circulation. Massage into the affected joint, in an outward circular direction and with upward strokes toward the heart.

Wheat germ oil is ideal for sprains and bruises because it is rich in antioxidant vitamins, aids in strengthening weakened capillaries, and prevents scar tissue. Arnica montana is an herb that is used to make a very healing infusion oil beneficial in treating many first-aid injuries, including bruises and inflammations.

First-Aid Massage Oil

10 drops lavender essential oil
8 drops rosemary essential oil
4 drops ginger essential oil
3 drops peppermint essential oil
1 tablespoon wheat germ oil
1 tablespoon arnica infusion oil

In an amber glass bottle, add the essential oils, then the wheat germ and arnica oils. If the latter two oils are not available, any vegetable oil will do. Shake gently and label. Apply three to four times daily, preferably after compress treatments, in the morning upon rising, and before bedtime.

Stomach Ulcers

THE CURE FOR WHAT'S EATING YOU

More than 12 million people in the United States are walking around with the sudden pain and frequent burning of an ulcer. Many of them don't even know they have one—until some monumental upset lands them in the hospital.

Peptic or stomach ulcers are areas of erosion within the mucous membrane lining of the stomach. Until about ten years ago, it was commonly believed that stomach ulcers were caused by too much acid, which eroded the delicate stomach lining. That changed when scientists linked a bacteria known as *Helicobacter pylori* with stomach ulcers. As many as 70 percent of people with stomach ulcers are infected with *H. pylori*.

This, however, does not rule out other suspects long linked to ulcers—most notably, emotional stress. It appears that it is not necessarily the amount of stress that determines digestive problems but rather how well stress is managed.

Some drugs, like aspirin, aminophyllin, and nonsteroidal analgesics, can irritate the stomach lining, and prolonged usage has been linked to ulcer formation. Drinking acid-producing products, like coffee, black tea, and cola beverages, and smoking tobacco are also associated with an increased risk of stomach ulcers. Genetics plays a part, too.

AROMATHERAPY

Aromatic stomach aids. Essential oils traditionally utilized in stomach ulcer conditions are basil, cardamom, chamomile, lemon, marjoram, niaouli, peppermint, petitgrain, rose, rose geranium, rosemary (verbenone type), and ylang-ylang. Also, any of the relaxing essential oils, such as chamomile, lavender, marjoram, and ylang-ylang, will be beneficial in reducing stress levels and calming the mind and body.

DIET

Drink lemon water. Drink fresh lemon juice in warm water every morning—half a lemon squeezed into an 8-ounce glass of water—to balance your pH.

Drink cabbage juice. Drinking 2 to 3 cups of raw cabbage juice daily has been known to heal ulcers. It can be purchased at natural health-food stores or by mail order.

Get more fiber. Increase fiber in your diet by eating organic whole grains and fresh vegetables—in particular, cabbage and okra. These foods enhance mucous secretion and protect the stomach lining.

Balance your pH. Eat a diet rich in alkalinizing foods such as vegetables, sea vegetables (wakame, kelp, nori, hijiki), millet, quinoa and amaranth grains, Celtic Sea salt, herbs and herbal tea, lemons, limes, unsweetened cranberries, and cultured foods like natural sauerkraut, raw cultured vegetables, and kefir (cultured milk product).

Sprout your own raw seeds and nuts, which are very alkalizing and make an excellent

Acid-Forming Foods to Avoid

The human body is a living ecosystem within itself. A healthy body and strong immune system depend on several factors. One of these factors is the pH balance of body fluids. They should be slightly alkaline (7.4 pH). An acidic state—the opposite of alkaline—is considered unhealthy and promotes yeast, viruses, bacteria, parasites, and possibly cancer cells, to grow. The following foods are highly acid forming and are most likely to compromise your health in many ways:

Artificial sweeteners
Beans and soy products
Refined flour products
Roasted nuts and nut butters
Sugar, candy, sodas
Wine, beer, and alcohol

protein snack with live enzymes. Acid-forming foods should not constitute more than 20 percent of your diet; otherwise, they will create an acidic pH balance in your body.

Practice food combining. Give your digestive system a rest by practicing effective food combining. Because the stomach needs to produce different enzymes to digest different proteins, fats, and carbohydrates, it makes good sense to eat them at the correct times.

Basically, you want to eat fruit alone; only eat protein with nonstarchy vegetables; and eat grains with starchy and/or nonstarchy vegetables. This will free up energy for healing and stop stressing your body to produce enormous amounts of digestive enzymes to process your meals.

HERBS

Herbal healers. Botanical medicine can stimulate enzyme production, balance pH, promote healing of the gastric lining, as well as stimulate the immune system. All and all, herbs have much to offer in the healing and prevention of stomach ulcers.

Licorice root and cayenne pepper are perhaps the most widely used herbs for ulcer conditions. Licorice compounds have a long historical use for effectively treating acute stomach ulcers. Cayenne pepper stimulates the secretion of hydrochloric acid (HCL), aids the digestion of protein, and prevents bleeding.

Primary herbs that are very effective for remedying stomach ulcers are aloe vera, barley grass, calendula, cayenne, cramp bark, dandelion root, echinacea, fennel seed, garlic, goldenseal root, licorice root, and slippery elm. Aloe vera, brewer's yeast, cardamom seed, catnip, ginger root, peppermint, and red raspberry are considered acid/alkaline balancing herbs. Herbs that stimulate hydrochloric acid are cayenne, gentian root, goldenseal, milk thistle, Oregon grape root, sienna, and turmeric. Use these herbs in teas, tinctures, or capsule formulations. Take according to product label directions.

MASSAGE

Give yourself a belly rub. Almost any vegetable oil can be used as the carrier for the essential oils in this blend; calendula infusion oil, however, is known in herbal medicine to aid in ulcer healing, so I highly recommend using it in this recipe. Vitamin E is an antioxidant that helps to prolong the shelf life of the vegetable oil, in addition to its other healing benefits.

I suggest you use this massage oil daily, preferably at the same time each day, and incorporate its application into your daily regimen, perhaps following your morning shower. This way you will be getting consistent daily absorption of these anti-ulcer plant oils. All the essential oils listed in the recipe help in stressful conditions and are also antimicrobial.

⟋ Ulcer-Healing Massage Oil ⟍

10 drops lavender essential oil
5 drops geranium essential oil

> 5 drops lemon essential oil
>
> 4 drops chamomile essential oil
>
> 400 international units vitamin E
>
> 2 tablespoons vegetable oil
>
> (preferably calendula infusion oil)

Count out the recommended amounts of the essential oils into an empty amber glass bottle. Add the vitamin E, then the vegetable oil. Shake gently to mix. Label contents. Warm the oil prior to massage, to increase its absorption ability. Do this by placing the bottle of oil in a hot-water bath. Apply the massage concentrate oil to the abdomen, concentrating on the upper abdominal region over the stomach.

Real-Life Cure

HIS ULCER IS GONE!

With a high-stress job and a diet high in acid-forming foods, it's no surprise that Byron came down with a peptic ulcer at the age of forty-seven. Remaining under a doctor's care, he came to see me for natural healing therapy.

The first thing we did was examine his diet. I suggested he get off acid-forming foods and experiment with more alkalinizing foods like seaweed. He cut out coffee and took up herbal tea. I suggested he drink cabbage juice, and, to my surprise, he loved it.

The next important thing was searching for a stress reduction plan—one that worked for *him*. Over a four-month period we modified and re-evaluated different stress reduction plans as well as experimented with various aromatherapy blends. The Ulcer-Healing Herbal Tea (featured on page 456) became his blend of choice, which he used faithfully twice a day in the beginning, then once a day, and now several times per week. His greatest challenge was making time for his stress-relief program and staying away from coffee. He became a great fan of the cabbage juice and the massage oil.

After nine months of aromatherapy and lifestyle changes, Byron was off all prescription drugs, and his doctor told him his ulcer had healed. He continues regular follow-up visits with his physician and is aware of his tendency to develop ulcers, should he return to his former lifestyle and dietary habits.

Slow, rhythmic, clockwise motion is desired. Following the application, inhale the essences by cupping your hands over your nose and mouth. Take several long, deep, relaxed breaths.

TEAS AND TONICS

Tasty tea treat. Since herbs are such stomach saviors, it only makes sense that herbal teas should become part of your ulcer-fighting regime. These ulcer herbs are best for teas: calendula, catnip, echinacea, fennel seed, ginger root, licorice root, meadowsweet, and peppermint. Use Sage Honey to sweeten, since sage is proving useful as a possible ulcer-healing agent. I've included the recipe on page 446.

❦ Ulcer–Healing Herbal Tea ❢

1 part ground marshmallow root
1 part ground licorice root
1 part slippery elm
½ part ground echinacea root
½ part peppermint herb
Sage Honey to taste (page 446)

Mix the herbs in a bowl. Pour 1 cup of boiling water to 1 teaspoon of herb. Let steep for 15 minutes. Drink on an empty stomach, 2 to 3 cups daily. These herbs have been used traditionally for healing stomach ulcers and decreasing stomach acids, as well as for binding proteins. The Sage Honey is recommended for its astringent properties in preventing bleeding and healing ulcers. Directions on how to make it are on page 446.

When to Call the Doctor

Bleeding, perforation, and blockage are all complications of an ulcer that can be potentially dangerous if not treated immediately. If you have an ulcer and experience vomiting, dizziness, and bowel abnormality, see your doctor at once.

Also, if you have chronic indigestion and stomach pain after eating, see a health-care practitioner for a complete evaluation to rule out an ulcer.

Stress

ᘓ

The Big Chill-Out

Stress is a condition that needs no definition. It's all around us; it's within us. Nobody can escape it.

Babies experience stress when they are hungry or can't relate a need. Children experience stress as a result of both peer and adult pressures to succeed in school and sports. Adults experience the most stress: Work, family, financial, and health concerns can load us down with stress.

Stress in and of itself, however, is not the problem. Stress only becomes a problem when we don't handle it well. Think of it like a bad reaction.

Some of the most common signs of stress include headache, neck and back pain, palpitations, indigestion, stomach pain, loose bowels, lethargy, nervousness, decreased libido, low initiative, irritability, aggression, concentration difficulties, insomnia, high blood pressure, teeth grinding, and recurrent infections such as colds.

Stress can cause personality changes in some people. They overeat, argue, burst into tears, drink too much, sleep too much, and talk too fast. As if that's not enough, chronic stress can lead to a host of health problems: angina, asthma, depression, heart disease, high blood pressure, immune problems, and ulcers, just to name a few. Besides the health risks it poses, stress can impact virtually every aspect of life: your marriage, your relationships, your job, and your overall enjoyment of life.

Scientists have spent millions of dollars studying stress and its consequences. Clearly, reacting to stress with distress is damaging to our psyche and physical well-being. There are lots of antidotes to combat stress, including prescription drugs, which are addictive and *not* a good idea. But all these antidotes have one common denominator: relaxation. When you're stressed out, you need to chill out.

Grown-Up Stress Makers

It's probably no surprise to hear that job pressures and money problems are the top two causes of stress for American adults. They are followed by family responsibilities, housework, health concerns, child care, and caring for aging parents.

AROMATHERAPY

Take it from nature. A pleasant smell or aroma in and of itself has the ability to relieve stress. Fill your lungs with an aroma you love, and you can practically feel stress escape as you exhale.

Mother Nature has given us particular scents that possess properties that are natural relaxants. Fortunately, nearly all essential oils contain these properties, but the ones most noted for stress reduction are the fresh citrus scents, the deep-calming woods and resins, and the mood-altering floral aromas. They include basil, bergamot, cedarwood, chamomile, clary sage, cypress, frankincense, geranium, grapefruit, jasmine, juniper, lavender, lemon, lemongrass, lime, marjoram, melissa, myrtle, neroli, orange, palmarosa, patchouli, petitgrain, pine, rose, sandalwood, vetivert, and ylang-ylang.

BREATH WORK

Start the day with a blast of calm air. Dedicate a few minutes a day to promoting calmness and clarity of mind and to feeling invigorated. Sit straight in a chair with your arms hanging at your sides. Tilt your head back and place your hand over your abdomen. Breathe deeply through your nose. Be aware of your chest and abdomen filling with air. Pause for a few seconds and then exhale through your mouth, sighing loudly and letting your head and body fall forward. Repeat several times, concentrating on expelling stress with each exhalation and breathing in peace, love, and light.

In addition to the above exercise, you can refer to the breathing exercises given in Part One. Be sure to breathe slowly and deeply, preferably in combination with an essential oil. It is good practice to perform deep breathing exercises throughout the day: upon rising in the morning (during a basic stretch routine), in the car while driving, and in the evening prior to dinner and retiring to bed. The benefits of deep breathing are multiplied sevenfold when used with aromatherapy.

Diet

Stay clear of stimulants. Avoid caffeine, sugar, table salt, and nicotine. These are all stimulants and the antithesis of calming agents.

Eat energy foods. Eat a healthy diet that includes raw nuts and seeds, flax oil, whole grains, fresh fruits and vegetables, pure water, and herbal tea. You will be building the body, not draining it of energy.

Bring healthy snacks to the office or have them handy during the day. Low fat granola, dried fruit, fruit and vegetable juices, organic yogurt, raw vegetables, rice cakes, popcorn, and whole grain crackers are some excellent choices that will provide you with energy and fight fatigue. Eat regularly planned meals in a relaxed environment.

Eat for relaxation. Bananas, rice, milk, turkey, spinach, and pasta contain tryptophan, an amino acid that encourages relaxation. Get some at every meal.

Herbs

Help from nature. Herbs that are nourishing and calming to the nervous system are black cohosh, catnip, celery seed, chamomile, evening primrose, gotu kola, hops, kava kava, kelp and sea vegetables, lady's slipper, lemon balm, motherwort, passionflower, royal jelly, skullcap, and valerian root. Mineral-rich herbs mainly help balance the body's pH but also have been found to help relieve stress. These include alfalfa, bilberry, burdock root, Irish moss, kelp and sea vegetables, marshmallow root, oat straw, and parsley leaf.

Do It in the Dark

A great antidote for stress-caused sensory overload is to take a neutral spa bath in complete darkness. By making the bathwater the same temperature as your body (about 98 degrees), you will create a sense of sensory deprivation, since as the nerve endings in your skin will be nonsensitized (sensing neither hot nor cold derivations). Be ready for a profound experience. Have a flashlight handy.

HYDROTHERAPY

Retreat and rejuvenate. Aromatic baths are one of my favorite ways to unwind. The warmth of the water, in addition to the relaxing benefits of essential oils, melts away muscle tension and helps to quiet the mind.

Concentrate on your breathing while soaking. Breathe by inhaling deeply and slowly. Visualize being at your favorite place; it may be an herb garden, flower garden, or the ocean. Exhale through your nose, pushing out all the day's stress and negative energy. Repeat this several times if you wish, until you find yourself in a peaceful, restful place.

I recommend taking your bath right after work or before retiring. Darken the room and light a few candles. Close the bathroom door and hang a DO NOT DISTURB sign on the knob. If you have a tension headache, rub a few drops of lavender on your temples before soaking in the spa bath.

⟨⟨ Stress–Relief Retreat ⟩⟩

7 drops lavender essential oil
2 drops lemongrass essential oil
1 drop basil essential oil
4 tablespoons Celtic Sea or Dead Sea salt

Add the essential oils to the salt and add to a full bath. Warm to hot water temperature is suggested (approximately 92 to 104 degrees is perfect). Soak for 20 to 30 minutes.

Help for Nervous Nellies. This bath is designed for the heavy-duty triple: stress combined with nervous tension and anxiety. Dim the lights in the bathroom for a soothing ambiance or burn a single candle for simplicity and focus. Take deep, relaxing breaths and, on the exhale, consciously release each and every tension and stress you have carried with you throughout the day. Play some relaxing music or nature sounds if this appeals to you or opt for the solace silence brings.

Cool, Calm, and Collected Mineral Salts

4 tablespoons Celtic Sea salt
¼ cup powdered sea kelp (optional)
9 drops lavender essential oil
3 drops clary sage essential oil
1 drop marjoram essential oil

Pour the salt into a small dish and, if desired, mix in the kelp. Add the essential oils and mix with the back of a spoon. After the bathwater has been drawn, pour the sea mixture into the water and disperse with your hands.

INHALATION

Mellow out at work. I created these three synergies to be used in a diffuser or aroma lamp at the office. All are uplifting, purifying, and proven to be effective.

❧ I Love My Job ❧

A synergy for workplace bliss.

9 parts lavender essential oil
3 parts lemon essential oil
2 parts geranium essential oil

❧ Anti–Stress Synergy ❧

An effective calming essence blend for everyday stress.

2 parts bergamot essential oil
4 parts lavender essential oil
1 part ylang-ylang essential oil

❧ Deep–Relaxation Blend ❧

Encourages a profound state of calm with a sense of lightness.

6 parts lavender essential oil
2 parts marjoram essential oil
1 part mandarin essential oil

Measure out the oils with an eyedropper. One part is equivalent to one eyedropper full. Store in an amber glass bottle with a secure top. Label. Use in a diffuser, aroma lamp, or room spray.

LIFESTYLE

Self-care is key. One of the hardest things to do when you are under stress is also one of the most important things you should do: Take time for yourself. Do the things you love, like take a walk along the ocean or in the park. Take a cold shower or hot aromatic bath. Give yourself a solo massage, which can be done easily on your neck, head, and feet.

Prayer, meditation, hypnosis, singing, gardening, walking along the beach, and flying a kite are among the things people do to relax. All are very different ways people can choose to unwind. You get the idea. Whatever it is you love to do, just do it!

Get organized. Being late, a sloppy desk, misplacing documents, and not being prepared are leading stressors on the job. Take a class or find a book that teaches good organizational skills. Just the time an organized life saves is an automatic stress reducer.

Take up a hobby. But who has the time? You do—or will—when you practice the tips in this section. A hobby you love will add to your relaxation and enjoyment of life.

Start a new daily habit. Give yourself permission to relax on a daily basis. Most stressed people have a difficult time doing this. Many get sick (unconsciously) in order to give themselves permission to take a much needed break from work.

MASSAGE

The ultimate relaxer. Massage, especially aromatherapy massage, is total relaxation. And no excuses that you don't have the time! Some companies now have massage therapists on site at various times of the week offering employee massages.

This is my favorite relaxation massage oil. Mix it and request that your masseuse use it for your massage. Don't be fooled by its simplicity. It's wonderful!

ᛩ Massage–Away–Stress Oil ᛩ

10 drops lavender essential oil
2 drops neroli essential oil or rose essential oil
2 tablespoons sweet almond oil or vegetable oil

In a shallow dish or bottle, combine the essential oils. and the warm sweet almond oil or vegetable oil. Mix well. Apply to the skin with slow rhythmic hand strokes, working toward the heart. Be sure to pay special attention to the hands, feet, and neck.

SOUND AND MUSIC THERAPY

Tunes for the tense. Sound and music therapy is soothing vibrational medicine for the psyche and soul. Surely, you have noticed how different musical pieces affect you, either positively or negatively, depending on your mood and preferences. The music listed below was chosen for its calming effect on the mind and body.

In general, brass, percussion, and heavy sounds of bass notes affect the physical body, while woodwinds and strings affect the emotional and mental body. Seek out the music that balances and calms you and play it softly in the background to create your personal vibrational healing. Here are a few of my favorites:

Halpern-Kelly—*Ancient Echoes*
Lee—*Celestial Spaces for Koto*
Copland—*Quiet City; Appalachian Spring*
Vivaldi—*Oboe Concertos*
Windham Hill Artists—*Winter's Solstice Collections*
Young—*The Mystery of Destiny*
Deuter—*Wind and Mountain*
Harmonix Ensemble—Herbal Harmonic series, especially *Kava Kava*
Bekker—*Spa*

TEAS AND TONICS

No worries, mate. Brew a cup of herbal tea to sip while soaking in your aromatic stress-release bath. This blend is very soothing to the nervous system. It can be consumed several times per day or taken an hour before bedtime to encourage a restful sleep.

Stress–Free Herbal Tea

2 parts chamomile flowers
2 parts lemon balm herb
1 part catnip herb
1 part lavender flowers
1 part peppermint leaf
1 part rose petals
1 part lemongrass (optional)
Pinch of nutmeg to taste
Vanilla Honey to taste (page 221) (optional)

Combine the dried herbs, flowers, and spices in a glass jar. Label. To prepare 1 cup of herbal tea, use 1 to 2 teaspoons per cup of hot water. Steep for 5 minutes. Sweeten with the Vanilla Honey if desired.

YOGA AND MOVEMENT

Let go of tension. Yoga requires that you fully concentrate on the pose, which in turn relaxes the mind and encourages rhythmic breathing. Yoga postures aid in stretching muscles, building strength, and achieving balance. By performing the following posture, you will automatically release stress, open your body, and gradually become balanced. Allow yourself at least 10 minutes to perform this pose on both sides. For a less agile pose, you can opt the Easy Pose or Corpse Pose given in the Burnout and Anxiety sections.

Tree pose. Stand with your feet parallel and shoulder-width apart, looking straight ahead. Shift your weight to your right leg, keeping your knees soft. Turn your left knee out to the side and bring your left heel toward your right ankle. Hold your arms out to the sides for balance. Slide your left foot up the inside of your right calf, then farther up until it rests on your inner thigh. Press your left knee backward and your left hip forward. When you feel balanced, raise your arms up to the prayer position in front of your chest. Inhale deeply and relax, then raise your arms overhead with palms touching. Breathe deeply six times. Repeat on the other side.

For more information and remedies, see Anxiety *and* Burnout.

Stretch Marks

∿

SUSTAINING SUPPLE SKIN

Stretch marks are *not* the exclusive domain of pregnant women.

Known medically as *striae gravidarum,* stretch marks appear as thin, pinkish to deep red streaks or striations of fibers over skin stretched and taut from rapid weight gain. Pregnancy is the obvious front runner for getting stretch marks. But they also have been seen in teenage girls who have experienced rapid weight gain with the onset of puberty and men who have experienced rapid weight gain. But now there is a new category of people prone to stretch marks: bodybuilders. Men (and women) who gain an enormous amount of muscle over a relatively short period of time get them, too.

Areas of the body that are prone to skin striations are the abdomen, breasts, hips, thighs, buttocks, and upper arms. Some health practitioners contend that stretch marks are caused by hereditary influences because they are more common among fair complexioned people. Dry skin also can contribute to stretch marks because dryness depletes the elasticity of the skin.

Stretch marks seldom disappear completely, but they do fade over time, leaving white to silver feathery lines on the skin. To help them diminish faster, here's what to do.

DIET

Eat healthy. Adequate nutrition supports healthy skin and prevents rapid weight gain. You will not want to gain too much weight too fast. Include barley grass, kelp, and other sea vegetables in your diet. They provide an abundant amount of minerals.

Get more fiber. There is some evidence that the straining involved in chronic constipation can increase the likelihood of developing stretch marks. To avoid constipation, eat a diet high in fiber. Make vegetables, fresh fruit, and whole grains the focus of your diet. Since inadequate hydration can make constipation worse, drink plenty of pure water, lemon water, herbal tea, and mineral water to stay regular.

HERBS

Herbs with flexibility. Botanicals greatly nourish the skin and support skin tone and elasticity by providing the body with crucial minerals. Among the effective herbs for skin healing and nutriment are the chlorophyll-rich plants such as alfalfa, barley, dulse, kelp, and parsley. Other mineral-rich and alkalizing herbs are aloe vera, burdock root, calendula, chamomile, dandelion root, marshmallow root, and yellow dock.

Herbs and other natural ingredients that aid in skin tone and healthy skin are borage seed and flaxseed (GLA sources), burdock root, evening primrose, ginger root, horsetail, lemongrass, nettles, pumpkin seed, royal jelly, and sage. These herbs can be used in a wide variety of ways, such as herbal teas, tinctures, or in capsule form.

MASSAGE

Regenerate and nourish. Aromatherapy in the form of massage is the primary treatment of choice for preventing and alleviating stretch marks. Gentle massage single-handedly can increase circulation and aid elasticity, but, when used in conjunction with essential oils, the benefits are greatly multiplied. Essential oils soften and moisturize the skin, which helps encourage supple skin.

Essential oils useful in preventing and decreasing the appearance of stretch marks are bergamot, chamomile (German and Roman), frankincense, jasmine, lavender, mandarin, myrrh, neroli, rose, rosewood, and tangerine.

When doing this massage, pay special attention to any areas of your body that feel taut, dry, or itchy. The itching is caused by the skin being overly stretched. Use a gentle but slightly firm touch, concentrating above and below the targeted area as well.

If you find the consistency of the lotion too heavy, add more vegetable oil. Depending on the climate in which you live, you may need to adjust the cocoa butter and oil ratio to get the perfect consistency. If you live in a cooler climate, you will require less cocoa butter, while those in a warmer and dryer climate will require more cocoa butter to make into a thick cream. Coconut oil or cocoa butter melts easily at about 70 degrees.

✍ E-Cream ✍

This lotion got its name because it contains vitamin E and essential oils.

2 tablespoons cocoa butter or coconut oil

2 tablespoons blend of vegetable, nut, and
seed oils (see list in Appendix B)

800 international units vitamin E (capsules)

4 drops jasmine essential oil

4 drops neroli essential oil

4 drops lavender essential oil

20 drops mandarin essential oil

12 drops carrot seed essential oil

Gently melt the cocoa butter over a low-heat source. Once melted, remove from heat and add the additional vegetables oils. Cut open the vitamin E capsules and squeeze the contents into the oils. Add the essential oils and mix well with a spoon. Pour the aromatic oil combination into a 4 ounce (or larger) jar. High-density plastic jars with a wide mouth work best. Label. Apply to tight, itchy areas of the body that are prone to stretch marks (buttocks, hips, thighs, etcetera). Apply daily, preferably after your daily shower or bath.

∞ Resiliency Balm Oil ∞

*This balm recipe is simpler to prepare since it does not contain cocoa butter,
which needs to be melted. However, it, too, is very effective due to the
beautifying effects of rose oil and other essential oils.*

4 drops rose essential oil (rose otto)
12 drops lavender essential oil
8 drops chamomile essential oil
(German or Roman)
800 international units vitamin E (capsules)
4 tablespoons blend of vegetable, nut,
and seed oils (see list in Appendix B)

Place the essential oils into a 4-ounce (or larger) bottle. High-density plastic bottles with a squirt top work best. Cut open the vitamin E capsules and squeeze the contents into the bottle. Pour the blend of vegetable oils into the bottle and shake well. Label. Apply to tight, itchy areas of the body that are prone to stretch marks (buttocks, hips, thighs, etc.). Apply daily with gentle massage.

Vital skin that glows. To achieve healthy skin, you need to regularly stimulate and exfoliate it. One way to do this is through regular dry skin brushing to increase circulation. It also assists the functions of sweat and oil glands that lubricate and moisturize the skin, strengthens collagen and elastin fibers, and breaks down cellulite deposits. See page 40 for instructions.

Sunburn

ᴅᴇᴇᴘ-ʜᴇᴀᴛ ʀᴇʟɪᴇꜰ

The sun is the perfect health conundrum. How can something so good for you—in fact, something that is necessary to both your physical and emotional well-being—be so bad for you at the same time?

When we try to get too much of a good thing.

Sure, we need the power of the sun to get life-essential vitamin D. Sure, we need daylight and sunshine to lift our mood and spirit and ward off seasonal affective disorder. The problem is not the sun at all, but our desire to bask our bodies bronze under its harmful ultraviolet rays.

Most bodies don't have the ability to tan—even less the ability to tan safely. But all of us have the ability to burn, and that carries two serious consequences: It accelerates the skin's aging process and greatly increases the chance of developing skin cancer.

A burn that turns the skin red and is hot to the touch can be a first-degree burn, meaning that the outer layer of the skin, the epidermis, has been damaged. Typically the epidermal layer peels within five days, becomes itchy and pink, and is well on its way to total healing in about one week. There is usually no resulting scar from a first-degree burn. Prolonged exposure to harmful UV rays can cause sunburns that go deeper into the skin, making your risk of skin cancer increase.

UVAs are the longer sun rays that can penetrate clouds and car and home windows. These rays are strongly linked to the formation of wrinkles and malignant melanoma, a fatal form of skin cancer. UVB rays are the shorter wavelength rays. They are responsible for rapid sunburns, wrinkles, age lines, and cataracts of the eye.

As a cancer nurse working in Seattle, I saw many fishermen, avid golfers, and construction workers who had developed skin cancers on unprotected areas of their bodies such as the neck, back of the hands, and ears. You probably wouldn't think that Seattleites could get skin cancer since they don't see the sun for months at a time! But even clouds don't protect us from the harmful UVA rays.

More than 50 percent of skin damage resulting from overexposure to the sun occurs before the age of eighteen. It is crucial that we protect our children by preventing sunburns. But if you have one, here's what to do.

AROMATHERAPY

Soothe the burn. The primary essential oil for treating sunburns is lavender. Other essential oils useful in treating general burns are chamomile, eucalyptus, geranium, lavender, neroli, rosemary, and tea tree.

Spray on relief. This sunburn relief spray will be most welcome. It can be stored in the refrigerator for extra cooling relief for "hot" spots.

✺ After-Sun Healing Spray ✺

½ cup distilled water
¼ cup witch hazel lotion
¼ cup aloe vera gel or juice (whole-leaf extract best)
8 drops lavender essential oil
2 drops chamomile essential oil
1 drop geranium essential oil
1 teaspoon honey

In an 8-ounce (or larger) spray bottle, add the water, witch hazel, and aloe. In a small bowl, combine the essential oils and honey and mix very well with the end of a spoon. Add the aromatic honey to the water mixture. Shake well to completely mix. Label the bottle with directions for use. Shake well before applying to the skin. Avoid the eye area. Apply freely several times per day.

HERBS

Say aloe. Aloe vera, an anti-inflammatory and healing herb, has been used for centuries to heal burns. It can be added to aromatic baths, compresses, and lotions. Research studies show that using aloe vera before sunning protects the immune system from the deleterious effects of UV ray exposure. It is not uncommon to find aloe vera in sunscreen products marketed today.

Give aloe extra action. Lavender and tea tree essential oils can be added to aloe vera for extra healing power. Use 6 drops of essential oil per 1 tablespoon of aloe vera.

HYDROTHERAPY

The ultimate burn bath. The ultimate answer to treating your sunburned skin is to soak in a bath with an abundance of healing herbs, soothing essential oils, and aloe vera. This recipe is a bit more complicated than others because you have to prepare a strong herbal infusion (tea). However, if your body is screaming for it, you best make it! It will be worth the extra effort.

Lavender, chamomile, and peppermint essential oils are the perfect combination to take to the bath for sunburns. Lavender and chamomile are calming to the skin and nervous system and anti-inflammatory, while peppermint (in very small doses) is cooling. For small children, divide the quantity of essential oils by half. The infusion of herbs is optional if you are short on time. The optimal bath water temperature for burns and inflammations is cool to tepid, which is approximately 70 to 92 degrees.

> ### Folk Remedy: Cider Vinegar
>
> An old-time folk remedy for sunburn calls for a simple spray made with apple cider vinegar. Use 1 tablespoon of vinegar per 1 cup of pure water, hydrosol, or herbal tea. Put it in a clean spray bottle and use it freely. Store it in the refrigerator for extra cooling action.

✺ Sunburn-Relief Bath ✺

2 tablespoons of each of the following herbs:
   calendula, comfrey, raspberry leaf, slippery elm
1 quart boiling water

½ cup baking soda

½ cup apple cider vinegar or witch hazel lotion

½ cup aloe vera gel or juice

2 tablespoons honey

6 drops lavender essential oil

2 drops peppermint essential oil

2 drops chamomile essential oil

Make a strong infusion of the herbs by pouring boiling water over them in a bowl or pot and allowing it to steep for 20 to 30 minutes. Strain and set aside. Fill the bath with cool to tepid water. Add the herbal tea mixture to the bath, along with the baking soda, vinegar, and aloe. Mix the essential oils with the honey to combine well and add to the bathwater by stirring well with your hands. Soak for 20 minutes or longer. Gently pat dry. Follow with the After-Sun Healing Spray (recipe on page 471).

Mist-Me-Beach Balm

This oil, which combines lavender floral water and Rescue Remedy (a popular Bach flower essence), is soothing to sunburns and helps keep the skin moist. I recommend keeping a spray bottle in your beach bag and misting yourself with it.

Simply add 6 drops of Rescue Remedy to 6 ounces of authentic lavender floral water. Not only is it a cool refresher but it encourages relaxation, too!

MASSAGE

The olive-oil cure. Olive oil is an excellent oil to heal burns and scalds and has traditionally been used in this way for centuries. The extra virgin (first pressing) is high in vitamins and minerals. Wheat germ oil and vitamin E oil are both useful for sunburned skin, as they encourage healing of damaged tissues.

After sun spray. The following body oil recipe includes three fine healing oils in addition to the essential oils. The oil goes on easily when the skin is moist. First, spray the body with lavender flower water (hydrosol) or don't completely dry after bathing. Spread this oil on in a thin layer. It will help to seal in the moisture on the skin and glides on easily when applied in this way. Put on this oil after the skin has cooled for several hours or overnight.

✏ Après–Sun Aromatic Body Oil ✏

32 drops lavender essential oil
4 drops neroli essential oil
2 drops chamomile essential oil
5 tablespoons extra virgin olive oil
2 tablespoons calendula infusion oil
1 tablespoon wheat germ oil

In a 4-ounce amber glass bottle, add the essential oils. Add the olive, calendula, and wheat germ oils and shake gently to mix. Label contents. Apply to moistened skin two to three times daily until completely healed.

Note: It is recommended as day-after skin care and not for blistered or broken skin. For children, use half the amount of essential oils called for in the recipe, to create a lower dilution.

LIFESTYLE

Educate to prevent. Use a broad-spectrum sunscreen that blocks both UVA and UVB rays with an SPF of at least 15. Reapply after swimming or water play, according to product labeling. Be sure you protect your little ones with shade, adequate clothing, sun hats, sunglasses, and sunscreen.

Stay away from citrus. Citrus essential oils are phototoxic. Also, beware of perfumes made with real citrus oils. Several of the popular English colognes once contained large amounts of bergamot essential oil, which is known to have caused dark pigmentations on women's necklines, where they had sprayed their perfumes.

Beware of medicines. Certain medications, such as diuretics, antibiotics, and birth control pills, can increase sun sensitivity, making you more susceptible to sunburn.

Burn in a Bottle

The following essential oils are phototoxic, meaning they have the ability to make your skin more sensitive to the sun.

Do not use these oils prior to direct sunlight exposure. If you have a family history of skin cancer or if you have large moles or extensive dark freckles, these oils are not recommended for regular use. It is the fruit peel–derived oils that are considered phototoxic, especially if they have been produced by a process called cold-expression. If the essential oils are steam distilled, then they are not as photosensitive.

Angelica root	Lemon verbena
Bergamot (expressed)	Lime (expressed)
Celery	Lovage
Cumin	Orange (bitter, expressed)
Ginger	All absolutes and concretes
Grapefruit (expressed)	(not true essential oils sol-
Lemon (expressed)	vent extracted)

The following herbs can make you more sensitive to the sun. If you are taking them internally or in skin-care products, be aware of their potential for making you sun sensitive.

Agrimony	Parsley
Dong quai	Rosemary
Fennel	Rue
Khella	St. John's wort
Masterwort	Yarrow
Motherwort	

SALVES

A honey of a treatment. Honey is a great healing agent for a sunburn dressing because it is antibacterial and anti-inflammatory. When essential oils are combined with it, you multiply its effects. I recommend that you use lavender or chamomile essential oil, along with 1 drop of tea tree for dressings. Mix 3 drops of lavender essential oil or 1 drop of chamomile essential oil in 1 tablespoon of honey. Apply a thin layer of the aromatic honey to the gauze dressing and apply to the burn. Leave on for 4 to 6 hours, changing at least three times daily. Aloe vera gel, or the fresh juice from the plant, can be used in the same way.

Teething

∞

TAMING TENDER GUMS

Teething is often a baby's first experience with pain and discomfort so it is no surprise that they don't take it quietly. Crying and irritability are obvious signs of unhappiness about what's happening in their mouths. Also, their cheeks can become flushed and their gums can get red and swollen. All will be well in due time. But if baby is fussing and you feel on edge, here are a few things you can do.

AROMATHERAPY

Baby gums with chamomile. Thankfully, nature has provided us with the chamomile plant, one of the most powerful anti-inflammatory essences known. Essential oil of Roman chamomile, also known as true chamomile or sweet chamomile, is widely used and recommended by health practitioners for teething discomfort problems. It is very effective as a pain reliever when mixed with a vegetable oil and applied to sore and irritated gums.

Other useful oils considered safe for children while teething are German chamomile, lavender, and yarrow. Be sure to use a minute amount of essential oil when preparing any aromatherapy blend for your small child. They are very potent and should be used safely and correctly, according to directions.

This recipe is effective, safe, and well tolerated by babies. It should only be given to children six months and older.

✺ Teething Oil ✺

2 tablespoons extra virgin olive oil (organic preferably)
1 drop Roman chamomile (*Anthemis nobilis*) essential oil

Pour the olive oil in a small amber glass bottle. Add the chamomile oil. Cap, shake well to mix, and label. Rub a few drops onto the affected gum line every couple of hours for soothing relief. Store in the refrigerator. Because the oil will harden, take it out of the refrigerator a few minutes before use.

DIET

Bake a teeth treat. Here's a healthy and natural alternative to store-bought, sugar-coated teething biscuits. Babies love them, and you will be doing your very best as a parent in keeping your baby healthy.

✺ Tasty Teething Biscuits ✺

Make your teething biscuits into fun shapes with cookie cutters fashioned in dinosaur, doggy bones, chicken, or cat shapes. Be creative!

1 egg, beaten (organic)
3 tablespoons honey
1 tablespoon vegetable oil
¼ cup condensed milk (goat's or soy milk)
1 tablespoon wheat germ
1 tablespoon finely ground fennel seed
1 cup whole wheat flour or whole wheat pastry

Combine the wet ingredients in a bowl. Add the dry ingredients and mix until the dough is well combined and stiff. Roll out to about ¼-inch thickness and cut into rounds or shapes with a cookie cutter or the open end of a glass. Place on an ungreased cookie sheet. Let stand overnight for extra-hard biscuits. Bake at 350 degrees for 15 minutes or until lightly browned. Cool and store in an airtight container.

Tennis Elbow

GET BACK IN THE SWING

Tennis elbow is the popular name for tendonitis, a painful inflammation of the tendon sheath surrounding a joint. It got its name because as many as one-third of avid tennis players over the age of thirty get it.

Severe pain in the elbow joint and forearm, stiffness, swelling, and muscle strain surrounding the joint are typical symptoms of tendonitis. It's caused by repeated use and overuse of the elbow. You don't have to be a tennis pro to get it. Carpenters, gardeners, baseball players, golfers, bowlers, and even business professionals who carry heavy briefcases are targets for tennis elbow.

AROMATHERAPY

Tendonitis tamers. Many of the essential oils that are helpful with arthritis and bursitis are also effective for tendonitis, because all of these conditions necessitate anti-inflammatory and pain-relieving action. Oils useful for this ailment are benzoin, cajeput, caraway, cedarwood, chamomile, coriander, cypress, eucalyptus, ginger, juniper, lavender, lemon, marjoram, myrrh, peppermint, petitgrain, pine, rosemary, sandalwood, thyme, and vetiver. Essential oil therapy can be applied in a compress, massage oil, or bath treatment.

Get infused. St. John's wort (*Hypericum perforatum*) oil and arnica (*Arnica Montana*) oil are both infused oils, meaning they are prepared by infusing the fresh or dried plant in virgin olive oil to extract its beneficial herbal components. Both are powerful agents for painful tennis elbow. St. John's wort oil contains hypericin, which imparts a beautiful red color to the oil. When purchasing this oil, make certain it is a reddish color. If it is not, it most likely was not made correctly or has been diluted with other less expensive oils.

If you cannot find these oils at your local health-food store, you can mail order them. Alternatively, but not as effective as the infusion oils, you can opt to make your treatment oil with vegetable oil.

HERBS

Herbs for joints. Herbs with anti-inflammatory and pain-relieving properties include alfalfa, barley grass, devil's claw, garlic, kava kava, St. John's wort, white willow bark, wintergreen, yarrow, and yucca. Some herbs help by working to restore joint flexibility. These are alfalfa, aloe vera, bee pollen, black cohosh, chlorella, comfrey root, devil's claw, evening primrose, flaxseed, hawthorn, horsetail, licorice root, marshmallow root, oat straw, rose hips, royal jelly, St. John's wort, yarrow, and yucca. Herbal medicines such as these can be taken internally in tea, tincture, or capsule form, according to the product label.

This spice works like ice. The popular Indian cooking spice turmeric, taken in capsule form three times per day, has been found effective in relieving the discomfort of tendonitis due to its highly useful anti-inflammatory properties.

HYDROTHERAPY

Cool it. For immediate relief of pain and swelling, get ice or a cold water bath on a painful joint as soon as possible. To prepare a cold water bath, fill a basin with cold water and ice cubes and add 4 drops of the appropriate essential oils such as chamomile, eucalyptus, pine, or rosemary. Submerse the elbow or affected joint into the aromatic water for several minutes at a time, up to three times daily.

Compress it. This compress treatment is designed to help reduce inflammation. The apple cider vinegar helps alleviate soreness. While using the compress, keep the joint elevated if possible. Propping it up with a few pillows works well. During acute and severe tendonitis pain, compress treatments can be done three times per day.

✑ Tendonitis Compress ✑

3 drops eucalyptus essential oil
2 drops hyssop essential oil
1 drop rosemary essential oil
½ cup apple cider vinegar
1 cup cold water

Add the essential oils to the vinegar and then add to a bowl of cold water. Stir well to disperse. Soak a cloth in the aromatic water. Wring the cloth out and apply it to the affected joint. Place a cold pack or ice pack over it to keep it cold. Layer a towel over this. Change the compress when it becomes warm or dry. Leave it on for 20 to 30 minutes.

LIFESTYLE

Prevention the best tactic. Tennis elbow will go away by using the measures recommended above and resting the joint. But you should expect it to return if you don't take some corrective action.

- Practice good form, especially when serving and using your backhand return.
- Consider using a lighter racket that is loosely strung to alleviate some of the strain on your arm.
- Get support for your elbow by asking your doctor to fit you for an elastic support brace.
- Strengthen the forearm muscles, which will help. Exercises such as ball squeezing, arm rotation, wrist curls, and finger stretches have been recommended for tennis elbow conditions.
- Avoid carrying a heavy briefcase and instead opt for a shoulder bag or backpack.

MASSAGE

Help for chronic pain. For chronic complaints of tendonitis, a daily application of a therapeutic essential oil blend will help to alleviate discomfort and to prevent further swelling and pain. This oil contains arnica and St. John's wort, which are mentioned above.

⟋ Tennis Elbow Taming Oil ⟍

8 drops rosemary essential oil
8 drops eucalyptus essential oil
6 drops peppermint essential oil
2 drops chamomile essential oil
1 tablespoon arnica infusion oil
1 tablespoon St. John's wort infusion oil
½ teaspoon rose hip seed oil

Mix the essential oils in an amber glass bottle. Add the arnica, St. John's wort, and rose hip seed oils and shake gently to combine. Label the bottle with the contents and directions for use. To use, apply a small amount of this concentrated oil to the affected area. Be sure to apply to the area surrounding the affected joint, as muscle strain can be present as well.

Tonsillitis

TREATMENT ON THE SPOT

Back in the "old days," tonsillitis was an infection you only experienced once. That's because the common "cure" was to remove them. Tonsillectomies were so common, they were practically a rite of childhood.

Not anymore! And thank goodness.

Today, popular opinion says these structures, situated in the back of the mouth, are there for good reason; they are part of the body's defense for "filtering" germs. All my children have their tonsils, and I intend to keep it that way!

Tonsillitis, however, is still a common occurrence, especially among schoolchildren, and can range from mild to severe. Symptoms include pain, difficulty swallowing, fever, swollen glands, and the telltale white or yellow spots on the tonsils. Sometimes the swelling becomes so severe it impedes swallowing.

AROMATHERAPY

Throat-pleasing scents. Essential oils most useful for tonsillitis are ones that fight germs, reduce pain, and stimulate the immune system. These are bergamot, cajeput, clary sage, eucalyptus, geranium, German chamomile, ginger, lavender, myrrh, niaouli, oregano, peppermint, pine, sandalwood, tea tree, and thyme (linalool or thymol). They are best used in gargles, steam inhalations, throat sprays, and cool compresses.

Oregano to the rescue. Oregano (*Origanum vulgare* or *O. compactum)* essential oil is highly recommended for throat infections accompanied by swollen glands. It has been used traditionally for pain relief, inflammation, and various infections. As with all oils, make sure you are using the correct essential oil by double-checking the Latin name on the bottle's label. Do not confuse it with other types of oregano or with marjoram.

Oregano oil is a powerful antiseptic. However, it is known as a dermal irritant. It should always be diluted prior to use and is very effective in 1-percent concentrations or less. It is most often used internally rather than externally on the skin. Examples of uses include aromatic honey, tea, gargles, and throat sprays.

When to Call the Doctor

For recurrent tonsillitis, I recommend you see your doctor to address the underlying condition or weakness that may be promoting this condition. If your tonsils are extremely swollen and are interfering with breathing and the ability to swallow, seek medical attention immediately.

Gargle. This gargle will help decrease swelling and fight infection. The area in the back of the throat is very vascular—that is, it has a good blood supply. The longer you can hold the gargle, the more readily absorbed and effective the essential oils will be. To be most effective, avoid drinking or eating for 20 minutes following the gargle.

✧ Sore-Throat Gargle ✧

1 cup warm water
1 teaspoon Celtic Sea salt

1 drop thyme (linalool) essential oil

1 drop grape seed extract

Pour the warm water into an 8-ounce clean glass bottle. Measure out the Celtic Sea salt and add 1 drop each of the thyme essential oil and the grape seed extract. Add the salt to the bottle and shake well to combine. Label. Shake well before using. Take a mouthful, tilt your head back, and gargle for as long as you can tolerate. Then empty your mouth and repeat three times. This rinse can be used several times throughout the day.

Take time for tea. This preparation takes more time, but it's worth it.

Germ–Destroying Gargle

1 cup near-boiling water

1 cup warm sage or thyme herbal tea

1 tablespoon apple cider vinegar

1 tablespoon fresh lemon juice

1 teaspoon Sage Honey (page 446),
   Ginger Honey (page 48), or plain honey

1 drop geranium essential oil

1 drop lemon essential oil

1 drop ginger essential oil

1 drop oregano (*Origanum compactum*) essential oil

Brew the herbal tea in 1 cup of near-boiling water and strain. Add the vinegar and lemon juice. In a separate bowl add the honey and the essential oils and mix well. Add the aromatic honey to the warm tea. Gargle with this mixture several times, three times per day. Hold in the mouth and gargle for as long as possible before rinsing. Wait at least 20 minutes before eating or drinking anything immediately following the remedy.

HYDROTHERAPY

Go for cool comfort. Cool compresses help reduce the swelling in the tonsil region as well as in the glands near the jaw. In this recipe, essential oils and water work together to achieve the desired outcome: to decrease swelling and fight infection.

Continue using this for two days following the disappearance of symptoms.

✌ Cool–Comfort Compress ✌

> 2 cups cool (70 to 80 degrees) water
> 4 drops lavender essential oil
> 2 drops tea tree essential oil
> 1 drop chamomile essential oil
> 1 drop lemon essential oil

Pour the cool water into a bowl. Make sure the temperature is correct (cool, not cold to the touch) at approximately 70 degrees. Add the essential oils to the bowl of water and stir to disperse as much as possible. Soak a cloth in the water. Remove the cloth and squeeze out most of the moisture. Apply to the neck region directly under the lower jaw. The best position for this is the horizontal, lying position, with the head tilted back. Do not use a pillow. Keep the compress on for 15 to 20 minutes. Remoisten and apply again within a few minutes or when it becomes body temperature (warm).

TEAS AND TONICS

Sip your way to health. Herbalists often recommend drinking warm or cool herbal teas to decrease inflammation and fight infection. Herbal teas to prepare include echinacea, fresh ginger root, and sage. These can be sweetened with honey, an infection fighter itself. Lemon juice is beneficial in balancing the pH (alkalizing) of your body.

For more information and remedies, see Sore Throat.

Toothache

Rub for Relief

A toothache hurts *a lot*. It hurts to talk even because the air you're letting into your mouth rushes over the affected tooth as a reminder (as if you need one!) that it's time to see a dentist fast. In the meantime, here is what you can do.

Herbs

Chew on clove. Clove is the spice most helpful for the miserable pain of a toothache. Clove contains pain-killing properties, and oil of clove was used in early dentistry for its analgesic ability. Rub ground cloves over the painful tooth at the gum line. You should feel relief in a minute or two. Or chew a few whole cloves. The whole spice is always more potent than the ground version because it contains more essential oil.

Roots for the root. Other herbs that are helpful in relieving a toothache are catnip, chamomile, feverfew, hops, rosemary, skullcap, valerian root, white willow bark, and wintergreen. They can be made into herbal tea or taken by tincture or capsule. Follow the package directions.

Teas and Tonics

Sage advice. A strong herbal infusion of sage can be made and used as a mouthwash for tooth pain. Swish the warm tea vigorously and leave in your mouth for longer than usual before rinsing (about 1 to 2 minutes). A pinch of ground clove can be added to this wash for extra pain relief.

⁄ᴏ Sage Tea for Toothache ᴏ⁄

1 cup water
2 teaspoons fresh or dried sage leaf

Bring the water to a boil and add the sage herb. Cover and steep for 10 minutes. Strain and pour into a glass. Swish and gargle while warm. The leftover infusion may be stored in the refrigerator. Use freely as needed throughout the day.

Varicose Veins

⁄ᴏ

SOOTHE SORE LEGS

Varicose veins are dilated, purple and blue, distorted, ropelike bulges that appear most commonly in the legs. While unsightly, they are usually harmless, which is why many women deal with the problem by hiding them behind slacks.

Varicose veins can be caused by a weakness in the vein's structure, primarily the wall and the valves of the blood vessel. The veins become dilated and filled with blood that is insufficiently returning to the heart. Typical symptoms include discomfort, itching, and a feeling of heavy or tired legs.

Women are four times more likely to develop varicose veins than men, which is one reason for suspecting a link to hormone levels. More than half of women over age fifty experience some degree of this condition. These veins are more common in women who have had children.

The natural approach to treatment is to tone the vein walls by improving circulation and strengthening. Just as it has taken months, and even years, for this condition to present itself, it will also take time for treatments to become effective. Combinations of the following are the best approach.

AROMATHERAPY

Cypress is most essential. Essential oil of cypress and lemon are most well known for their positive effects on varicose veins. These essential oils are vasco-constrictive, astringent, and toning.

Other vein efforts. Essential oils that are vaso-constrictive, meaning they constrict blood vessels, reduce inflammation, and are slightly diuretic, are used to help treat varicose veins. These include basil, bergamot, cajeput, cedarwood, chamomile, clary sage, cypress, geranium, ginger, helichrysm, juniper, lavender, lemon, neroli, niaouli, patchouli, peppermint, rosemary, sandalwood, spikenard, tea tree, and yarrow. You can use these essential oils in compresses, baths, and massage preparations.

DIET

Eat more fiber. Straining at stool caused by constipation has been linked to varicose veins. It can also exacerbate a current condition. To ease bowel problems, increase dietary fiber by eating more fresh vegetables, fruit, and whole grains such as bran and legumes.

Drink at least a minimum of 6 to 8 glasses of pure water daily to help bowel motility. Try the Restorative Flax Tea recipe on page 186 for its laxative effects as well as the Guaranteed-to-Work Bran Muffins on page 192.

Get more berries and cherries. Fruits high in bioflavonoids are especially helpful for alleviating or preventing this condition because they strengthen blood vessel walls, making them less prone to varicosities. Foods high in bioflavonoids include blackberries, blueberries, and cherries. Vitamin C in the berries also prevents broken capillaries and keeps varicose veins from getting worse.

HERBS

Herbs that help. Anti-inflammatory herbs will help decrease the swelling and discomfort of varicose veins. These herbs can be used in the form of herbal teas, capsules, or tinctures. Take them according to the manufacturer's directions on the package. They include alfalfa, aloe vera, calendula, chamomile, comfrey root, echinacea root, marshmallow root, and yarrow.

Astringent herbs are also very effective for alleviating swelling and include bayberry bark, cranesbill, plantain, red raspberry, St. John's wort, white oak bark, and witch hazel bark and leaf.

Herbs known as circulatory tonics are bilberry, cardamom, cayenne, ginger root, Ginkgo biloba, hawthorn leaf and berry, peppermint, red clover, Siberian ginseng, and shizandra berry. These herbs can be taken in tea, tincture, or capsule form.

HYDROTHERAPY

Kick your feet up. A cold compress made with witch hazel (or vinegar) is easy to prepare and brings welcome and immediate relief after a long day on your feet. Refrigerate the witch hazel lotion so it is cold for application. The cold temperature aids in decreasing swelling and helps with the aches associated with varicose veins.

If you have only one varicose vein to treat, then the ½ cup amount will be plenty. If you have several veins to cover, then use more witch hazel and several pieces of flannel if in different locations.

✍ Comfort-for-Veins Compress ✎

6 drops cypress essential oil
1 drop lemon essential oil
1 drop bergamot essential oil
½ to 1 cup cold distilled witch hazel lotion

Add the essential oils to the witch hazel and swish the liquid well to disperse. Soak a cloth and wring most of the liquid from it. Apply to the areas needing treatment. Lay an ice pack over this and wrap with a towel. Leave on for 20 minutes. Change the compress once it becomes body temperature or begins to dry. Apply the compress as needed. Follow with the Vein-Soothing Oil on page 490 specifically designed for weak vein walls.

No hot baths. Avoid hot baths—temperatures above 100 degrees—because hot water can dilate and weaken veins even more.

LIFESTYLE

Stand up or sit down. Long periods of sitting or standing can exacerbate varicose veins and contribute to aches and pains. Standing continuously for hours, for example, exerts more than ten times the pressure on the leg veins! Take frequent breaks and change your posture as much as possible throughout your working routine.

Real-Life Cure

SHE PRACTICED WHAT I PREACHED AND WON

Lila was a sixty-two-year-young student of mine who decided to put her newly learned knowledge to the ultimate challenge: her varicose veins. She had several veins on one leg that particularly concerned her because of their unsightliness—two on the back of the thigh, above the knee joint, and one on her ankle. They were starting to cause her a lot of discomfort after long periods of sitting or standing.

Lila and I discussed in detail the essential oils, especially cypress and lemon oils, that could work for her, and I showed her how to make the formulas I've outlined in this section. She wanted to try them all! Although energetic and active in social and civic activities, she was not much into exercise, which I figured had likely contributed to her 15 to 20 pounds of excess weight. I encouraged her to start walking at least three times a week.

Lila was committed and over the next three months worked religiously on her regimen. After one month, she began to see a big change in the appearance of her veins. After thirteen weeks, her skin was markedly improved, specifically in the area directly over the veins. Her veins had become smaller and less bulging. Plus she had lost nearly half of her excess weight.

These days she's a confirmed believer in aromatherapy and natural medicine. "I'm proof that it works!" Lila says.

Get support. Support hose have been a savior to women with varicose veins. By providing counterpressure to the legs, support hose encourage blood flow and support weakened areas. Also avoid tight-fitting clothes that can impede circulation.

Drop a few. Extra weight puts extra stress on the circulatory system. Lose those extra pounds, if warranted.

MASSAGE

Daily treatment. If used daily, this is the ultimate treatment for toning weak veins. It may sound complicated due to the various carrier oils I have included, but it is deceivingly simple to make. If you cannot find the infusion oils, any vegetable oil will suffice, although it will not have the toning, anti-inflammatory, and healing properties of those oils suggested.

Mullein oil helps relieve pain and inflammation. Arnica oil, made from *Arnica Montana* flowers, is also used for inflammation. Apricot kernel oil is high in vitamins A and B and is a light, easily absorbed seed oil that helps heal delicate, damaged, and inflamed skin. You can see how these carriers are doing more than just transporting the essential oils into the skin. They are healing agents in themselves!

✍ Vein-Soothing Oil ✍

15 drops cypress essential oil

10 drops lavender essential oil

5 drops bergamot essential oil

400 international units vitamin

E capsules (optional)

1 tablespoon mullein infusion oil

1 tablespoon arnica infusion oil

1 tablespoon apricot kernel oil

In an amber glass bottle, add the essential oils. If desired, cut the end of the vitamin E capsules and squeeze contents into bottle. Add the various carrier oils and shake gently to mix completely. Label contents. Apply in small amounts to the affected areas with a gentle touch, using upward massage strokes. Use a light touch, as you do not want to damage this delicate tissue further. The goal is to encourage blood and lymph flow toward the heart and aid in absorption. Apply twice daily.

Yoga and Movement

Start moving. Get regular exercise, like walking, at least three times per week for 20 minutes or more, to benefit all the systems of the body. Exercise helps push the blood back to the heart and strengthens the entire body.

Do the butterfly. Yoga in general is helpful for any condition that requires relaxation as part of its healing remedy. The Wall Butterfly Pose on page 266 is helpful to those with varicose veins because it helps relieve pressure and swelling. It's also simple to perform.

When to Call the Doctor

Varicose veins in and of themselves are not a problem. Even though they are classified as a medical condition, varicose veins are mostly a cosmetic problem. There can be cause for concern, however, if a vein ruptures or clots. A vein that becomes very painful and one that turns into a red lump are both signs that you should see your doctor. Red varicose veins may be indicative of phlebitis, a serious circulatory condition that needs immediate medical attention.

Warts

🖉

Thick Skinned No More

Warts are abnormal growths that mysteriously appear on the skin. Though there is plenty of folklore as to what causes warts, the truth is that nobody knows for certain. What is known is that they are caused by a virus and are contagious.

Common warts are typically hard, flesh-colored growths of varying sizes that appear on the hands, knees, or face. They can be rough, raised, and scaly. They can disappear as mysteriously as they appear, but some can be so stubborn that they have to be removed surgically. Before going to that extreme, however, try these natural remedies.

Aromatherapy

Spot treatment. To make an aromatherapy remedy for warts, simply mix a few antiviral essential oils such as bay laurel, black pepper, cypress, eucalyptus, geranium, lavender, lemon, and tea tree together and place 1 to 2 drops on a Band-Aid. I suggest purchasing a box of small, round bandages at your local pharmacy.

Alternatively, you can use a cotton swab to apply this oil directly to the wart. Avoid getting the essential oils on the surrounding healthy tissue. Use either application two to three times daily until the wart has disappeared.

Aromatic corroding action. Essential oils used for treating warts are escharotic, that is, they are corrosive in nature. They include helichrysm, lavandin (a lavender hybrid), lemon, tea tree, thyme, and yarrow. Here is a synergy that I have seen used successfully on many occasions for stubborn warts.

✑ Good-Bye Wart Synergy Blend ✑

1 part lemon essential oil
1 part lavender essential oil or lavandin
1 part tea tree essential oil
1 part helichrysm essential oil (optional)

Use 1 dropperful to equal 1 part in the above recipe. This will make 60 drops total. This should be enough, depending on the size of your dropper measure. Store the synergy blend in a small amber glass bottle and label.

To use, simply put 1 to 2 drops of this synergy on the inside of a bandage and apply directly over the wart.

HERBS

Garlic: head healer. Raw garlic is possibly the most powerful substance against warts. It's a simple remedy, and I have used it on family and friends who were daring enough to try it. Because essential oil of garlic is extremely strong, I prepare this easy treatment by using fresh, organic raw garlic. Slice a thin piece of garlic and place it over the wart. Hold the garlic in place with a small Band-Aid, changing the Band-Aid and garlic twice daily. I have personally seen it dissolve several common growths in a very short period of time.
Caution: In rare cases, garlic can be an irritant to sensitive skin.

When to Call the Doctor

Warts that are discolored or painful should be examined by a physician for correct diagnosis and treatment. As with a mole, be sure to report any changes in a wart to your doctor, as this could be a warning sign of something more serious.

Follow-up herbs. Other virus-fighting herbs used against warts are astragalus, comfrey root, echinacea, grapefruit seed extract, lomatium, myrrh gum, and St. John's wort. Herbs that stimulate and enhance the immune system are ashwaganda, astragalus, boneset, echinacea, pau de arco, red root, reishi and shiitake mushrooms, sea vegetables and chlorophyll-rich plants, and Siberian ginseng. These herbs can be taken internally (tincture or capsule form) or applied externally as a cream or ointment.

Appendix A

Essential Oil References

BOTANICAL NAMES AND ORIGINS OF ESSENTIAL OILS

It is imperative that you use the correct essential oil when preparing personal products, spa treatments, and inhalation blends. I have referenced all the essential oils by their common, familiar names throughout the book for simplicity; however, be certain you are using the right oil by comparing with this list of Latin botanical names. There are numerous varieties of plants within the same family, sometimes possessing major chemical and property differences. Also, the most common country of origin is included for reference and interest. Before purchasing your oil, check this reference list.

The oils used in this book were chosen for their wide range of benefits, safety, and well-documented therapeutic applications. They will create a strong foundation from which to work in using essential oils for prevention, treating everyday health challenges, and creating pleasurable healing home spa treatments.

Purchase the highest-quality and authentic therapeutic essential oils. Choose organic, ethically wild harvested, and ecologically farmed oils whenever possible. Safeguard and store your oils responsibly and they will provide healing benefits and last for many, many years.

Angelica—*Angelica archangelica* (Europe)
Aniseed—*Pimpinella anisum* (Hungary)

Basil—*Ocimum basilicum* (India)

Bergamot—*Citrus bergamia* (Italy)

Black Pepper—*Piper nigrum* (India)

Cajeput—*Melaleuca minor, M. cajeputi* (Malaysia)

Cardamom—*Elettaria cardamomum* (Guatemala)

Carrot Seed—*Daucus carota* (Hungary)

Cedarwood Atlas—*Cedrus atlantica* (Morocco)

Celery—*Apium graveolens* (India)

Chamomile German—*Matricaria recutita, M. chamomilla* (Egypt)

Chamomile Roman—*Anthemis nobilis* (England)

Citronella—*Cymbopogon nardus* (Java)

Clary Sage—*Salvia sclarea* (Hungary)

Clove—*Eugenia caryophyllata* (Indonesia)

Coriander—*Coriandrum sativum* (Russia)

Cumin—*Cuminum cyminum* (Egypt)

Cypress—*Cupressus sempervirens* (Spain)

Eucalyptus—*E. citriodora, E. globulus, E. radiata, E. smithii* (Australia)

Fennel Sweet—*Foeniculum vulgare* (Java)

Frankincense—*Boswellia carteri* (Saudi Arabia)

Geranium—*Pelargonium graveolens* (Madagascar)

Ginger—*Zingiber officinale* (China)

Grapefruit—*Citrus paradisi* (USA)

Helichrysm—*Helichrysm italicum* (France)

Hyssop—*Hyssopus officinalis* (Hungary)

Jasmine—*Jasminum officinale* (Egypt)

Juniper—*Juniperus communis* (Italy)

Lavender—*Lavendula officinalis, L. angustofolia* (France)

Lemon—*Citrus limon* (Brazil)

Lemongrass—*Cybopogon citratus* (India)

Mandarin—*Citrus reticulata* (Italy)

Marjoram Sweet—*Origanum marjorana* (Egypt)

Myrrh—*Commiphora myrrha* (Africa)

Neroli—*Citrus aurantium* (France)

Niaouli—*Melaleuca viridflora* (Spain)

Nutmeg—*Myristica fragrans* (Sri Lanka)

Orange—*Citrus sinesis* (USA)

Palmarosa—*Cymbopogon martini* (India)

Patchouli—*Pogostemon patchouli* (Indonesia)

Peppermint—*Mentha piperita* (USA)

Petitgrain—*Citrus aurantium* (Paraguay)

Pine—*Pinus sylvestris* (Hungary)

Ravensara—*Ravensara aromatica* (Madagascar)

Rose—*Rosa centifolia, R. damascena* (France, Bulgaria)

Rosemary—*Rosmarinus officinalis* (Spain)

Sandalwood—*Santalum album* (India)

Spikenard—*Nardostachys jatamansi* (India)

Spruce—*Picea mariana* (Canada)

Tagetes—*Tagetes minuta* (Africa)

Tangerine—*Citrus reticulata* (USA)

Tea Tree—*Melaleuca alternifolia* (Australia)

Thyme—*Thymus vulgaris* (France)

Valerian—*Valeriana officinalis* (China)

Vetiver—*Andropogon zizanioides* (Java)

Ylang-ylang—*Canaga odorata* (Comoros)

MEASUREMENT EQUIVALENTS

When making your own purchases or using other books or references for essential oils, you may come across measurements different than those used in this book. The following estimated equivalents have been simplified in measuring quantity and dilution ratios in order to make a complicated and time-consuming task easy and straightforward.

cc = ml

1 cc = 20 drops

5 cc = 1 teaspoon = 100 drops

10 cc = 2 teaspoons = 200 drops

15 cc = 1 tablespoon = 300 drops

30 cc = 1 ounce = 2 tablespoons = 600 drops

½ eyedropper holds approximately 10 drops

1 full eyedropper holds approximately 20 drops

1-ounce bottle = 30 cc = 2 tablespoons = 600 drops

2-ounce bottle = 60 cc = 4 tablespoons = 1,200 drops

4-ounce bottle = 120 cc = ½ cup = 8 tablespoons = 2,400 drops

8-ounce bottle = 240 cc = 1 cup = 16 tablespoons = 3,600 drops

WHERE TO FIND ESSENTIAL OILS AND BLENDING SUPPLIES

All of the essential oils discussed in this book are available through the Internet and mail order from the following companies as 100-percent pure, unadulterated, genuine, and authentic essential oils of therapeutic and medicinal quality.

Flora Medica

Integrative Aromatherapy™ and Genuine and Authentic Essential Oils
Post Office Box 18
Issaquah, WA 98027
Phone/Fax: 1-877-FMEDICA
Website: www.floramedica.com

AROMATHERAPY AND HOLISTIC EDUCATION:

Valerie Cooksley, RN, Nursing Director and faculty member, cofounded the Institute of Integrative Aromatherapy, which offers professional training in holistic and clinical essential oil therapy. She presents a five-month diploma program, specialty workshops, and mentors the home-study diploma course. Educational contact hours are available for nurses and massage therapists.

The Institute of Integrative Aromatherapy

Phone/Fax: 1-877-363-3422
Website: www.Aroma-RN.com

Books of Interest

The Body Ecology Diet, Donna Gates, B.E.D. Publications, 1996.

Creative Healing, An Introduction to Joseph B. Stephenson's "Hands On" Healing, Patricia B. Bradley, Joseph B. Stephenson Foundation, Inc., 1994.

The Stephenson Method of Natural Care, Creative Healing, Patricia B. Bradley, Joseph B. Stephenson Foundation, Inc., 2000.

Music Resource

Gaiam—The Relaxation Company
360 Interlocken Boulevard, Suite 300
Broomfield, CO 80021
Phone: 1-800-788-6670
Website: www.gaiam.com

Appendix B

Blending Resources

∞

VEGETABLE, NUT, AND SEED OILS

Vegetable, nut, and seed oils that are used as carrier oils in *Feel Good Remedies* should be natural, organic, and cold pressed (unrefined) whenever possible. The less processed an oil is, the higher nutrient content, thus offering beneficial nourishment to your skin. The oils that are marked by an asterisk (*) are suggested as 10 to 15% part of an oil blend. These tend to be more costly, may be heavier waxes, or are very concentrated oils that can be readily diluted further in other vegetable, nut, and seed oils. Infusion oils are labeled below and include those produced by maceration, a form of infusing the fresh or dried plant material in a base oil, usually virgin olive, to extract their healing properties. Jojoba, wheat germ, and Vitamin E are ingredients that can also be used for their natural antioxidant properties to prolong the shelf life of your home spa blend.

Almond	Borage*	Cocoa butter*
Apricot kernel	Calendula (infusion)	Coconut
Arnica (infusion)	Calophyllum*	Comfrey (infusion)
Avocado	Canola	Evening primrose*
Black cumin	Carrot seed*	Flax seed
Black currant*	Castor	Grapeseed

Hazelnut	Olive	Shea butter*
Hemp seed	Palm	Soybean
Hypericum (infusion)	Passionfruit	Squalene*
Jojoba*	Peach kernel*	St. John's Wort
Kokum butter*	Peanut	Sunflower
Kukui nut*	Pecan nut	Sweet almond
Linden blossom (infusion)	Pistachio nut	Tamanu*
Macadamia	Rice bran	Turkey red
Mango butter	Rosehip*	Vitamin E*
Mullein (infusion)	Safflower	Walnut
Neem	Sesame	Wheat germ*

OTHER NATURAL INGREDIENTS USED IN VARIOUS TREATMENTS IN *FEEL GOOD REMEDIES*:

Aloe vera gel	Grains
Apple cider vinegar	Grapefruit seed extract
Baking soda	Herbs (fresh, dried, infusions)
Beeswax	Homeopathic remedies
Celtic Sea salt	Honey
Comfrey ointment	Hydrogen peroxide (3%)
Dairy (cream, milk, yogurt, eggs)	Hydrolates (floral waters)
Epsom salt	Mineral clay
Essential oils	Myrrh tincture
Flower Essences	Seaweed (fresh, dried, gel)
Glycerine	Witch hazel lotion

GENERAL TREATMENT BLENDING CHART

While specific amounts are indicated throughout *Feel Good Remedies,* this chart denotes the various equivalents of carrier to essentials oils for various types of spa treatments found in this book.

METHOD	CARRIER/AMOUNT	ESSENTIAL OIL/DROPS
Full Body Spa Treatments		
Body Mud Mask	about 1 cup	8 to 10
Body scrub	about ½ cup	8 to 10
Dry brush	—	1 to 3
Body lotion*	8 ounces	80
Body oil*	4 ounces	50
Spa bath*	full tub	6 to 10
Shower	wet washcloth	6 to 8
Sauna	1 to 3 cups water	3
Jacuzzi	full tub	3 to 5 drops per person (not to exceed 15 total)
Body wrap	12 ounces	10 to 15
Full Beauty Spa Treatments		
Facial mist	4 ounces	6 to 8
Facial scrub	3 to 4 teaspoons	2 to 3

*Caution: Children, elderly, and pregnant women should divide essential oil amounts by at least half.

Facial masks	3 to 4 teaspoons	3 to 5
Facial steam	4 to 6 cups	2 to 3
Facial oil	3 teaspoons	5
Concentrated massage oil*	2 ounces	50
Chest rub*	2 ounces	30 to 50
Ointment/salve	2 ounces	80 to 100
First aid/undiluted	—	1 to 2
Compress	4 to 8 ounces	4 to 6
Poultice	¼ to ½ cup	2 to 4
Foot/hand bath*	small tub	4 to 6
Hair/scalp oil	1 ounce	20
Shampoo/conditioner	8 ounce	80 to 100
Make Room for Me/Inhalation therapy		
Steam/vapor	4 to 6 cups	2 to 3
Humidifier	full	3 to 10
Room mist	4 ounce	10 to 20

*Caution: Children, elderly, and pregnant women should divide essential oil amounts by at least half.

Aroma lamp	¾ full	3 to 5
Light bulb ring	—	1 to 2
Smelling salts	½ oz. bottle salt	10 to 15
Tissue/handkerchief	—	1 or 2
Miscellaneous		
Vacuum machine	bag or filter	2 or 3 drops
Organic household cleaner	8 ounces	80 to 100 drops

Bibliography

Airola, Paava O. *Health Secrets from Europe.* New York: Parker Publishing Co., 1970.

Andrews-Miller, Sharleen. *The Art and Science of Herbal Medicine Making.* January 1998, Notes.

Arasaki, S., and Arasaki, T. *Vegetables from the Sea.* Tokyo: Japan Publications, Inc., 1983.

Baker, Elizabeth. *The Unmedical Miracle—Oxygen.* Drelwood Communications, 1994.

Biological Medicine: Mirror of Nature. Marco Pharma International, LLC, Roseburg, Or.: 1999.

"Biowaves." *The Sound Therapy Gazette.* July 1, 2000.

Bradley, Patricia. *Creative Healing.* Joseph B. Stephenson Foundation, Inc., 1988.

Buhner, Stephen Harrod. *Herbal Antibiotics.* Pownal, Vt.: Storey Books, 1999.

Chopra, Deepak. *Magical Mind, Magical Body.* Harmony Books, 1990.

De Langre, Jacques. *Seasalt's Hidden Powers.* Magalia, Calif: Happiness Press, 1994.

Dewhurst-Maddock, Olivea. *The Book of Sound Therapy.* New York: Simon and Schuster, 1993.

Donsbach, Kurt W. *Oxygen, Oxygen, Oxygen.* Rockland Corp., 1994.

Feinstein, Alice, ed. Prevention*'s Healing with Vitamins.* Emmaus, Penn.: Rodale Press, 1996.

Gates, Donna. *The Body Ecology Diet.* Atlanta: B.E.D. Publications, 1996.

Goldman, Jonathan. *Healing Sounds: The Power of Harmonics.* Rockport, Mass.: Element, Inc., 1992.

Grieve, Maud. *A Modern Herbal.* New York: Barnes & Noble Books, 1996.

Hendricks, Gay. *Conscious Breathing: Breathwork for Health, Stress Release, and Personal Mastery.* New York: Bantam Books, 1995.

Hover-Kramer, Dorothea. *Healing Touch: A Resource for Health Professionals.* Delmar Publishers, 1996.

Kaminski, Patricia, and Katz, Richard. *Flower Essence Repertory.* The Flower Essence Society, Earth-Spirit, Inc., 1994.

Lidell, Lucy. *The Sivananda Companion to Yoga.* New York: Simon and Schuster, 1985.

Lingerman, Hal A. *The Healing Energies of Music.* Wheaton, Ill.: The Theosophical Publishing House, 1983.

Lipton, Bruce. *The Biology of Complimentary Medicine.* Santa Cruz, Calif., 2001.

Maurer, Charles F. "Spiral Journey." *Prayer and Individual Health,* October 2000.

Minkler, James. *Energy Balancing for Natural Health.* Mont.: 2000.

Rama, Swami, Ballentine, R., and Hymes, A. *Science of Breath: A Practical Guide.* Pa.: Himalayan International Institute of Yoga Science and Philosophy, 1979.

Rector-Page, Linda, N.D., Ph.D. *How to Be Your Own Herbalist.* 1991.

Richburg, Inga Marie. *Gentle Healing with Homeopathy.* New York: Sterling Publishing Co., 1997.

Schechter, Steven. *Fighting Radiation and Chemical Pollutants with Foods, Herbs and Vitamins.* Vitality, Ink., 1991.

Sheppard-Hanger. *The Aromatherapy Practitioner Reference Manual.* Tampa, Fl.: Atlantic Institute of Aromatherapy, 1995.

Tvedten, Stephen L. "The Use of Vinegar and Hydrogen Peroxide to Disinfect." *Alternative Medicine,* January 2002.

Wade, Carlson. *Health Secrets of the Orient.* New York: Parker Publishing Company, Inc., 1973.

Walden, Patricia. *Yoga Journal's Yoga for Beginners.* Calif.: Healing Arts Home Video, Healing Arts Publishing, Inc., 1990.

West, Kim. "Americans Take Health Into Their Own Hands." *HerbalGram,* 52, 2001.

Wildwood, Christine. *Flower Remedies.* Rockport, Mass.: Element, 1995.

Index